Mosby's

EMT-Intermediate and Paramedic Certification Preparation and Review

Mosby's

EMT-Intermediate and Paramedic Certification Preparation and Review

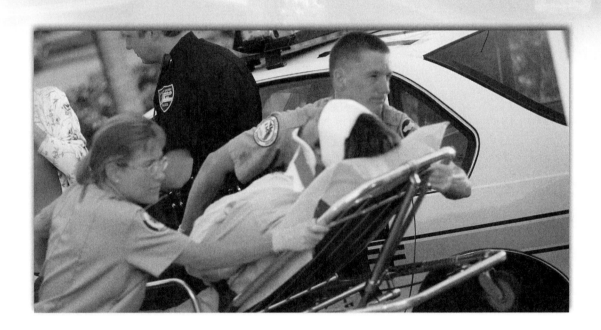

Daniel Mack, NREMT-P

Assistant Chief
Miami Township Fire & EMS
Clermont County, Ohio

Keith Wesley, MD, FACEP

EMS Medical Director
Chippewa Valley Emergency Care
Eau Claire, Wisconsin

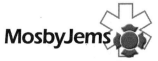

MosbyJems

An Affiliate of Elsevier Science

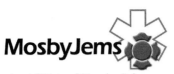

An Affiliate of Elsevier Science

11830 Westline Industrial Drive
St. Louis, Missouri 63146

MOSBY'S EMT-INTERMEDIATE AND
PARAMEDIC CERTIFICATION
PREPARATION AND REVIEW

ISBN 0-323-01927-7

NOTICE

Emergency medical services is an ever-changing field. Standard safety precautions must be followed, but as new research and clinical experience broaden our knowledge, changes in treatment and drug therapy may become necessary or appropriate. Readers are advised to check the most current product information provided by the manufacturer of each drug to be administered to verify the recommended dose, the method and duration of administration, and contraindications. It is the responsibility of the licensed prescriber, relying on experience and knowledge of the patient, to determine dosages and the best treatment for each individual patient. Neither the publisher nor the authors assumes any liability for any injury and/or damage to persons or property arising from this publication.

Library of Congress Cataloging-in-Publication Data

Mack, Daniel, 1960-
   Mosby's EMT-intermediate and paramedic certification preparation and review/Daniel Mack, Keith Wesley.
      p. cm.
   Includes index.
   ISBN 0-323-01927-7
   1. Medical emergencies—Examinations, questions, etc. 2. Emergency medical technicians—Licenses—United States—Study guides. I. Title: EMT-intermediate and paramedic certification preparation and review. II. Wesley, Keith. III. Title.
RC86.9.M343 2004
616.02´5´076—dc21

2002045241

Publishing Director: Andrew Allen
Associate Developmental Editor: Lisa M. Neumann
Publishing Services Manager: Deborah L. Vogel
Design Coordinator: Teresa Breckwoldt
Internal Design: Judith Schmitt
Cover Design: MW Design

Printed in the United States of America

Last digit is the print number: 9   8   7   6   5   4   3   2   1

INTRODUCTION

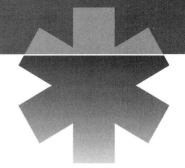

USING THIS REVIEW MANUAL

The questions in this manual appear primarily in a multiple-choice format. This type of question tests not only the knowledge of the correct answer, but also the ability to understand why the answer is incorrect. Other formats, such as matching and fill-in-the-blank, are also used in this manual. These types of questions accomplish two things. First, they allow the reviewer to perform different question analysis functions. In the field, the EMS personnel must analyze information in a variety of ways; the answer isn't there to choose from a list. Second, the use of different question formats breaks the monotony of nothing but multiple-choice questions. Keep in mind, however, that the National Registry test and certain other state tests contain only multiple-choice questions.

This review manual is not meant to take the place of a textbook or instructor, nor is it intended to simulate an actual test. There are key differences between a review manual and a test; each serves a different purpose. Because of the limited amount of space on an EMS test, there are relatively few questions in comparison with the amount of information presented in the EMT-Intermediate and EMT-Paramedic course. The test cannot be all encompassing. Many tests are computer generated; questions are chosen randomly from a large bank of test questions. There is no way for the student to know exactly what will be covered. On the other hand, a review manual presents the opportunity for all or most of the critical items presented in the EMT-Intermediate or EMT-Paramedic curriculum to be covered. This allows the user to review specific areas of the material or, if questions are chosen randomly, a variety of information.

GETTING THE MOST FROM PRACTICE QUESTIONS

Questions on specific subjects are grouped together, allowing the user to focus on specific problem areas. This will also help the reader identify areas where additional study is needed. As you read each question, see if you can answer it without looking at the answer choices. If you answer correctly, read the rationale for the answer anyway. There may be additional helpful information included in the answer rationale. If you answer a question incorrectly, look for a pattern. Try to determine why the answer was incorrect:

Is there a particular subject area you are having difficulty with, or is the missed question isolated?

If you are having difficulty with an entire subject area or portion thereof, place emphasis on studying this section of your EMS text.

Did you not know or did you forget the information being tested? Were you unfamiliar with the subject content?

Spend extra time reviewing this material. If your time is limited, do not waste valuable study time reviewing information you already know. Concentrate on the parts of the EMS text that cover the topics you feel the least familiar with. Look for key points and definitions. Try to remember concepts, not rote answers.

Did you misunderstand the content or concept when reading the EMS text or covering the material in class, or did you draw a wrong conclusion when studying the topic?

Talk with your instructor or a knowledgeable EMT-Intermediate or Paramedic. Try to explain the subject using your own words and ask why your explanation is incorrect. Ask for help in adjusting any misunderstanding and don't be afraid to consult other EMS texts to compare the information presented. Each EMS text has its strong points. You may find that a different textbook presents clearer, easier to understand information on the particular subject.

Did you actually know the correct answer but simply misread the question or answer choices?

It may be that you need to take more time to carefully read the question and answer choices. Recognizing that you have difficulty reading and comprehending test questions may be as important as identifying where additional study of the materials is needed.

Did you read too much into the question?

The only information you are expected to consider is the information presented in the stem. Do not try to determine what happened before or might happen after the fictional "event" the question refers to.

Were you overconfident?

A positive attitude is good, but overconfidence can cause even the most competent student to fail.

HELPFUL TIPS FOR SURVIVING EMS TESTS

Very few people enjoy taking tests. Test taking can be even more stressful for EMS students taking an initial certification test or for certified EMT-Intermediates or Paramedics taking a recertification test. Most of us got into this field because of a desire to be an EMT-Intermediate or Paramedic. It was or is a personal goal we wanted to meet. For many EMS students, some time has elapsed since high school or college. When we were in school, the daily expectation of tests or quizzes kept us in a "test taking" frame of mind. It has likely been quite a while since we had to take such a critical test, and to make matters worse, we find ourselves faced with a test that will decide the course of our EMS career path. But remember: you've come this far, and you *can* pass the test. Although you may never enjoy test taking, it can be less stressful if you follow some simple, helpful hints. The more relaxed you are, the more clearly you will think. Those who created the test do not want you to fail, but they do want you to be challenged. Keeping a level head and using your sense of reasoning and problem solving will allow you to meet that challenge.

BEFORE THE TEST

- Schedule time for both personal and group study. Each has its advantages. When you study alone, you have a chance to go over material you are unsure of. When you study in a group, you can learn from your partners and help others.
- Get plenty of rest. It's hard to think clearly if you're tired.
- Dress comfortably. Wear layered clothing so you can add or remove clothing if the testing room is too hot or too cold.
- Avoid overeating or eating foods that may be hard to digest, such as spicy or greasy foods. Instead, eat foods low in fat or with complex carbohydrates, such as nuts, pasta, or yogurt. If your test is in the morning, eat breakfast (if this is what you normally do).
- Avoid too much caffeine, which can affect attention and concentration. Do not drink alcohol prior to the test (there will be plenty of time for this after the test).
- Although you should not self-medicate, there are a number of medications your doctor can prescribe if you have severe test anxiety that hampers your performance.

- Although you may think that cramming for the test the night before will help, in general, this is not the case. Cramming tends to clutter the mind and confuse the test taker.
- Give yourself enough time to reach the test location and try to arrive early. Running late for a test will only increase your anxiety level. Also, by arriving early, you will have an opportunity to choose your seat wisely. Although this may not seem important, a seat in an area that is too hot, too cold, too noisy, or uncomfortable for any other reason can cause additional anxiety.
- Try to relax. If you have some favorite relaxation techniques, use them prior to starting the test. Relaxation and stress reduction exercises can also be practiced during the test provided they do not distract the other students. A simple exercise is to sit up straight and close your eyes. Take five deep breaths, counting each one and exhaling completely each time. As you count each breath, focus on relaxing all the muscles in your body.
- Have confidence in your ability to pass the test. Maintain a positive "I-can-pass-this-test" attitude. Put forth your best effort. Imagine how good you'll feel when you receive word that you have passed.
- If you have had a history of not doing well on written examinations, there is a possibility you may have a reading or learning disability. Professionals at the counseling center at your local training facility, community college, or university can help you determine if this is the case. If you do have a diagnosed learning disability, they can provide you with strategies to help compensate for it. Also, in some cases, certifying agencies will allow reasonable accommodations, such as longer testing times, if you have a documented learning disability.

TIPS FOR TAKING MULTIPLE-CHOICE TESTS

- Carefully read all of the directions prior to starting the test to be sure you understand what you are supposed to do. If you don't understand the test instructions, ask the test proctor for clarification.
- Carefully read the entire question before attempting to answer it. Important background information is often contained in the sentences leading up to the actual question. You don't want to lose any points because you have misread a question.
- After reading the entire question, try to answer it without looking at the choices. Then look at the choices to see if your answer is the same as or close to one of the choices.
- Read *all* of the choices. Even if the first choice seems to be the correct answer, read the other choices so you do not overlook a better choice.
- Give all the words in the question and the answer choices equal attention. A missed or misread word

can mean the difference between a correct answer and an incorrect answer.

- In most cases, ensuring scene safety, ensuring an open airway, and correcting life-threatening problems take precedence. Look for answers that deal with these aspects of patient management.
- If you are unsure of an answer, leave the corresponding number on the answer sheet blank and proceed to the next question. Be careful not to get answer numbers out of sequence. Don't forget to go back to unanswered questions after completing the exam.
- Don't take a question personally. Don't get upset over a question or answer choice you don't like. This will only increase your anxiety and tension.
- Be sure the number on the answer sheet corresponds to the number of the question. Check periodically to ensure that the question number and answer number correspond.
- It is usually best to trust your first answer choice. Only change an answer if you think you must.
- If time permits or if you are having difficulty deciding on an answer, read the question using each of the answer choices given. Reading the question and each answer choice together in their entirety allows you to focus on choices that make sense both logically and grammatically.
- The answers to multiple-choice questions do not follow a pattern, so don't try to find one. Trying to find a pattern will only add to any confusion you may already feel.
- Be cautious of using test-taking "tricks" such as "when in doubt mark 'c'" or "there will never be more than three of the same letter in a row." People who design high-stakes tests know about these tricks and design exams to reduce their effectiveness.
- If you do not immediately recognize the correct answer, eliminate any choice that you are sure is incorrect so you have fewer answers to choose from. If you can narrow the number of choices to two plausible answers, you have greatly increased your chances of getting the question right.
- Look for absolutes, such as "never," "always," or "every." These types of words may indicate that the choice is wrong.
- Look for key words in the question such as "immediately," "initially," "first," or "most." These may help you identify which answer choice is the best.
- Carefully read any question using the words "not" or "except." These types of questions are used to determine if you can tell what should not be done or if you know an exception. Many test developers try to avoid such questions, but some still use them.
- Be wary of any distractors that contain words or information you have never seen, even if they seem to be plausible choices.

- Base your answers on what you learned from the text, not an experience other practicing EMT-Intermediates or Paramedics may have had with different patients.
- If you are allowed to use a sheet of paper to solve problems, take advantage of it.
- Generally, it is best to answer every question. However, some tests are scored with a system that does not penalize for unanswered questions but does penalize incorrect responses to discourage guessing. On this type of test it is better to leave questions blank if you are not very sure of the correct answer. Be sure you understand the system that will be used to grade the exam you are taking.

MANAGING YOUR TIME

- Know how much time is allotted for the test and how many questions you must answer. For instance, for both the EMT-Intermediate and Paramedic level tests, the National Registry allows 3 hours to complete 180 questions (which averages out to 1 minute per question). In most cases, you will be given more time than you are likely to need. Relax and do not be overly time conscious early on.
- Use all the allotted time. Only knowledge is being tested, not your ability to finish early.
- When taking the exam, try to answer the easiest questions first. Save the harder questions for last. Doing so will allow you to spend more time on the harder questions.
- Make sure you go back to all the questions you have left blank. If unanswered questions count against you, take a guess if you still don't know the answer.
- If you have time left at the end of the exam, review your answers. Sometimes the content of a later question or answer may remind you of information that could affect a previous answer.
- Check your answer sheet. Be sure each choice marked on the answer sheet corresponds to the choice you want. Even if you know the answer to a question, marking errors can cause the choice to be scored as incorrect. Also check to be sure you did not leave any questions unanswered.

A word of caution applies when this or any review manual is used. Do not view this book as a review manual to pass the National Registry test or any other particular test. If you are taking the National Registry test, some questions may be presented differently. Do not become overly confident simply because you have completed a review manual. Passing tests does not make you a good EMT-Intermediate or Paramedic. Instead, if you try to be the most knowledgeable and best EMT-Intermediate or Paramedic you can be, passing the test will be an added bonus. We wish you the best in your endeavors to become, or remain, the best EMT-Intermediate or Paramedic you can be.

NOTE TO THE READER

This review manual contains questions taken from the EMT-Intermediate and Paramedic National Standard Curriculum. The questions cover both EMT-Intermediate and Paramedic level material. Because the actual material covered in the EMT-Intermediate course varies from state to state, readers are advised to disregard any questions that do not apply to the course they are taking.

The authors and publisher have made every attempt to ensure that the drug dosages and patient care procedures presented in this text are accurate and represent accepted practices in the United States. They are not provided as standards of care. It is the reader's responsibility to follow patient care protocols established by medical direction physicians and to know current standards for the delivery of emergency care.

 Paramedic Only Questions

This manual includes some questions on subjects that are found only in the EMT-Paramedic National Standard Curriculum. These questions are clearly identified by a "star of life" icon around the question number. If you are an EMT-Intermediate or are currently enrolled in an EMT-Intermediate course, this information may or may not have been presented in your class. However, knowing this information may prove helpful when working in the field. Also, it can provide you with a better understanding of why patients with medical problems present in a particular way or why certain care works best. This can increase your confidence and your abilities as an EMT-Intermediate. Therefore it is the decision of the reader as to whether these questions should be reviewed when using this book.

ACKNOWLEDGMENTS

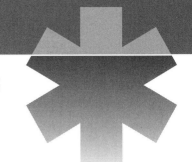

No book such as this could be accomplished without the hard work of dedicated reviewers who looked at questions for hours on end. It is only with the input of these unsung heroes that a manual can be of any quality. A special word of thanks goes to:

Kathleen A. Ballman, RN, CEN, EMT-P
Director, Bethesda Hospital Paramedic Program
TriHealth
Cincinnati, Ohio

Margot Daugherty, RN, BSN, CEN, NREMT-P
EMS Coordinator
Bethesda North Hospital
Cincinnati, Ohio

William J. Doss, EMT-P
Paramedic/Firefighter
Miami Township Fire and EMS
Clermont County, Ohio

Janet Fitts, RN, BSN, CEN, EMT-P
Education Specialist
Prehospital and Emergency Nursing Education
Pacific, Missouri

John Eric Powell, PhD(c)
Research Coordinator
Department of Emergency Medicine
University of Tennessee Medical Center
Knoxville, Tennessee

S. Rutherfoord Rose, PharmD, FAACT
Associate Professor of Emergency Medicine
Director, Virginia Poison Center
Virginia Commonwealth University Health System
Richmond, Virginia

To the staff at Elsevier
To Claire Merrick
I value our relationship and the support you have given me over the years with various projects. You've helped me to fulfill a lifelong dream. ~D.M.

Thanks for taking a chance on a new author. Your support has been invaluable. Here's to more success in the future. ~K.W.
To Lisa Neumann
I know it's been a learning experience, but you've been a joy to work with. I hope we didn't make it too complicated. (By the way, where's that speaker phone you ordered?) ~D.M.

No project would be possible without the constant encouragement and prodding of an excellent editor. Lisa, you're the best. ~K.W.
To Laura Bayless
Thanks for your hard work in getting the project started and working with us during the initial difficult times. We got off to a slow start, but you can't stop a train once it gets rolling. ~D.M
To Derril Trakalo
Thanks for helping to make these projects successful. It's only through good marketing that we can get useful books into the hands of those who need them. (By the way, if there are any books or videos that you don't want to ship back . . .) ~D.M.
To Derril and Kelly Trakalo
Thank you for all your efforts in marketing and the karaoke lessons. ~K.W.

CONTENTS

HUMAN SYSTEMS AND PATHOPHYSIOLOGY

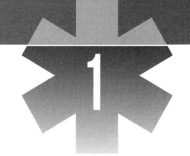

1. Directional terms are used to refer to the human body in the anatomical position. Which of the following refers to people in the anatomical position?
   a. lying supine on their back
   b. lying prone on their stomach
   c. standing erect with the feet and palms facing the examiner
   d. standing erect with the feet turned outward and the palms resting at their side

2. The body structure relationships are classified into anatomical planes. Referring to Figure 1-1, match the following terms to their appropriate plane: transverse, frontal, midsagittal, sagittal.

3. Imagine a line drawn down the center of the body and one across the waist. The position of body parts and the sites of injury are relative to these lines. Fill in the blank using the appropriate term.

1. cephalad	6. posterior
2. caudal	7. medial
3. proximal	8. lateral
4. distal	9. superior
5. anterior	10. inferior

   a. The wrist is _____ to the elbow.
   b. The head is _____ to the shoulders.
   c. The chest is on the _____ surface of the body.
   d. The breast is _____ to the sternum.
   e. Moving cephalad is to move (toward, away from) the head.
   f. The dorsal surface is _____.
   g. The navel is _____ to the nipples.
   h. Moving caudal is to move (toward, away from) the head.
   i. The knee is _____ to the ankle.
   j. The little finger is _____ to the thumb.

4. Body cavities are lined with a serous membrane. The membrane that comes into contact with the wall of the cavity is called the *visceral pleura*.
   a. true
   b. false

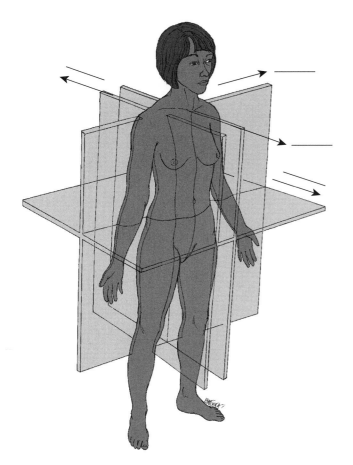

Figure 1-1

5. Referring to Figure 1-2, label the cavities using the following terms: abdominal cavity, pelvic cavity, pleural cavity, pericardial cavity.

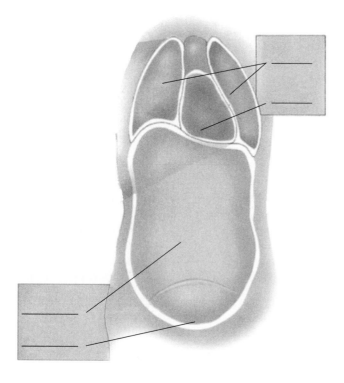

Figure 1-2

6. The structure that lies between the left and right pleural cavities is the:
a. parietal pleura
b. mediastinum
c. diaphragm
d. none of the above

7. The three *main* parts of all human cells are the cytoplasmic membrane, cytoplasm, and:
a. glycoproteins
b. nucleus
c. mitochondria
d. ribosomes

8. The two major classes of free-living cells are subdivided by the way genetic material is organized inside them. The two main types are:
a. eukaryotes and prokaryotes
b. "true nucleus" and "before nucleus"
c. mycoplasms and chondrocytes
d. both a and b are correct

9. A structure that has a specific function and is composed of two or more different types of tissues is called a(n):
a. cell
b. system
c. organelle
d. organ

10. The capsule of the kidneys, the parietal pleura, and the outer layer of blood vessels are composed of what tissue type?
a. epithelial
b. muscle
c. connective
d. nervous

11. All of the following are true cellular adaptations *EXCEPT:*
a. atrophy
b. hypertrophy
c. hyperplasia
d. dysplasia

12. Your patient is a long-time cigarette smoker and has developed nonciliated squamous epithelial cells in the bronchial lining. What form of cell adaptation would you consider this change to be?
a. dysplasia
b. metaplasia
c. hyperplasia
d. atrophy

13. Hypoxic injury to cells only results from poor respiratory function, which limits the amount of oxygen to the body, such as a suffocation injury, asthma, or other pulmonary obstructive diseases.
a. true
b. false

14. Which of the following is not considered to be a cause of chemical injury to cells?
a. chemotherapy drugs
b. carbon monoxide
c. ethanol
d. all of the above have the potential to cause injury

15. By producing toxins that can injure or destroy cells and tissues, bacteria are able to proliferate in the body. The toxins most likely to activate an inflammatory process and produce fever directly would be:
a. exotoxins
b. epitoxins
c. hypertoxins
d. endotoxins

16. The body uses a group of proteins called the complement system to coat bacteria and kill them directly or assist in the body's disposal of them. What condition causes the complement system to work against the body, rather than act as a defense mechanism?
    a. hypersensitivity
    b. septicemia
    c. bacteremia
    d. the complement system always works for the body

17. Viruses are responsible for many human diseases. Like bacteria, they produce endotoxins and exotoxins to infect the living cells of host tissues.
    a. true
    b. false

18. Viruses act on cells by:
    a. engulfing cells, thereby causing cellular death by hypoxia
    b. rapidly moving through the body in the extracellular fluid
    c. attaching to the cellular membrane and utilizing the nutrients of the cell to reproduce
    d. invading the cell membrane and replicating viral nucleic acids, or causing the cell to burst

19. Cellular membranes are injured by direct contact with cellular and chemical components of the immune or inflammatory process. The resultant injury occurs when:
    a. macrophages cause a large collection of viral particles to form causing vessel blockages
    b. viruses cause an abnormal release of capsid, which deteriorates the nutrients in the cell
    c. the cellular membrane is injured or the sodium/potassium transport mechanism fails
    d. the actions of monocytes, neutrophils, and macrophages cause the eventual destruction of cellular metabolism

20. Hyperglycemia in an example of an injurious nutritional imbalance.
    a. true
    b. false

21. Injured cells and some healthy cells accumulate substances such as fluids and electrolytes. Irreversible damage occurs to cells when:
    a. phagocytes migrate toward cells and engulf them
    b. they are unable to rid excessive amounts of sodium or calcium
    c. macrophages fix to tissues and ingest lipids
    d. none of the above are a cause of damage to cells

22. After cell death, structural changes occur. The process of self-destruction of the cells is known as:
    a. catabolism
    b. anabolism
    c. autolysis
    d. necrosis

23. Water is distributed throughout the body in various compartments. The largest compartment is the _____ compartment, which contains approximately 75% of all body water.
    a. extracellular
    b. intravascular
    c. intracellular
    d. interstitial

24. Total body water and its distribution will vary with age and patient condition. Based on the average normal percent of water by body weight, which of the following patients is most likely to develop electrolyte disorders?
    a. 30-year-old male
    b. 79-year-old female
    c. 3-month-old male
    d. b and c are correct

Questions 25 through 27 refer to the following scenario:

Your patient is a 70-year-old female who has fallen at work and complains of wrist pain. You arrive to find the patient sitting in a chair behind the counter of a gift store. She is alert, oriented, and in no obvious distress. She has pain in her wrist with some deformity but denies all other injury. During your detailed physical exam, you note that she has significant edema in her ankles. She denies any medical problems and states she annually sees her physician for checkups. She has no shortness of breath and her lungs are clear.

25. The accumulation of water (edema) in her ankles most likely is due to:
    a. the trauma of the fall
    b. prolonged standing
    c. an immune response
    d. an obstruction of the lymph system

26. The patient has edema in her ankles, which can cause relative dehydration. This patient most likely compensates for the edema by which of the following mechanisms?
  a. net filtration
  b. oncotic force
  c. Starling's hypothesis
  d. release of ADH

27. Management of this patient may include all of the following *EXCEPT*:
  a. splinting and elevating the affected wrist, applying ice for pain
  b. transporting the patient in position of comfort, rather than the shock position
  c. administering 40 mg of furosemide to aid in removing the fluid from her ankles
  d. monitor vital signs for any indications of impending shock

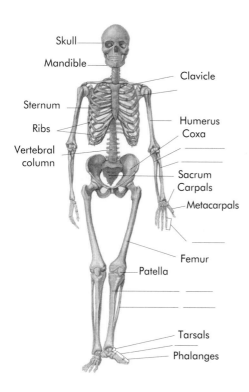

Figure 1-3

28. Referring to Figure 1-3, label the following bones: scapula, radius, ulna, phalanges, tibia, fibula, metatarsals.

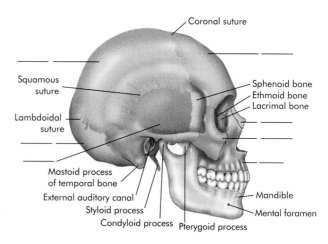

Figure 1-4

29. Referring to Figure 1-4, label the following bones: parietal, temporal, occipital, frontal, nasal, zygomatic, maxilla.

30. Match the body movement with its definition.

  1. flexion   4. abduction
  2. extension   5. pronation
  3. adduction   6. supination

  a. _____ rotation of the forearm so that the anterior surface is down
  b. _____ movement away from the midline
  c. _____ bending
  d. _____ rotation of the forearm so that the anterior surface is up
  e. _____ stretching out
  f. _____ movement toward the midline

31. The difference between isometric and isotonic muscle contraction is that isometric contraction does not reduce the length of the muscle.
  a. true
  b. false

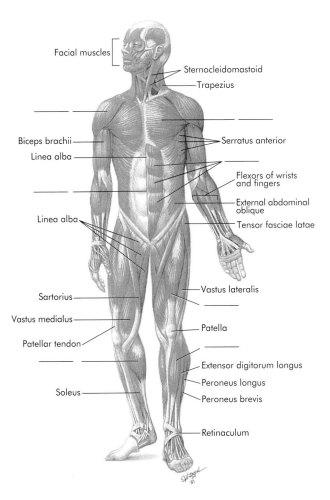

Figure 1-5

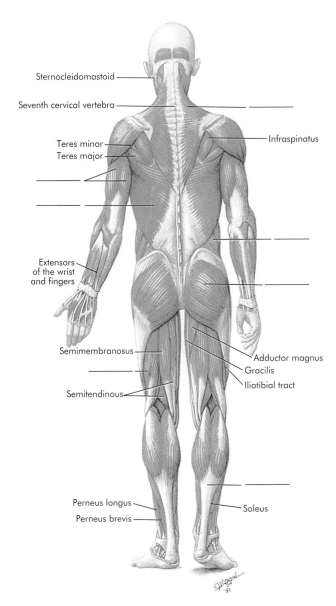

Figure 1-6

⚕ **32.** Referring to Figure 1-5, label the following muscles: deltoid, pectoralis major, brachioradialis, rectus abdominis, rectus femoris, tibialis anterior, gastrocnemius.

⚕ **33.** Referring to Figure 1-6, label the following muscles: trapezius, triceps, latissimus dorsi, external abdominal oblique, gluteus maximus, biceps femoris, Achilles tendon.

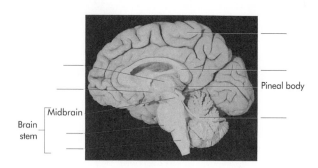

Figure 1-7

34. The central nervous system is composed of the brain, brain stem, and spinal cord. Referring to Figure 1-7, label the following parts of the brain and brain stem: thalamus, hypothalamus, cerebral cortex, cerebellum, pons, medulla, corpus callosum.

35. What is the difference between the afferent and efferent pathways in the peripheral nervous system?
    a. afferent pathways carry impulses to the muscles and organs
    b. afferent pathways are part of the autonomic nervous system
    c. efferent pathways are part of the somatic nervous system
    d. none of the above

36. Match the brain area with its function.

    1. medulla   4. thalamus
    2. pons   5. cerebellum
    3. hypothalamus   6. cerebrum

    a. _____ muscle coordination and equilibrium
    b. _____ regulation of body temperature, water balance, and sleep
    c. _____ primary control of respiration
    d. _____ regulation of heart rate, respirations, and vasomotor control
    e. _____ emotions
    f. _____ consciousness and memory

37. Which of the following accurately describes the structure of neurons?
    a. Neurons are composed of two portions, the cell body and the dendrite.
    b. Dendrites transmit impulses away from the neuron cell body.
    c. Neurons have three portions: the dendrite, cell body, and the axon.
    d. Axons in the CNS are surrounded by Schwann cells for insulation.

38. Regarding afferent, efferent, and connecting neurons:
    a. afferent neurons are motor nerves
    b. efferent neurons transmit impulses away from the brain
    c. connecting neurons join afferent neurons to efferent neurons
    d. afferent neurons transmit impulses away from the brain

39. Neurons transmit impulses throughout the nervous system. To facilitate this process:
    a. myelinated neurons transmit impulses faster than unmyelinated neurons
    b. acetylcholine is the only neurotransmitter involved at the synapse
    c. the interruptions between Schwann cells in unmyelinated neurons are called nodes of Ranvier
    d. none of the above

40. Regarding the autonomic nervous system assign the effect to either sympathetic (S) or parasympathetic (P) control.
    a. Accelerates the heartbeat   S   P
    b. Increases peristalsis   S   P
    c. Dilates the pupil   S   P
    d. Causes "goose bumps"   S   P
    e. Stimulates urination   S   P
    f. Increases sweat secretion   S   P

41. There are three types of blood cells circulating in the body: red blood cells, white blood cells, and platelets. The most common type of white blood cells are the:
    a. lymphocytes
    b. neutrophils
    c. monocytes
    d. eosinophils

42. The pericardium surrounding the heart is composed of two layers, an outer _____ layer and an inner _____ layer.
a. serous, fibrous
b. visceral, parietal
c. fibrous, visceral
d. fibrous, parietal

43. Blood flows from the superior vena cava into the atria and subsequently into the right ventricle after passing the _____ valve.
a. mitral
b. pulmonic
c. tricuspid
d. aortic

Normal blood flow

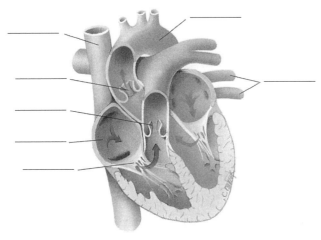

Figure 1-8

44. Referring to Figure 1-8, match the structure to the blanks: superior vena cava, aorta, right atrium, tricuspid valve, pulmonary valve, pulmonary veins, aortic valve.

45. Match the part of the heart's conduction system with its location.

1. interventricular septum
2. wall of right atrium
3. myocardium
4. interarterial septum

_____ a. sinoatrial node
_____ b. atrioventricular node
_____ c. bundle of His
_____ d. Purkinje system

46. When listening to the heartbeat we hear the typical "lub dub." During the "lub" sound, what is happening in the heart?
a. the aortic valve is closing
b. the mitral and tricuspid valves are closing
c. the ventricle is relaxing
d. the coronary arteries are being perfused

47. The lymphatic system is a passive circulatory system for the transportation of lymph. What is lymph?
a. fluid filled with white blood cells to fight infection
b. platelets to improve blood clotting
c. digestive juices for the gastrointestinal tract
d. excess extracellular fluid

48. The gastrointestinal tract is divided into several sections. Which of the following lists is in the correct order starting from ingestion to excretion?
a. esophagus, stomach, ileum, duodenum, colon
b. stomach, duodenum, jejunum, ileum, colon
c. esophagus, duodenum, stomach, colon, ileum
d. stomach, duodenum, ileum, jejunum, colon

49. The appendix lies in the small intestines resting in the right lower quadrant.
a. true
b. false

50. Which of the following is *not* a function of the liver?
a. iron metabolism
b. storage of reserve blood cells
c. detoxification of the plasma
d. production of bile for digestion

51. The colon is involved in which of the following processes?
    a. absorption of water and salts
    b. absorption of vitamin K from bacteria
    c. conversion of chyme to feces
    d. all of the above

52. The functional unit of the kidney is the:
    a. glomerulus
    b. loop of Henle
    c. nephron
    d. renal cortex

53. The first step in the production of urine within the nephron is:
    a. filtration of the blood in the glomerulus
    b. reabsorption of water, glucose, and other nutrients in the loop of Henle
    c. active secretion of hydrogen and salts in the collecting tubules
    d. none of the above

54. The formation of urine is controlled by:
    a. sympathetic stimulation
    b. parasympathetic stimulation
    c. hormones
    d. blood pressure

55. Water movement between the intracellular fluid and the extracellular fluid occur by each of the following mechanisms *EXCEPT*:
    a. dispersion
    b. diffusion
    c. osmosis
    d. mediated transport

56. Several things can lead to accumulation of fluid in the interstitial space. During an immune response the primary mechanism is:
    a. increased capillary hydrostatic pressure
    b. decreased oncotic pressure
    c. increased capillary permeability
    d. lymphatic vessel obstruction

57. The primary hormone involved in water retention is:
    a. aldosterone
    b. antidiuretic hormone (ADH)
    c. atrial natriuretic hormone
    d. none of the above

58. Aldosterone stimulation is controlled by the concentration of what ions in the urine?
    a. potassium and sodium
    b. chloride and sodium
    c. potassium and chloride
    d. hydrogen

59. Which of the following best describes the renin-angiotensin system?
    a. the kidney secretes renin, which is converted by the liver to angiotensin, which increases blood flow to the kidney
    b. renin is secreted and stimulates the formation of angiotensin I, which is converted in the lung to angiotensin, a potent vasoconstrictor that raises blood pressure
    c. renin stimulates the production of ADH
    d. all of the above

60. Hyperkalemia, an elevated serum potassium level, has all of the following signs and symptoms *EXCEPT*:
    a. irritability
    b. weakness
    c. hyperactive reflexes
    d. cardiac conduction disturbances

61. Calcium is a critical ion involved in neuromuscular control and bone formation. Which of the following is the most specific symptom of hypocalcemia?
    a. nausea
    b. diarrhea
    c. paresthesias
    d. none of the above

62. Hypomagnesemia occurs in alcoholics, diabetics, and diseases that cause hypocalcemia and hypokalemia. Signs and symptoms of hypomagnesemia include all the following *EXCEPT*:
    a. tremors
    b. seizures
    c. cardiac dysrhythmias, particularly torsades
    d. depressed deep reflexes

63. The acid-base balance is part of the process of the body to maintain:
    a. homeostasis
    b. equilibrium
    c. neutral pH
    d. oxygenation

64. As the concentration of hydrogen ions increases, the pH lowers.
    a. true
    b. false

65. The primary buffer used by the body to respond to acidosis is:
a. carbonic acid
b. bicarbonate
c. carbon dioxide
d. none of the above

66. The body is better able to respond to alkalosis than acidosis.
a. true
b. false

67. What organ system has the greatest ability to respond to changes in the acid-base balance?
a. the renal system
b. the cardiovascular system
c. the respiratory system
d. the gastrointestinal system

68. What is the respiratory response to acidosis?
a. hypoventilation
b. hyperventilation
c. slower but deeper respirations
d. slower but shallower respirations

69. The renal system is also involved in acid-base balance. However, it is less responsive than the respiratory system because it is slower.
a. true
b. false

70. During hypoventilation carbon dioxide levels rise, resulting in:
a. metabolic acidosis
b. metabolic alkalosis
c. respiratory acidosis
d. respiratory alkalosis

71. Which of the following would result in respiratory acidosis?
a. central nervous system depression from opiate overdose
b. acute anxiety
c. pain
d. breathing 100% oxygen

72. Metabolic acidosis occurs when excess hydrogen ions circulate in the bloodstream. Conditions that could result in this excess include:
a. shock
b. severe diarrhea
c. renal failure
d. all of the above

73. When metabolic acidosis develops, the body responds by increasing the respiratory rate resulting in a compensatory respiratory alkalosis.
a. true
b. false

74. The best way to think of metabolic and respiratory acid-base balance is:
a. metabolic response has to do with the release of carbon dioxide
b. respiratory response has to do with the production of buffers
c. metabolic response is acid production, respiratory response is carbon dioxide movement
d. all of the above

ANSWERS TO CHAPTER 1: HUMAN SYSTEMS AND PATHOPHYSIOLOGY

1. c. The anatomical position is used as a point to which the position of an organ, injury, or complaint can be referenced. Although it does not appear natural, the person stands with the feet, palms, and forearms facing the examiner.

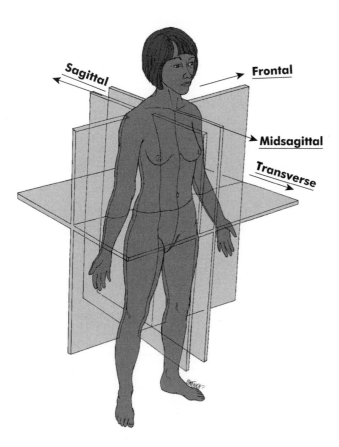

Figure 1-1

2. The body structure relationships are classified into anatomical planes. Referring to Figure 1-1, match the following terms to their appropriate plane: transverse, frontal, midsagittal, sagittal.

3. Imagine a line drawn down the center of the body and one across the waist. The position of body parts and the sites of injury are relative to these lines. Fill in the blank using the appropriate term.

1. cephalad	6. posterior
2. caudal	7. medial
3. proximal	8. lateral
4. distal	9. superior
5. anterior	10. inferior

a. The wrist is _4_ to the elbow
b. The head is _9_ to the shoulders
c. The chest is on the _5_ surface of the body
d. The breast is _8_ to the sternum
e. Moving cephalad is to move (toward) the head
f. The dorsal surface is _6_
g. The navel is _10_ to the nipples
h. Moving caudal is to move (away from) the head
i. The knee is _3_ to the ankle
j. The little finger is _7_ to the thumb

4. b. False. The membrane in contact with the body cavity wall is the parietal pleura and the membrane in contact with the organs is the visceral pleura. The primary difference is that the parietal pleura has nerve fibers, whereas the visceral pleura does not.

5. Referring to Figure 1-2, label the cavities using the following terms: abdominal cavity, pelvic cavity, pleural cavity, pericardial cavity.

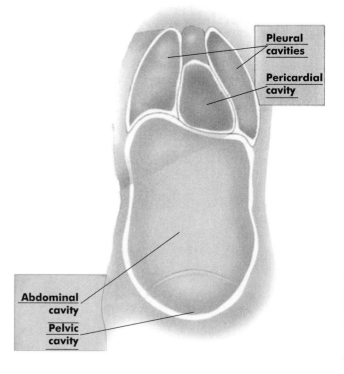

Figure 1-2

6. b. The mediastinum is contained within the thoracic cavity resting between the lungs and contains the heart, thymus, and trachea.

7. b. The nucleus is a relatively large structure that is usually located near the center of the cell. The cell nucleus is surrounded by a nuclear membrane, which encloses a special type of protoplasm known as nucleoplasm. Glycoproteins are chemically modified proteins to which carbohydrate molecules are attached. Mitochondria are the organelles responsible for cellular energy production. Ribosomes are the portion of the cells where proteins are synthesized.

8. d. Eukaryotes are the "true nucleus" and prokaryotes are "before nucleus." Mycoplasms are prokaryotes, and chondrocytes are cartilage cells.

9. d. Each organ has a specific function or functions. The cell is the basic unit of the body. Systems are made up of structures that adapt to perform functions necessary to life, such as the respiratory system. Organelles are components of the cell and have specific cellular functions.

10. c. Connective tissue is the most abundant and widely distributed type of tissue in the body. Epithelial tissue covers surfaces or forms structures derived from body surfaces. There is little or no intercellular material between the cells of this tissue. Muscle tissue is a contractile tissue responsible for movement. Nervous tissue is characterized by the ability to conduct electrical signals, which are known as action potentials.

11. d. Dysplasia is not considered a true cellular adaptation but rather an atypical hyperplasia. Dysplasia refers to abnormal changes of mature cells. Atrophy is a decrease or shrinkage in cellular size that affects cell function. Hypertrophy is an increase in the size of cells without an increase in numbers. Hyperplasia is an excessive increase in the number of cells that results in an increase in the size of a tissue or organ. Metaplasia is the conversion into a form that is not normal for that cell or the replacement of normal tissue cells by other cells that may be better able to tolerate adverse environmental conditions.

12. b. Metaplasia converts the normal ciliated epithelial cells to nonciliated squamous epithelial cells, which are more resistant to irritation. This can be reversed when one quits smoking cigarettes. Dysplastic changes are considered precancerous and also can result from chronic irritation or inflammation. They are frequently found adjacent to cancerous cells. Examples of hyperplasia would include formation of a callus. Atrophy is most common in skeletal muscle, the heart, secondary sex organs, and the brain.

13. b. Although hypoxic injury may result from decreased oxygen in the air or diseases of the respiratory system, it also can result from altered hemoglobin function, decreased red blood cells, trauma, and narrowing or blockages of arteries. Prolonged ischemia leads to infarction or cell death. Hypoxic injury is the most common cause of cellular injury.

14. d. Chemotherapy drugs target the genetic material of cells, whereas other toxins such as carbon monoxide affect the cytochrome system found in the mitochondria, which ceases oxidative metabolism in the cell. Ethanol, carbon monoxide, lead, and complex toxins either injure cells directly or are metabolized and create a toxin that affects the cells.

15. d. Endotoxins are contained in the cell walls of some bacteria and are released during treatment with antibiotics or when cell walls disintegrate. The bacteria that cause meningitis are an example of this type. Bacteria that produce endotoxins are also called *pyrogenic bacteria*, because they produce fever through release of cell membrane toxins. Fever is caused by the release of endogenous proteins (pyrogens) that act on the thermoregulatory centers of the hypothalamus. These pyrogens are released from macrophages or circulating white blood cells that are attracted to the injury site. Exotoxins are a byproduct of bacteria, rather than a component. Exotoxins made by bacteria have highly specific effects. Streptococci would be an example of exotoxin-producing bacteria.

16. a. A rare but life-threatening pathogenic mechanism of bacterial toxins is hypersensitivity. Hypersensitivity develops after reexposure to a toxin, causing an inflammatory response. Occasionally, the response is so extreme that the host is killed instead of the bacteria. The complement system can activate blood clotting and cause white cells to aggregate and form clumps leading to blockage of small vessels in the lungs and clots in small arteries elsewhere in the body. Septicemia (bacteremia) is the result of the failure of the body's defense mechanisms causing a proliferation of microorganisms in the blood.

17. b. Viruses lack many of the mechanisms that allow bacteria and other cells to grow and multiply. They require nucleic acid (either DNA or RNA) to reproduce. Viruses have no organelles and therefore have no metabolism.

18. d. Viruses usually consist of a protein coat called *capsid* that encloses a core of nucleic acid. Cells are thought to engulf the viruses by surrounding them with part of the cell membrane. Once inside the cell, the virus loses its capsid and begins to replicate viral nucleic acids. Some viruses cause the cell to burst, whereas others replicate without destroying the cells.

19. c. When the cell membrane is injured or the transport system begins to fail, an increase in intracellular water occurs, causing cellular swelling. If cellular swelling continues, the cell may eventually rupture. Cellular and chemical components of the immune and inflammatory response can injure the cell membrane but do not cause blockages of vessels.

20. a. Cells require adequate amounts of essential nutrients to function normally. Pathophysiological cellular effects occur when the required nutrients are not provided through diet and transported to cells. Other examples would include malnutrition, scurvy, and rickets.

21. b. If sodium, water, or calcium continue to accumulate, the cells become irreversibly damaged. Phagocytes normally migrate to injured tissue and engulf dying cells and abnormal substances. When lipids accumulate in the cells, the macrophages can ingest excessive extracellular lipids and cellular debris from injured cells.

22. c. Autolysis occurs when the lysosome begins to have membrane breakdown, releasing lysosomal enzymes that begin to digest the cell. The nucleus shrinks and dissolves or breaks into fragments. Catabolism is a chemical process in which energy is released in the cells by breaking down complex substances into simple compounds. Anabolism is any process that produces energy in which simple substances are converted into more complex matter. Necrosis is the death of cells or tissues through injury or disease.

23. c. Intracellular fluid is the fluid found inside of the body cells. The extracellular compartment contains the remaining 25% of all body water. It contains the extracellular fluid, all the fluid that is found outside the cells. The intravascular compartment is a division within the extracellular compartment. It contains the intravascular fluids, which are found in the circulatory system. Interstitial fluids are found outside the cell membrane but not within the circulatory system.

24. d. As the body ages, the loss of body mass and the body's inability to regulate fluid lower total body water (TBW) to approximately 45% to 55% of body weight. Because of decreased ability to regulate fluid levels, the elderly and the very young are at high risk for dehydration. The elderly are often alone and illness and decreased oral intake result in dehydration and electrolyte imbalances. Infants have less fat than adults and therefore have a higher TBW. It is estimated that the TBW in infants is 75% to 80%. Body mechanisms to regulate fluid loss are immature, so the infant can rapidly become dehydrated as a result of fever, diarrhea, or vomiting. Average adult males have an estimated TBW of 65% to 70%.

25. b. An increase in hydrostatic pressure (the pressure inside the capillaries, caused by the force against the vessel walls created by contractions of the heart) can result from obstruction of the venous system. Water and salt retention, prolonged standing, and restrictive clothing at waist or extremities can cause the increase. This forces more water into the interstitial space than the body can handle and eliminate. Trauma causing burns or hemorrhage can cause a loss of plasma proteins. The result of the loss is that oncotic force is decreased to the point that water lost through the hydrostatic pressure is not regained. During an immune response, increased capillary permeability occurs and allows plasma proteins to leak into the capillaries. Lymphatic system obstruction can occur after infection or surgery. Interference with this system causes a backup of fluids into the interstitial space.

26. d. When the osmoreceptors in the anterior hypothalamus detect changes in the concentration of plasma, they stimulate the release of ADH (antidiuretic hormone). Further, baroreceptors located in the carotid sinus, kidney, and aortic arch detect changes in pressure. The changes will again stimulate the release of ADH, helping to maintain homeostasis by regulating water retention and distribution. Net filtration is the total loss of water from blood plasma across the capillary membrane into the interstitial space. Oncotic force is a form of osmotic pressure that is exerted by the solute concentration. Starling's hypothesis describes the actions that equal net filtration.

27. c. Dependent edema that does not exhibit cardiovascular symptoms does not require treatment in the field. The most appropriate immediate treatment for the ankle edema is to elevate the edematous extremities.

28. Referring to Figure 1-3, label the following bones: scapula, radius, ulna, phalanges, tibia, fibula, metatarsals.

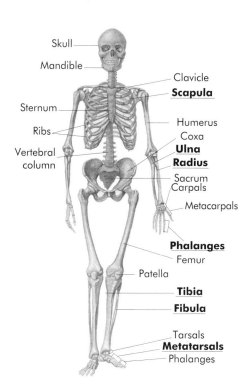

Figure 1-3

29. Referring to Figure 1-4, label the following bones: parietal, temporal, occipital, frontal, nasal, zygomatic, maxilla.

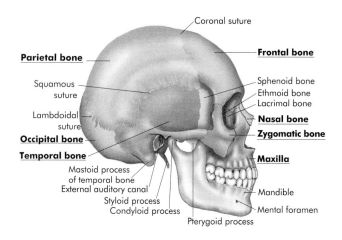

Figure 1-4

30. a. pronation; b. abduction; c. flexion; d. supination; e. extension; f. adduction.

31. a. During isometric contraction the tone increases but the muscle does not shorten. During isotonic contraction the length of the muscle shortens as the contraction occurs. Isometric muscles are involved in maintaining posture while isotonic muscles are involved in movement.

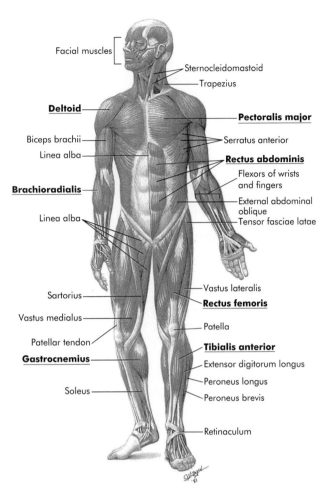

Figure 1-5

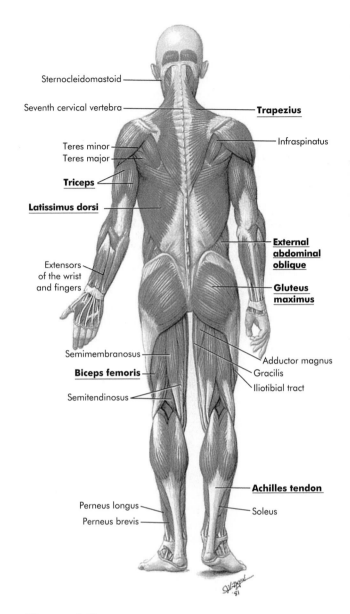

Figure 1-6

32. Referring to Figure 1-5, label the following muscles: deltoid, pectoralis major, brachioradialis, rectus abdominis, rectus femoris, tibialis anterior, gastrocnemius.

33. Referring to Figure 1-6, label the following muscles: trapezius, triceps, latissimus dorsi, external abdominal oblique, gluteus maximus, biceps femoris, Achilles tendon.

34. The central nervous system is composed of the brain, brain stem, and spinal cord. Label the following parts of the brain and brain stem in Figure 1-7: thalamus, hypothalamus, cerebral cortex, cerebellum, pons, medulla, corpus callosum.

35. c. Efferent pathways transmit action potentials from the CNS to the organs such as muscles and glands then are further divided into the somatic nerves, which innervate the muscles and the autonomic nervous system. Afferent

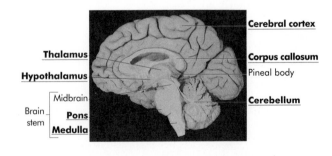

Figure 1-7

pathways carry signals from sensory organs to the CNS.

36. a. cerebellum; b. hypothalamus; c. pons; d. medulla; e. thalamus; f. cerebrum.

37. c. The neuron consists of three parts: a neuron cell body, which contains the nucleus; one or more branching dendrites, which transmit impulses to the cell body; and the elongated axon, which transmits the impulse away from the cell body. The axons in the peripheral nervous system are surrounded by Schwann cells, which act as insulation and are referred to as myelinated, whereas those in the central nervous system have no Schwann cells and are called unmyelinated.

38. b. Afferent neurons transmit sensory impulses to the spinal cord and brain, whereas efferent neurons transmit motor impulses away from the brain and spinal cord. Connecting neurons join a series of afferent or efferent neurons.

39. a. Myelinated neurons are surrounded by Schwann cells, which leave periodic gaps of exposed axon called nodes of Ranvier, which increase the speed of conduction down the axon. Besides acetylcholine, there are multiple neurotransmitters including norepinephrine, epinephrine, and dopamine.

40. a. S, b. P, c. S, d. S, e. P, f. S

41. b. Neutrophils constitute 50% to 75% of the white blood cells and function primarily to scavenge and destroy foreign matter and bacteria. Lymphocytes are the smallest white blood cells and play an important role in immunity by producing antibodies. Monocytes are the largest and are involved in chronic infections in tissue. Eosinophils are involved in the allergic response.

42. a. The pericardium has an outer *fibrous* layer, which is the parietal pericardium and an inner *serous* layer, which is the visceral pericardium.

43. c. The tricuspid valve separates the right atria and right ventricle. The pulmonic valve separates the right ventricle from the pulmonary artery. The mitral valve separates the left atria from the left ventricle. The aortic valve separates the left ventricle from the aorta. "Try to do right" helps us to remember the tricuspid valve is on the right side.

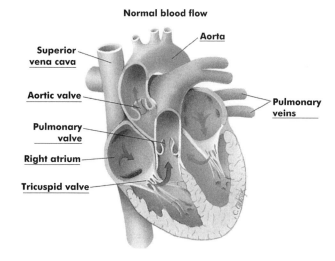

Normal blood flow

Aorta
Superior vena cava
Aortic valve
Pulmonary veins
Pulmonary valve
Right atrium
Tricuspid valve

Figure 1-8

44. Refering to Figure 1-8, match the structure to the blanks: superior vena cava, aorta, right atrium, tricuspid valve, pulmonary valve, pulmonary veins, aortic valve.

45. a. wall of right atrium; b. interarterial septum; c. interventricular septum; d. myocardium.

46. b. During the heartbeat cycle the first heart sound, "lub," occurs during systole when the ventricle contracts and the atrioventricular (mitral and tricuspid) valves close. During diastole the ventricle relaxes and the aortic and pulmonic valves close. Coronary artery perfusion occurs during diastole.

47. d. Excess extracellular fluid enters the lymphatic system to be returned to the circulatory system by way of the thoracic duct.

48. b. From the mouth the GI tract enters the esophagus, which empties into the first portion of the small bowel, the duodenum. The small bowel has three sections, the duodenum, the jejunum, and the ileum. The ileocecal valve separates the small intestines from the large intestine or colon, which has three sections—the ascending, transverse, and descending—which terminate in the rectum.

49. b. False. The appendix extends from the cecum, which is in the first portion of the ascending colon or large intestines.

50. a. The liver produces about a liter of bile per day and detoxifies drugs and foreign material in the bloodstream. Iron binding for red blood cells occurs here as well as the production of clotting agents and other important proteins. The liver is the major site of reserve glycogen stores for energy.

51. d. Chyme is the products of digestion that enter the colon. The colon removes excess water and salts for hydration. Bacteria in the colon produce vitamin K, which is necessary for blood clotting.

52. c. The nephron is the structural and functional unit of the kidney, which forms urine in a three-step process. It is composed of the glomerulus, the ascending and descending loop of Henle, and the collecting tubule.

53. a. The three-step process of urine production occurs first through filtration, second by reabsorption, and third by secretion.

54. c. Aldosterone, ADH, and atrial natriuretic hormone exert influence on the nephron to regulate urine production by controlling the movement of salts and water.

55. a. Diffusion occurs from constant, random movement of molecules through a medium such as water. Osmosis occurs from movement of water across semipermeable membranes in response to the concentration of molecules on each side of the membrane. Mediated transport requires the use of energy to move large molecules against a gradient.

56. c. During an immune response, as during an allergic reaction, histamine is released, which causes increased permeability of the capillaries, which allows for movement of white blood cells into the interstitial space to fight the allergen. Increased capillary hydrostatic pressure results from venous occlusion or salt retention. Decreased oncotic pressure occurs when the body is low in albumin, an important protein. Lymphatic vessel obstruction can occur from infection of the lymph glands or surgical removal.

57. b. ADH is stimulated when the osmolality (concentration) of the blood rises and is sensed by the hypothalamus. Aldosterone and atrial natriuretic hormone are involved but to a lesser extent and through a different mechanism.

58. a. When the urine concentration of potassium rises and sodium lowers, ADH secretion is stimulated by production of renin from the kidney.

59. b. The renin-angiotensin system results in blood pressure elevation, which increases renal blood flow, then ADH acts to increase water reabsorption. Patients with renal hypertension from atherosclerosis of the renal artery have increased angiotensin production leading to further hypertension and water retention. It is treated with angiotensin-converting enzyme (ACE) inhibitors, which reduce the conversion of angiotensin I to angiotensin.

60. c. Hyperkalemia causes irritability of the CNS and cardiac conduction pathways. Weakness and hyporeflexia are hallmarks of the condition.

61. c. Hypocalcemia causes increased neural irritability because the low calcium levels do not allow the neurons to depolarize correctly, resulting in abnormal sensations and uncontrolled muscle contractions and cramps.

62. d. Elevated magnesium levels result in irritability of the central nervous system. This results in hyperactive reflexes, tremors, seizures, and cardiac dysrhythmias. Torsades, a form of ventricular fibrillation, has been shown to be related to hypomagnesemia from chronic malnutrition.

63. a. Homeostasis functions to keep the hydrogen ion concentration within a fairly narrow range to ensure proper functioning of the organs. Any significant deviation from this normal range results in compensatory actions by the body correct the cause of the deviation.

64. a. True. Lower pH equals acidosis, which is an increase in hydrogen ions; higher pH equals alkalosis or a decrease in hydrogen ion concentration.

65. b. Bicarbonate binds to the hydrogen ions and forms carbonic acid, which then dissolves into water and carbon dioxide.

66. b. False. There is twenty times as much bicarbonate in the body as carbonic acid. Therefore the body is more responsive to correcting acidosis than alkalosis. This makes sense because the normal process of metabolism creates acids as by-products.

67. c. The respiratory system plays the primary role of controlling acid-base balance by controlling the removal of carbon dioxide.

68. b. Carbon dioxide is removed from the body by increasing the respiratory rate. This allows greater amounts of carbonic acid to be created, thus freeing up more bicarbonate to combine with hydrogen ions. The net result is a rising of the blood pH.

69. a. True. The kidney's role in acid-base balance is complex and involves the excretion of hydrogen ions and the retention of bicarbonate. This process can take 10 to 20 hours to respond to a change in the blood pH and is involved more in the long-term compensation of acidosis.

70. c. As carbon dioxide rises carbonic acid levels increase and hydrogen ions are released. Because this process occurs as a result of lung impairment it is called respiratory acidosis.

71. a. Both central nervous system depression and obstructive lung disease can result in hypoventilation, leading to respiratory acidosis.

72. d. When the body is in shock, cell injury and death occur, which release acids into the system. Diarrhea results in loss of bicarbonate from the body. Renal failure results in the inability of the body to excrete hydrogenions.

73. a. True. The increased respiratory rate drives carbon dioxide out of the system, resulting in a respiratory alkalosis. This assists the body in removing the excess acids, causing the metabolic acidosis. Unfortunately, although it is compensatory, it will not completely reverse the metabolic acidosis until excess metabolic acid production is decreased.

74. c. To simplify the understanding of the metabolic and respiratory compensations during acid-base balance, think of the respiratory system as blowing off or retaining carbon dioxide and the metabolic response as creating or removing hydrogen ions in the system.

Pharmacology, Venous Access, and Medication Administration

1. A difference between generic names and trade names is that:
   a. a generic name is the same as a brand name, but a trade name is assigned by the government
   b. a medication can have only one generic name but several trade names
   c. generic names are given to a medication by the company that makes it, but trade names are assigned by the government
   d. generic names are generally simple sounding, but trade names are a form of the medication's chemical name

2. The copyright name designated by a drug company is the:
   a. trade name
   b. chemical name
   c. official name
   d. nonproprietary name

3. The generic name of a medication:
   a. is a proprietary name chosen by the drug company
   b. is often an abbreviated form of the chemical name
   c. must be different from the official name
   d. is followed by the initials *USP* or *NF*

4. Drugs are most often classified by all the following *EXCEPT*:
   a. body system
   b. class of agent
   c. route of administration
   d. mechanism of action

5. Under the Controlled Substances Act of 1970, the drugs with the greatest restrictions are:
   a. Schedule I
   b. Schedule II
   c. Schedule III
   d. Schedule IV

6. The amount of medication to be administered to the patient is known as the:
   a. dose
   b. concentration
   c. form
   d. action

7. The term that describes a medical or physiological factor that makes it harmful to administer a medication to a patient is:
   a. an untoward effect
   b. a dosing regimen
   c. a contraindication
   d. a specification

8. The method by which a medication affects the human body is the:
   a. mode of operation
   b. mechanism of action
   c. symbiotic effect
   d. standard reaction

9. The term *side effect* refers to:
   a. an undesirable action of a drug
   b. a life-threatening reaction to a drug
   c. a reason not to administer a drug to a patient
   d. the way the body metabolizes the medication

10. A disadvantage of using the oral route of medication administration is:
    a. the medication is absorbed faster than when it is injected
    b. very few medications may be given orally
    c. absorption rates are slower than when the medication is injected
    d. oral medications have a shorter shelf life

11. An advantage of using the pulmonary route of medication administration is:
    a. any liquid medication that can be given intravenously can be administered via the pulmonary route
    b. because the vascular network in the lungs is limited, absorption rates are much slower than that of the intravenous route
    c. the effect of the medication is local and limited to the pulmonary system
    d. absorption rates into the bloodstream are rapid

12. Four medications that may be administered by the endotracheal route include:
    a. atropine, Benadryl, cordarone, dopamine (ABCD)
    b. adenosine, Benadryl, lidocaine, epinephrine (ABLE)
    c. glucagon, adenosine, morphine, epinephrine (GAME)
    d. lidocaine, atropine, naloxone, epinephrine (LANE)

13. Under the Controlled Substances Act of 1970, morphine is listed as a:
    a. Schedule I substance
    b. Schedule II substance
    c. Schedule III substance
    d. Schedule IV substance

14. A process whereby a medication is chemically converted to a metabolite is known as:
    a. excretion
    b. distribution
    c. biotransformation
    d. absorption

15. The primary organ for excretion of toxic or inactive metabolites is the:
    a. liver
    b. stomach
    c. kidney
    d. gallbladder

16. The blood-brain barrier:
    a. inhibits barbiturates from passing to the brain
    b. allows most antibiotics to pass to the brain
    c. permits only water-soluble drugs to pass to the brain
    d. permits only lipid-soluble drugs to pass to the brain

17. Given the following list of common medications used by EMS personnel, note whether they are most commonly administered via the enteral route, parenteral route, pulmonary route, or topical route.

    _____ activated charcoal

    _____ adenosine

    _____ albuterol

    _____ amiodarone

    _____ aspirin

    _____ atropine

    _____ lidocaine

    _____ metaproterenol

    _____ morphine

    _____ naloxone

    _____ nitroglycerin paste

    _____ nitroglycerin spray

    _____ nitrous oxide

    _____ racemic epinephrine

    _____ viscous lidocaine placed on a nasotracheal tube

18. An agent that inhibits or counteracts effects produced by other medications is:
    a. an agonist
    b. a receptor
    c. an antagonist
    d. a chronotrope

19. The range of plasma concentration that is most likely to produce the desired drug effect with the least likelihood of toxicity is the:
    a. minimum effective concentration
    b. peak plasma level
    c. therapeutic index
    d. therapeutic range

20. The term *bioavailability* refers to:
    a. the amount of medication circulating in the bloodstream and available for uptake by the body's cells
    b. the amount of medication that is still active after it reaches its target tissue
    c. the amount of medication available prior to absorption by body tissues
    d. how readily available a drug is from natural sources

21. A maintenance dose is:
   a. the maximum amount of medication that may be given without harmful effects to the patient
   b. a bolus of a medication initially administered to rapidly attain a therapeutic plasma concentration
   c. medication given orally to enhance the effects of another medication
   d. the amount of a medication needed to maintain a steady therapeutic plasma concentration

22. Common factors that alter the response to drug therapy and that EMS personnel should consider before administering a medication include all the following *EXCEPT* the:
   a. medication's manufacturer
   b. patient's age
   c. patient's gender
   d. patient's weight

23. Cholinergic fibers release:
   a. levophed
   b. dobutamine
   c. acetylcholine
   d. dopamine

24. Adrenergic fibers release:
   a. acetylcholine
   b. norepinephrine
   c. dobutamine
   d. antidiuretic hormone

25. The sympathetic nervous system primarily dominates during:
   a. periods of emotional calm
   b. periods of physical calm
   c. asystole
   d. stressful events

26. The two main types of cholinergic receptors are:
   a. alpha and beta
   b. dopaminergic and dobutaminergic
   c. nicotinic and muscarinic
   d. thoracolumbar and craniosacral

27. Parasympathetic response primarily relates to:
   a. the body's ability to function under stress
   b. vegetative functions
   c. increased stimulation of heart rate and force of contraction
   d. decreased stimulation of digestive functions

28. The most common nonsteroidal antiinflammatory drug encountered by EMS personnel in the field is:
   a. acetaminophen
   b. aspirin
   c. morphine
   d. prednisone

29. Your patient had a kidney transplant approximately 4 months ago. A common type of medication prescribed to transplant patients is:
   a. an anticholinergic
   b. an antiarrhythmic
   c. a vasodilator
   d. an immunosuppressant

30. The primary benefit to giving aspirin to patients experiencing a myocardial infarction is that it acts as:
   a. an antidysrhythmic
   b. a thrombolytic
   c. an antiplatelet
   d. an analgesic

31. An example of a medication that is both an arteriolar and venous dilator is:
   a. nitroglycerin
   b. adenosine
   c. diltiazem
   d. procainamide

32. Under the Vaughn-Williams and Singh Classification System, amiodarone is classified as a:
   a. Class I antidysrhythmic
   b. Class II antidysrhythmic
   c. Class III antidysrhythmic
   d. Class IV antidysrhythmic

33. Examples of calcium-channel blockers commonly seen and in some EMS systems used by paramedics include:
   a. procainamide and lidocaine
   b. amiodarone and bretylium
   c. propranolol and phenytoin
   d. diltiazem and verapamil

Venous Access and Medication Administration

34. A membrane that allows some substances to enter but restricts the passage of others is a:
   a. gateway membrane
   b. semipermeable membrane
   c. aqueous membrane
   d. osmotic membrane

35. Most of the water in the body can be found in the form of:
   a. extracellular fluid
   b. intravascular fluid
   c. intracellular fluid
   d. special fluids

36. Interstitial fluid is an example of:
   a. intravascular fluid
   b. extracellular fluid
   c. intracellular fluid
   d. intraocular fluid

37. Match the following prefixes with their associated meaning: deci-, centi-, kilo-, micro-, milli-.
   _____ 1000 times greater
   _____ 1/10th
   _____ 1/100th
   _____ 1/1000th
   _____ 1/1,000,000th

38. When performing an intramuscular injection, the angle of entry should be:
   a. 30 degrees
   b. 45 degrees
   c. 60 degrees
   d. 90 degrees

39. A 45-degree angle of entry would be used when performing:
   a. intradermal injection
   b. subcutaneous injection
   c. intravenous injection
   d. intraosseous injection

40. The greater the gauge number of a needle, the:
   a. longer the length of the needle
   b. thicker the wall of the needle
   c. smaller the lumen of the needle
   d. greater the strength of the needle

41. Intramuscular needles are generally:
   a. ¼ to ½ inch in length
   b. ½ to 1 inch in length
   c. 1 to 2 inches in length
   d. 2 to 3 inches in length

42. When giving a subcutaneous injection, the volume of fluid is generally:
   a. less than 0.5 mL
   b. 0.5 to 1.0 mL
   c. 1.0 to 1.5 mL
   d. 1.5 to 2.0 mL

43. The maximum volume of fluid normally injected intramuscularly into the deltoid muscle is:
   a. 0.5 mL
   b. 1 mL
   c. 3 mL
   d. 5 mL

44. A medication commonly given sublingually is:
   a. aspirin
   b. albuterol
   c. diphenhydramine
   d. nitroglycerin

45. Two medications commonly administered via inhalation are:
   a. albuterol and isoetharine
   b. adenosine and ipratropium
   c. metaproterenol and diphenhydramine
   d. epinephrine and isoproterenol

46. The three main indications for obtaining vascular access in the field are:
   a. to administer fluids, to administer medications, and to obtain specimens
   b. to administer parenteral nutrition, to administer medications, and to provide access for inserting a transvenous pacemaker
   c. to administer medications, to administer parenteral nutrition, and to administer fluids
   d. to obtain specimens, to provide access for inserting a transvenous pacemaker, and to administer medications

47. A 67-year-old male is in cardiac arrest. The ECG monitor shows pulseless electrical activity and the patient has been intubated. The IV site of choice for this patient is:
   a. a long saphenous vein
   b. a dorsal hand vein
   c. the dorsalis pedis
   d. the antecubital fossa

48. The most common site of choice for obtaining intraosseous access is the:
   a. middle of the femur
   b. proximal tibia
   c. patella
   d. epiphyseal plate

49. Contraindications for initiating intraosseous access include all of the following *EXCEPT*:
   a. burns that may be infected by the access
   b. patient with a pulse and spontaneous respirations
   c. fracture proximal to the insertion site
   d. history of congenital bone disease

50. When inserting the intraosseous needle:
    a. point the needle toward the epiphyseal plate
    b. discontinue the procedure if a "pop" is felt or heard
    c. use a boring or screwing motion
    d. continue until increased resistance is felt

51. When administering medications via the endotracheal route, the medication should normally be:
    a. 2 to 2½ times the IV dose
    b. 5 mL or less in volume
    c. half the IV dose
    d. diluted with lactated Ringer's solution

52. The IV solution used most frequently in the prehospital setting is:
    a. 25% dextrose in water
    b. normal saline
    c. colloid solution
    d. 0.45% sodium chloride

53. In general, the amount of crystalloid solution that must be administered to replace every 1 L of blood lost by a patient is:
    a. 2 L of IV crystalloid solution
    b. 3 L of IV crystalloid solution
    c. 4 L of IV crystalloid solution
    d. 5 L of IV crystalloid solution

54. With the use of a microdrip IV administration set, the number of drops needed to deliver 1 mL of fluid is:
    a. 10
    b. 15
    c. 60
    d. 100

55. When an adult trauma patient is being managed, the preferred IV catheter size to use is a:
    a. 14 or 16 gauge
    b. 16 or 18 gauge
    c. 18 or 20 gauge
    d. 20 or 22 gauge

56. You are ordered to administer 30 mL of an IV drip medication over a period of 20 minutes. Using a microdrip IV administration set, the necessary flow rate would be:
    a. 30 drops per minute
    b. 60 drops per minute
    c. 90 drops per minute
    d. 120 drops per minute

57. A common reason an IV may not flow is:
    a. the IV bag is too high
    b. the flow regulator is open
    c. the tourniquet is still on
    d. the tip of the IV catheter is in the lumen of the vein

58. Normal saline is an example of:
    a. an inotonic solution
    b. a hypotonic solution
    c. a hypertonic solution
    d. an isotonic solution

59. Crystalloid solutions include:
    a. D_5W, normal saline, albumin
    b. lactated Ringer's, D_5W, normal saline
    c. normal saline, dextran, lactated Ringer's
    d. hetastarch, D_5W, lactated Ringer's

60. When an IV is started, if the first puncture attempt is unsuccessful, the second puncture should:
    a. be distal to the first
    b. use a larger gauge needle
    c. always use a smaller needle
    d. be proximal to the first

61. If it is necessary to access an indwelling vascular device:
    a. draw out 5 mL of blood before flushing the device
    b. wipe the connection site with alcohol and immediately pierce the device
    c. use the largest bore IV needle available if the device must be pierced
    d. use a hemostat to ensure adequate occlusion, if the catheter must be clamped

62. You are instructed to administer 5 mg of a medication to a patient. If the medication comes in a 1-mL vial with a concentration of the 10 mg/mL, the amount to be administered is:
    a. 0.25 mL
    b. 0.5 mL
    c. 1 mL
    d. 2 mL

63. You are told to mix 2 g of medication in an IV bag containing 500 mL of fluid. After mixing the medication, the concentration in the IV bag is:
    a. 1 mg/mL
    b. 2 mg/mL
    c. 3 mg/mL
    d. 4 mg/mL

64. After mixing the medication, you are instructed to administer 2 mg of medication a minute. If a microdrip IV set is being used, the drip rate should be:
a. 15 drops per minute
b. 30 drops per minute
c. 45 drops per minute
d. 60 drops per minute

65. A 10-mL multidose vial contains 50 mg of medication. Your protocol instructs you to give 30 mg of medication to your patient. The amount of fluid that should be drawn from the vial is:
a. 2 mL
b. 4 mL
c. 6 mL
d. 8 mL

66. Two emergency medications that may be administered rectally are:
a. diazepam and lorazepam
b. albuterol and dopamine
c. naloxone and diphenhydramine
d. epinephrine and vasopressin

ANSWERS TO CHAPTER 2: PHARMACOLOGY, VENOUS ACCESS, AND MEDICATION ADMINISTRATION

1. **b.** A difference between generic and trade names is that a medication can have only one generic name but several trade names. A generic name is assigned by the government and is usually a simple form of the medication's complex chemical name. A trade name, or brand name, is given to a medication by the company that sells the medication.

2. **a.** The trade name of a medication is a copyright name designated by the drug company that sells the medication. The first letter of a trade name is capitalized.

3. **b.** The generic name of a medication is often an abbreviated form of the chemical name. The generic name is the official name approved by the U.S. Food and Drug Administration (FDA).

4. **c.** Drugs are most often classified by the body system they affect, the class of the agent, or the agent's mechanism of action.

5. **a.** Schedule I drugs are controlled substances with the greatest restrictions. They have no accepted medical use and are used for research, analysis, or instruction only. Schedule I substances have high abuse potential and may lead to severe dependence. Examples include heroin, marijuana, and LSD.

6. **a.** The dose is the amount of medication that should be administered to a patient. The correct dose can vary, based on the patient's weight and age. Concentration refers to the quantity of a specified substance in a unit amount of another substance (i.e., number of milligrams of a medication in a milliliter of liquid).

7. **c.** A contraindication is a medical or physiological factor that makes it harmful to administer a medication that would otherwise have a therapeutic effect. In such situations, the medication may cause harm or it may provide no effect to improve the patient's condition or illness. An untoward effect is a side effect occurring after administration that proves harmful to a patient.

8. **b.** The mechanism of action is the way a medication affects the human body.

9. **a.** A side effect is an undesirable and often unavoidable effect of using therapeutic doses of a drug. It is not the same as a contraindication. Side effects may or may not be serious, but they are usually unwanted. Knowing the potential side effects of a medication can help prepare the EMS provider to deal with them if they occur.

10. **c.** Although many different medications may be given orally, including ones used by EMS personnel, the disadvantage of using the oral route of administration for a medication is that absorption rates are slower than when the medication is injected. Other disadvantages are that oral medications cannot be given to semiresponsive or unresponsive patients, and some medications are not absorbed well from the stomach.

11. **d.** Medications given via the pulmonary route are absorbed rapidly into the bloodstream. This is because of the large surface area and the rich capillary network adjacent to the alveolar membrane. Systemic and local effects from medications given via the pulmonary route may be seen. However, only certain medications can be given via this route.

12. **d.** Lidocaine, atropine, naloxone, and epinephrine all may be administered down an endotracheal tube. The dose should be 2 to $2\frac{1}{2}$ times higher than the IV dose. The names of these four medications can be remembered using the acronym *LANE*.

13. **b.** Morphine is a Schedule II substance. Schedule II substances have accepted medical uses but also have high potential for abuse, and their use may lead to severe physical or psychological dependence.

14. **c.** Biotransformation, or metabolism, is the process by which a drug is chemically converted to a metabolite. The purpose of biotransformation is to detoxify a drug and render it less active. Biotransformation can transform the drug into a more or less active metabolite, or it can make the drug more water soluble or less lipid soluble, which facilitates elimination. Excretion refers to the elimination of inactive or toxic metabolites. Absorption is the process by which drug molecules are moved from the site of entry into the body into the general circulation. Distribution is the transport of a

medication through the bloodstream to various tissues of the body and ultimately to its site of action.

15. c. The kidneys are the primary organs for excretion. The lungs, intestines, and sweat, mammary, and salivary glands also excrete metabolites.

16. d. The blood-brain barrier permits only lipid-soluble drugs (drugs easily soluble in fat), such as general anesthetics and barbiturates, to be distributed into the brain and cerebrospinal fluid. Antibiotics are poorly soluble in fat and have trouble passing across this barrier.

17. Given the following list of common medications used by EMS personnel, note whether they are most commonly administered via the enteral route, parenteral route, pulmonary route, or topical route.

<u>enteral route</u> activated charcoal
<u>parenteral route</u> adenosine
<u>pulmonary route</u> albuterol
<u>parenteral route</u> amiodarone
<u>enteral route</u> aspirin
<u>parenteral route</u> atropine
<u>parenteral route</u> lidocaine
<u>pulmonary route</u> metaproterenol
<u>parenteral route</u> morphine
<u>parenteral route</u> naloxone
<u>topical route</u> nitroglycerin paste
<u>enteral route</u> nitroglycerin spray
<u>pulmonary route</u> nitrous oxide
<u>pulmonary route</u> racemic epinephrine
<u>topical route</u> viscous lidocaine placed on a nasotracheal tube

18. c. An antagonist is an agent that binds to a receptor and prevents a physiological response or prevents other drugs from binding to the receptor. Agonists bind to a receptor and cause a physiological response. Receptors are protein molecules on the surfaces of cells to which drugs bind. Chronotropes are agents that affect the heart rate.

19. d. The range of plasma concentration that is most likely to produce the desired drug effect with the least likelihood of toxicity is the therapeutic range. Peak plasma level refers to the highest plasma concentration attained from a dose; therapeutic index is a measurement of the relative

safety of a drug; and minimum effective concentration relates to the lowest plasma concentration that produces the desired drug effect.

20. b. Bioavailability refers to the amount of medication that is still active after it reaches its target tissue. When administering a drug, the goal is to ensure sufficient bioavailability of the medication at the target tissue to produce the desired effect.

21. d. A maintenance dose is the amount of a medication needed to maintain a steady therapeutic plasma concentration. A loading dose is a bolus of a medication initially administered to rapidly attain a therapeutic plasma concentration.

22. a. Common factors that alter the response to drug therapy and which EMS personnel should consider before administering a medication include the patient's age, weight, and gender. Because stringent manufacturing standards must be adhered to, EMS personnel generally do not see any difference in patient response to medications based on who is the manufacturer.

23. c. Cholinergic fibers release acetylcholine. Acetylcholine is released from presynaptic neurons and stimulates receptors on postsynaptic neurons.

24. b. Adrenergic fibers release norepinephrine. Norepinephrine is the postganglionic neurotransmitter of the sympathetic nervous system.

25. d. The sympathetic nervous system dominates primarily during stressful events. It is commonly referred to as the "fight-or-flight" response.

26. c. The two main types of cholinergic receptors are nicotinic and muscarinic. Alpha and beta exist in the adrenergic system.

27. b. The parasympathetic nervous system is usually involved in activating vegetative functions such as digestion, defecation, and urination. Parasympathetic stimulation also decreases heart rate. It is often referred to as the "feed-or-breed" response.

28. b. Aspirin is the most common nonsteroidal antiinflammatory drug encountered by EMS personnel in the field. Other examples of nonsteroidal antiinflammatory drugs include ibuprofen (Advil, Motrin, and Nuprin) and naproxen (Aleve and Naprosyn).

29. d. Transplant patients are placed on immunosuppressants to prevent the rejection of foreign tissues. They reduce the activity of the body's immune system by suppressing the production and activity of lymphocytes.

30. c. Aspirin is an antiplatelet, that is, it interferes with platelet aggregation, thereby reducing the risk of further clot development. It does not prevent dysrhythmias or lower blood pressure. Unlike a thrombolytic, it does not dissolve clots after their development. Aspirin's analgesic effect is not a major factor when given to myocardial infarction patients.

31. a. Nitroglycerin is a potent vasodilator. It is both an arteriolar and venous dilator.

32. c. Amiodarone is a Class III drug. Class III antidysrhythmics produce potassium channel blockade, which increases contractility. They do not suppress automaticity and have no effect on conduction velocity.

33. d. Diltiazem (Cardizem) and verapamil (Isoptin) are examples of calcium-channel blockers. Calcium-channel blockers are classified as Class IV drugs. They depress the myocardial and smooth muscle contraction, decrease automaticity, and in some cases decrease conduction velocity.

Venous Access and Medication Administration

34. b. A semipermeable membrane allows some substances to enter but restricts the passage of others. The membrane regulates or restricts the flow of solutes on the basis of their size, shape, electrical charge, or other chemical properties.

35. c. Most of the water in the body can be found in the form of intracellular fluid (ICF). ICF accounts for 40% of total body weight. Extracellular fluid (ECF) accounts for 20% of total body weight. Special fluids include cerebrospinal fluid and intraocular fluid.

36. b. Interstitial fluid and plasma are examples of extracellular fluid, the water found outside of the cells. Intraocular fluid is an example of a special fluid.

37. Match the following prefixes with their associated meaning: deci-, centi-, kilo-, micro-, milli-.
kilo- 1000 times greater
deci- 1/10th
centi- 1/100th
milli- 1/1000th
micro- 1/1,000,000th

38. d. For an intramuscular injection, the needle should enter the skin at a 90-degree angle to reach deep muscle tissues.

39. b. For a subcutaneous injection, the angle of entry should be 45 degrees to reach the fatty tissues.

40. c. The greater the gauge number of a needle, the smaller the lumen of the needle. For example, the internal diameter of a 22-gauge needle is much smaller than that of an 18-gauge needle.

41. c. Intramuscular needles are generally 1 to 2 inches long to reach deep muscle mass.

42. a. When a subcutaneous injection is given, the volume of fluid is generally less than 0.5 mL.

43. b. Because the deltoid muscle is relatively small, it normally can accommodate only small doses of fluid, generally 1 mL or less (although some sources say the muscle will accommodate up to 2 mL of fluid). The dorsogluteal site can accommodate higher volumes. Large, well-developed muscles in this area may be able to accommodate as much as 5 mL of fluid. However, for many individuals, even volumes of 3 mL of fluid injected in this area may produce discomfort.

44. d. Nitroglycerin commonly is given sublingually. Sublingual nitroglycerin comes in both tablet and spray form. Nitroglycerin is also available in paste form and is administered topically, where it is absorbed slowly through the skin.

45. a. Albuterol (Proventil and Ventolin) and isoetharine (Bronkosol) are administered via inhalation. Such drugs may be administered via a metered-dose inhaler (MDI) or nebulizer. Metaproterenol (Alupent) and ipratropium (Atrovent) also are administered via inhalation.

46. a. EMS personnel most often obtain vascular access to administer fluids, medications, or obtain specimens.

47. d. In a cardiac arrest situation in an adult, the IV site of choice is the antecubital fossa. Leg and foot veins should be avoided because of the risk of medications not reaching the central circulation. Hand veins may not allow for large bore catheters and also do not allow medications to reach central circulation as quickly.

48. b. The most common site of choice for obtaining intraosseous access is the proximal tibia, one to two fingerbreadths below the tubercle on the anteromedial surface. An alternative site is the femur, two to three fingerbreadths above the lateral condyles in the midline. This location may be useful especially when initiating intraosseous access in small infants.

49. b. Contraindications for initiating intraosseous access include fracture of the insertion site or proximal to the site, congenital bone disease, burns that may be infected by the technique, traumatized extremity, and cellulitis. Patients should be unconscious but do not have to be in cardiac arrest.

50. c. The intraosseous needle should be inserted using a boring or screwing motion. Insert the needle pointing away from the epiphyseal (growth) plate. The needle should be inserted until it penetrates the bone marrow. A decrease in resistance or a slight "pop" is usually felt or heard when the needle enters the marrow.

51. a. When administering medications via the endotracheal route, the medication should normally be 2 to 2½ times the IV dose. The medication to be delivered should be diluted to form 10 mL of solution. Smaller volumes of solution may not be sufficient to reach the tracheobronchial tree.

52. b. Normal saline, D_5W, and lactated Ringer's solution are the preferred IV solutions in the prehospital setting.

53. b. In general, 3 L of crystalloid solution must be administered for every 1 L of blood lost. However, this does not mean that all this fluid should be administered before reaching the hospital. Also, caution must be exercised to avoid fluid overload, especially if the patient has a history of congestive heart failure.

54. c. When a microdrip IV administration set is used, 60 drops equals 1 mL of fluid. When using a macrodrip set (sometimes referred to as a *surgical set*) the number of drops needed to equal 1 mL of fluid depends on the manufacturer. They may be 10 drops to 1 mL, 15 drops to 1 mL, or 20 drops to 1 mL.

55. a. Large catheters, such as 14 or 16 gauge, should be used when starting an IV on an adult trauma patient, and the largest needle possible should be used if the trauma patient is a child. This allows for rapid delivery of IV solutions.

56. c. A flow rate of 1.5 mL/min is needed to administer 30.0 mL over 20 minutes. When a microdrip IV administration is used, 90 drops yield 1.5 mL of fluid.

57. c. Reasons an IV may not flow include the tourniquet being left on, the bag being too low, the regulator being closed, and the IV catheter not being in the lumen of the vein.

58. d. Normal saline and lactated Ringer's solution are isotonic solutions. 0.45% normal saline (one half normal saline) is hypotonic. D_5W, though technically isotonic, acts as a hypotonic solution because the glucose is actively transported into the cells and leaves excess free water behind.

59. b. Crystalloids, such as normal saline, D_5W, or lactated Ringer's solution, are the preferred IV solutions in the prehospital setting. Colloid solutions include blood and blood products such as albumin, and plasma substitutes such as dextran and hetastarch.

60. d. If the first IV attempt is unsuccessful, the second puncture should be proximal to the first if the IV attempt is in the same limb. Using a smaller needle is not always appropriate, such as if the patient needs certain medications or large amounts of fluid.

61. a. If it is necessary to cannulate an indwelling vascular device, draw out 5 mL of blood to remove heparinized blood and to ensure patency of the device. Special small-gauge, noncoring-type needles are normally used, not large-bore IV needles. Because of the high risk of infection, the connection site should normally be cleaned with povidone-iodine and allowed to dry. If the catheter must be clamped, use the clamp on the clamping sleeve provided to prevent nicking or severing the catheter.

62. b. Administer 0.5 mL. Because the dose to be delivered is less than the number of milligrams in the 1 mL vial, a "reasonable" calculation of volume is less than 1 mL.

$$\frac{\text{Desired dose (5 mg)}}{\text{Known dose on hand (10 mg)}} = 0.5$$

$$0.5 \times 1 \text{ mL} = 0.5 \text{ mL}$$

63. d. 2 g = 2000 mg. If 2000 mg of a medication are injected in a bag containing 500 mL of fluid, the resulting concentration is 4 mg/mL (2000 ÷ 500 = 4).

64. b. When a microdrip administration set is used, 60 drops = 1 mL. Therefore for a delivery of 0.5 mL every minute, the flow rate would be 30 drops per minute.

65. c. If 50 mg of medication is in a 10 mL multidose vial, the concentration of medication is 5 mg/mL (50 ÷ 10 = 5). If you are ordered to give 30 mg of the medication, the amount of fluid to be withdrawn would be 6 mL (30 mg ÷ 5 = 6 mL).

66. a. If IV access cannot be established, diazepam and lorazepam can be administered rectally.

AIRWAY MANAGEMENT AND VENTILATION

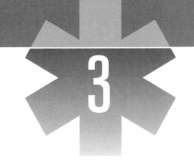

1. The point at which the trachea divides into the right and left main bronchi is called the:
   a. bronchial divisor
   b. cardiac bifurcation
   c. carina
   d. respiratory wye

2. The layer of tissue lining the chest wall is the:
   a. visceral pleura
   b. parietal pleura
   c. tracheal pleura
   d. bronchial pleura

3. The exchange of gases within the lungs takes place in the:
   a. bronchi
   b. pleural space
   c. alveoli
   d. trachea

4. The primary muscle associated with respiration is the:
   a. diaphragm
   b. quadricep
   c. pectoral
   d. deltoid

5. Lung compliance can best be described as:
   a. how easy it is to pass an endotracheal tube into the trachea
   b. the ratio of the peak inspiratory flow to the normal tidal volume
   c. the ability of lung tissue to absorb medications via the tracheobronchial tree
   d. the ease at which the lungs and thorax expand during pressure changes

6. Inspiration takes place when:
   a. intrapleural pressure is greater than atmospheric pressure
   b. atmospheric pressure is less than intrapulmonary pressure
   c. intrapulmonary pressure is greater than intrapleural pressure
   d. intrapulmonary pressure is less than atmospheric pressure

7. The part of brain that controls respirations is the:
   a. cerebrum
   b. cerebellum
   c. brain stem
   d. parietal lobe

8. If pulmonary circulation is inhibited, the blood leaving the lungs will have:
   a. a low oxygen content
   b. a lower than normal carbon dioxide content
   c. an abnormally high oxygen content
   d. a higher than normal pH

9. Normal tidal volume is:
   a. 2 to 4 mL/kg
   b. 5 to 7 mL/kg
   c. 8 to 10 mL/kg
   d. 11 to 13 mL/kg

10. Atelectasis is best described as:
    a. an abnormal condition characterized by the localized collapse of alveoli
    b. a buildup of fluid in the lungs
    c. an abnormal increase in the number of alveoli
    d. a condition characterized by the loss of lung elasticity

11. Minute volume is:
    a. tidal volume multiplied by respiratory rate
    b. inspiratory reserve volume minus expiratory reserve volume
    c. vital capacity multiplied by tidal volume
    d. total lung capacity minus functional residual capacity

12. The abbreviation FiO_2 refers to the:
    a. percentage of hemoglobin saturated with oxygen
    b. percentage of oxygen in inspired air
    c. ratio of carbon dioxide to oxygen in venous blood
    d. ratio of oxygen to carbon dioxide in arterial blood

13. Hypoxia refers to:
    a. inadequate oxygen at the cellular level
    b. a deficiency of oxygen in arterial blood
    c. a total absence of oxygen
    d. an inability of cells to utilize oxygen for cellular metabolism

14. The primary breathing stimulus in a healthy adult is:
    a. an increase in blood oxygen levels
    b. a decrease in blood CO_2 levels
    c. an increase in blood CO_2 levels
    d. a decrease in blood oxygen levels

15. Chemoreceptors involved in chemical control of respiration are found in the:
    a. trachea, bronchi, and alveoli
    b. aorta, superior vena cava, and inferior vena cava
    c. heart, lungs, and brain
    d. medulla, carotids, and aorta

16. A modified form of respiration that aids in clearing bronchi and bronchioles of foreign materials and mucus particles is the:
    a. cough
    b. sneeze
    c. gag reflex
    d. sigh

17. Tidal volume is:
    a. the sum of the vital capacity and residual volume
    b. the amount of gas that remains in the respiratory system after forced expiration
    c. the amount of gas that can be forcefully inspired after normal inspiration
    d. the volume of gas inhaled or exhaled during a normal breath

18. The normal respiratory rate for an adult is:
    a. 8 to 16 times per minute
    b. 12 to 20 times per minute
    c. 15 to 25 times per minute
    d. 20 to 30 times per minute

19. Pulmonary changes that occur as a result of the aging process include:
    a. a decrease in the size of alveolar ducts and sacs
    b. a slight fall in PO_2 and significant rise in arterial PCO_2
    c. an increase in chemoreceptor sensitivity
    d. increased thoracic rigidity and decreased elastic recoil

20. Match each abnormal respiratory pattern listed with its description: agonal, Biot's, Cheyne-Stokes, Kussmaul.

    _____ abrupt, irregular alternating periods of apnea and breathing of a constant rate and depth

    _____ abnormally deep, rapid sighing respiratory pattern

    _____ slow, shallow, irregular respirations

    _____ a repetitive breathing pattern characterized by a gradually increasing rate and depth of respirations followed by a gradual decrease in rate and depth of respirations with an accompanying period of apnea

21. Pulsus paradoxus can be defined as:
    a. an unusual increase in pulse rate that occurs when a patient is having respiratory difficulty
    b. bradycardia that occurs when a patient becomes hypoxic
    c. an abnormal presentation in which the radial pulse can be felt in one wrist but not in the other
    d. an abnormal decrease in blood pressure that occurs with inspiration

22. The tanks most commonly used in portable oxygen units are:
    a. "A" and "B" tanks
    b. "D" and "M" tanks
    c. "E" and "G" tanks
    d. "D" and "E" tanks

23. When using supplemental oxygen with a pocket mask or bag-valve-mask device, the proper flow rate is:
    a. less than 3 lpm if the patient has a history of respiratory illness
    b. 6 lpm if the patient is only in respiratory arrest
    c. 12 lpm if the patient is a child
    d. 15 lpm in all cases

24. A nasal cannula will oxygenate patients:
    a. even if they breathe through their mouth
    b. only if they breathe through their nose
    c. as well as a nonrebreather mask
    d. even if a nasal obstruction is present

25. Oxygen may be administered to a laryngectomy patient by:
    a. inserting supply tubing into the stoma
    b. placing a cannula in the patient's nose
    c. placing a child or infant mask over the patient's stoma
    d. placing a mask on the patient and instructing him to breathe only through his mouth

26. The proper oxygen flow rate for a nonrebreather mask is:
    a. 3 lpm if there is a history of asthma
    b. 6 lpm if the patient will not tolerate high flow
    c. 9 lpm if the patient complains of dry mouth
    d. 15 lpm in most cases

27. The reservoir of a nonrebreather mask should:
    a. fully deflate with each patient ventilation to allow the depth of breaths to be assessed
    b. be inflated before placing the mask on the patient
    c. be filled with the patient's expired air
    d. be removed if the patient insists that he or she is not getting enough air

28. A nasal cannula can be used if:
    a. the patient will not tolerate a nonrebreather mask
    b. the patient complains of a dry mouth
    c. a low oxygen tank pressure is discovered
    d. the patient is breathing primarily through the nose

29. There is no advantage to using nasal cannulas with oxygen flow rates greater than:
    a. 2 lpm
    b. 4 lpm
    c. 6 lpm
    d. 9 lpm

30. A technique that can be used to administer oxygen to a conscious child who will not tolerate a mask is to:
    a. increase the flow rate to a cannula
    b. administer oxygen using a blow-by technique to increase the concentration of the surrounding air
    c. place an adult mask over the child's entire face
    d. place a pediatric-sized mask tightly over the child's face and restrain the patient's hands

31. Your patient has taken an intentional overdose of benzodiazepines and is semiconscious. The patient has snoring respirations when his airway is not manually positioned. The airway of choice for this patient is the:
    a. oropharyngeal airway
    b. nasopharyngeal airway
    c. dual lumen airway
    d. endotracheal airway

32. When a single rescuer is using a bag-valve-mask or flow-restricted, oxygen-powered ventilation device:
    a. use an adjunctive airway only in adult patients
    b. use an adjunctive airway only for infants or children
    c. always use an adjunctive airway if the patient tolerates it
    d. use only a nasopharyngeal airway

33. To determine the proper size of an oral airway to be inserted, measure from the:
    a. patient's Adam's apple to the corner of the mouth
    b. angle of the patient's jaw to the Adam's apple
    c. angle of the patient's jaw to the clavicle
    d. patient's earlobe to the corner of the mouth

34. To insert an oral airway in an adult, insert the airway:
    a. upside down, then rotate it 180 degrees
    b. by pushing the tip along the tongue
    c. until the flange lies immediately behind the teeth
    d. so that the flange lies 1 inch beyond the lips

35. To determine the proper size of a nasopharyngeal airway to be inserted, measure from the:
    a. patient's upper lip to the Adam's apple
    b. tip of the patient's nose to the earlobe
    c. patient's nostril to the chin
    d. corner of the patient's mouth to the Adam's apple

36. When inserting an nasopharyngeal airway:
    a. force the airway if resistance is met
    b. attempt to insert the airway in the left nostril first
    c. do not try the other nostril if resistance is felt when inserting the airway in the first nostril
    d. lubricate the airway with a water-based jelly first

37. EMS providers should assist with ventilation of an adult patient if the breathing rate falls below:
    a. 8 breaths per minute
    b. 12 breaths per minute
    c. 14 breaths per minute
    d. 16 breaths per minute

38. A bag-valve-mask should be connected to oxygen:
    a. only if the patient is cyanotic
    b. only when ventilating infants or children
    c. only if the patient has no history of breathing problems
    d. whenever it is available

39. The advantage of using a bag-valve-mask versus a flow-restricted, oxygen-powered ventilation device when ventilating an intubated patient is:
    a. a higher concentration of oxygen can be delivered
    b. the rate of ventilation is slower
    c. the operator can manually monitor lung compliance
    d. it requires no training to use

40. A flow-restricted, oxygen-powered ventilation device should *not* be used on:
    a. infants and small children
    b. any trauma patient
    c. patients who are breathing
    d. patients without a gag reflex

41. A major problem associated with the use of a bag-valve-mask if a patient is not intubated is:
    a. difficulty maintaining a good seal with the mask
    b. inability to deliver an adequate concentration of oxygen
    c. inability to see if the patient has vomited
    d. that it is difficult for two operators to use

42. If a patient with an oral airway in place becomes conscious and develops a gag reflex, the best course of action is to:
    a. restrain the patient and keep the airway in place
    b. remove the airway and suction the patient if necessary
    c. remove the airway and insert a smaller one
    d. replace the oral airway with an endotracheal tube

43. A suction unit should provide a vacuum of:
    a. no more than 100 mm Hg of negative pressure
    b. no more than 200 mm Hg of negative pressure
    c. no less than 300 mm Hg of negative pressure
    d. no less than 400 mm Hg of negative pressure

44. Two common types of suction catheters used by EMS personnel are:
    a. hard and rigid
    b. French and soft
    c. hard and soft
    d. English and tonsil tip

45. When suctioning a patient:
    a. insert the catheter without suction
    b. suction only while advancing the catheter
    c. do not be concerned with wearing gloves because there should be no physical contact with the patient
    d. be careful not to rotate the catheter

46. The maximum length of time an adult patient should be suctioned is:
    a. 5 seconds at a time
    b. 15 seconds at a time
    c. 20 seconds at a time
    d. 25 seconds at a time

47. When suctioning the oropharynx, a soft suction catheter should be inserted no further than the:
    a. larynx
    b. first set of molars
    c. trachea
    d. base of the tongue

48. When performing tracheobronchial suctioning through an endotracheal tube, all of the following are correct *EXCEPT*:
    a. preoxygenate the patient with 100% oxygen
    b. inject 15 to 20 mL of sterile saline down the tube to loosen secretions
    c. place the patient on a cardiac monitor
    d. advance the catheter to about the level of the carina

49. When suctioning a laryngectomy patient:
    a. never inject fluid down the trachea
    b. instruct the patient to inhale while suctioning
    c. do not insert the catheter more than 3 to 5 inches into the trachea
    d. remove the suction catheter immediately if the patient coughs

Endotracheal Intubation

50. The leaf-shaped, flexible cartilage that hangs over the larynx to protect the trachea is the:
    a. pharynx
    b. carina
    c. epiglottis
    d. vallecula

51. A potential complication that may occur during intubation is:
    a. bradycardia
    b. tachycardia
    c. tachypnea
    d. hyperpyrexia

52. The laryngoscope should be held in:
    a. the left hand
    b. the intubator's dominant hand
    c. the right hand
    d. either hand

53. To raise the epiglottis out of the way, insert the tip of a curved laryngoscope blade into the:
    a. glottic opening
    b. vallecula
    c. carotid sinus
    d. carina

54. The type of laryngoscope blade that should be positioned under the epiglottis to expose the glottic opening is the:
    a. curved blade
    b. MacIntosh blade
    c. straight blade
    d. curved or MacIntosh blade

55. When immediate placement of an endotracheal tube is required, the most common size tube used for an average-sized adult is the:
    a. 6.5 mm
    b. 7 mm
    c. 7.5 mm
    d. 8 mm

56. After an endotracheal tube is placed, the cuff should usually be filled with:
    a. 3 to 5 mL of air
    b. 5 to 10 mL of air
    c. 10 to 15 mL of air
    d. 15 to 20 mL of air

57. The advantage of the endotracheal tube over an EOA or dual lumen airway is that the endotracheal tube:
    a. is easier to place
    b. can be placed without the use of special instruments
    c. works well in semiconscious patients
    d. protects the airway from aspiration of gastric contents

58. One way to confirm proper placement of an endotracheal tube is to:
    a. listen for sounds in the lower abdomen
    b. observe for fluid in the tube
    c. note the numerical markings on the tube
    d. attach an end-tidal CO_2 detector to the tube

59. The most critical complication of endotracheal intubation is:
    a. right mainstem bronchus placement
    b. unrecognized esophageal placement
    c. broken teeth
    d. traumatic injuries to the tongue

60. You and your partner are in the early stages of attempting to resuscitate a ventricular fibrillation patient. The patient was already in your ambulance with a complaint of chest pain when he suddenly arrested. You are getting ready to place an endotracheal tube. When performing intubation, the patient's head should be:
    a. hyperflexed
    b. placed in a neutral position
    c. tilted slightly forward
    d. placed in the sniffing position

61. A motorcyclist who was not wearing a helmet is lying in the middle of the road, where he landed after striking an oncoming vehicle. Fire department first responders have started CPR and your cardiac monitor is showing pulseless electrical activity. When performing intubation, his head should be:
    a. placed in the sniffing position
    b. hyperflexed
    c. in a neutral, in-line position
    d. slightly hyperextended

62. When properly placed in an endotracheal tube, the tip of the stylet should:
    a. not protrude from the end of the airway
    b. extend no more than $1/2$ inch out the end of the airway
    c. not extend past the middle of the airway
    d. extend approximately 1 inch out the end of the airway

63. When inserting the laryngoscope blade into the patient's mouth, insert the blade into:
   a. the middle of the mouth and allow the tongue to wrap around both sides of the blade
   b. the right side of the mouth and displace the tongue to the left
   c. the left side of the mouth and displace the tongue to the right
   d. the middle of the mouth and displace the tongue to the right

64. If after inserting an endotracheal tube and listening to lung sounds, sounds are only heard on the right side:
   a. deflate the cuff, pull the tube out, and reattempt intubation
   b. deflate the cuff and push the tube in slightly
   c. leave the tube in place and ventilate at a faster rate
   d. deflate the cuff and pull the tube back slightly

65. Most adult patients can be intubated using a:
   a. size 0 straight blade
   b. size 1 curved blade
   c. size 2 straight blade
   d. size 3 curved blade

66. Uncuffed endotracheal tubes should generally be used:
   a. only for infants below the age of 1
   b. for children between the age of 1 and 10
   c. for children over the age of 5
   d. for children under the age of 8

67. A technique for deciding what size endotracheal tube to insert in an infant or child is to match the tube size to the:
   a. diameter of the patient's little finger
   b. diameter of the patient's thumb
   c. diameter of the laryngoscope blade being used
   d. patient's age in years

68. While one rescuer attempts to intubate the patient, a second rescuer can assist by:
   a. performing chest compressions
   b. performing the Heimlich maneuver
   c. holding the laryngoscope
   d. performing the Sellick maneuver

Questions 69 through 75 deal with rapid sequence intubation (RSI).

69. The two types of neuromuscular blocking drugs are:
   a. sympathetic and parasympathetic agents
   b. depolarizing and nondepolarizing agents
   c. central and peripheral agents
   d. autonomic and somatic agents

70. The most common neuromuscular blocking agent initially used in the field to paralyze a patient requiring rapid sequence intubation is:
   a. pancuronium
   b. etomidate
   c. midazolam
   d. succinylcholine

71. A patient with a head injury or the possibility of increased intracranial pressure should be premedicated before paralysis with:
   a. atropine
   b. diphenhydramine
   c. lidocaine
   d. morphine

72. Fasciculations are best described as:
   a. uncontrollable muscle twitching caused by depolarizing agents
   b. bradyarrhythmias caused by depolarizing agents
   c. abnormal breathing patterns caused by nondepolarizing agents
   d. an increase in intracranial pressure caused by nondepolarizing agents

73. When performing rapid sequence intubation on a pediatric patient, the patient should be premedicated with:
   a. adenosine
   b. albuterol
   c. amiodarone
   d. atropine

74. Medications such as etomidate or diazepam are administered prior to and after rapid sequence intubation to:
   a. cause muscle paralysis
   b. provide pain relief
   c. produce amnestic effects
   d. prevent bradycardia

75. A neuromuscular blocking agent that may be used to provide long-term paralysis after confirmed placement and securing of an endotracheal tube is:
a. midazolam
b. promethazine
c. succinylcholine
d. vecuronium

Questions 76 through 78 deal with performing a cricothyrotomy.

76. When performing a needle cricothyrotomy, the needle should be inserted:
a. through the midline of the membrane at a 90-degree angle
b. to the right or left of the midline to allow insertion of two needles and at a 45-degree angle toward the patient's vocal cords
c. through the midline of the membrane at a 45-to 60-degree angle toward the patient's carina
d. to the right or left of the midline to allow insertion of two needles and at a 30-degree angle toward the patient's carina

77. While inserting the needle through the cricothyroid membrane:
a. use a twisting or boring motion
b. attach a syringe to the needle and apply negative pressure to the syringe while inserting the needle through the skin
c. maintain a flow of oxygen through the needle to prevent skin plugs from occluding the lumen of the catheter
d. have a second rescuer perform the Sellick maneuver

78. When transtracheal ventilation is performed on a patient with needle cricothyrotomy, the inspiratory-to-expiratory ratio should be:
a. 1 second of inspiration to 4 seconds of expiration if no upper airway obstruction is present
b. 1 second of inspiration to 2 seconds of expiration if upper airway obstruction is present
c. 2 seconds of inspiration to 1 second of expiration if no upper airway obstruction is present
d. 2 seconds of inspiration to 4 seconds of expiration if upper airway obstruction is present

ANSWERS TO CHAPTER 3: AIRWAY MANAGEMENT AND VENTILATION

1. **c.** The carina is the point at which the trachea divides into the right and left mainstem bronchi.

2. **b.** The parietal pleura is the layer of tissue lining the chest wall. The visceral pleura covers the lung tissue. The potential space between the parietal and visceral pleura is known as the pleural space.

3. **c.** The exchange of gases during respiration takes place in the alveoli. The alveoli, which resemble small grape clusters, are the "work stations" of the lungs. Gases cross the alveolar membrane and cellular membrane during the exchange.

4. **a.** The primary muscle associated with respiration is the diaphragm. It also separates the thoracic cavity from the abdominal cavity. Intercostal muscles also play a role in the mechanics of respiration.

5. **d.** Lung compliance can best be described as the ease at which the lungs and thorax expand during pressure changes. The greater the compliance, the easier the expansion. Some diseases or conditions (such as asthma, emphysema, bronchitis, and pulmonary edema) decrease lung compliance and therefore increase the energy required for breathing. Changes in lung compliance can sometimes be felt when manually ventilating a patient with a bag-valve-mask.

6. **d.** When intrapulmonary pressure is less than atmospheric pressure, air enters the lungs and inspiration takes place. When intrapulmonary pressure is greater than atmospheric pressure, expiration occurs.

7. **c.** The medulla and the pons, parts of the brain stem, control breathing.

8. **a.** If pulmonary circulation is inhibited, the blood leaving the lungs will have a low oxygen content. This is because normal gas exchange cannot take place.

9. **b.** Normal tidal volume is 5 to 7 mL/kg. In an average adult male, this is 500 to 600 mL.

10. **a.** Atelectasis is an abnormal condition characterized by the localized collapse of alveoli. This prevents the respiratory exchange of oxygen and carbon dioxide. Fluid in the lungs is known as pulmonary edema. In emphysema, the alveoli lose their elasticity and break down.

11. **a.** Minute volume is tidal volume multiplied by respiratory rate. For example, if the patient's tidal volume is 600 mL and he is breathing at a rate of 15 times per minute, the minute volume is 9 L (9000 mL) per minute.

12. **b.** Fio_2 refers to the fraction (percentage) of oxygen in inspired air. It is commonly documented as a decimal (e.g., $Fio_2 = 0.85$). A patient's Fio_2 increases with supplemental oxygen.

13. **a.** Hypoxia is inadequate oxygen at the cellular level. Hypoxemia refers to a deficiency of oxygen in arterial blood, and anoxia is a total absence of oxygen.

14. **c.** The primary breathing stimulus in a healthy adult is an increase in blood CO_2 levels, which in turn results in an increased acidity level of the blood. In the healthy human, oxygen levels play a relatively small part in regulating respiration.

15. **d.** Chemoreceptors in the medulla, carotids, and aorta sense changes in carbon dioxide and pH to help regulate respirations.

16. **a.** Modified forms of respiration include protective reflexes such as cough, sneeze, and gag reflex, sighing, and hiccoughing. Coughing aids in clearing bronchi and bronchioles of foreign materials and mucus particles.

17. **d.** Tidal volume is the volume of gas inhaled or exhaled during a normal breath. The sum of the vital capacity and residual volume is the total lung capacity. The residual volume is the amount of gas that remains in the respiratory system after forced expiration, and the inspiratory reserve volume is the amount of gas that can be forcefully inspired after normal inspiration.

18. **b.** The normal respiratory rate for an adult is 12 to 20 times per minute. Normal pediatric rates are faster.

19. **d.** A number of changes take place as patients age. Among the changes are increased thoracic rigidity and decreased elastic recoil. Additionally, enlarged alveolar ducts and sacs translate into less alveolar surface for gas exchange. As a person

grows older, the P_{O_2} falls, but there is no significant change in arterial P_{CO_2}. The functioning of the body's chemoreceptors also declines with age.

20. Match the abnormal respiratory pattern listed below with its description.

Biot's	abrupt, irregular alternating periods of apnea and breathing of a constant rate and depth
Kussmaul	abnormally deep, rapid sighing respiratory pattern
agonal	slow, shallow, irregular respirations
Cheyne-Stokes	a repetitive breathing pattern characterized by a gradually increasing rate and depth of respirations followed by a gradual decrease in rate and depth of respirations with an accompanying period of apnea

21. **d.** Pulsus paradoxus is an abnormal >10 mm Hg drop in systolic blood pressure that occurs with inspiration. Changes in pulse quality may be felt if pulsus paradoxus is present. It may be seen in COPD or pericardial tamponade patients.

22. **d.** "D" and "E" tanks are most commonly used in portable oxygen units. "M" and "G" tanks are commonly used for on-board ambulance oxygen systems.

23. **d.** When using supplemental oxygen with a pocket mask or bag-valve-mask, the flowmeter should be set to 15 lpm. If a pocket mask without oxygen inlet is all that is available, a nasal cannula may be worn by the rescuer performing ventilations to increase the concentration of delivered oxygen.

24. **a.** A nasal cannula will oxygenate patients even if they breathe through their mouth, provided they have a patent nasopharynx. The reason is that the oropharynx acts as a reservoir for the oxygen being delivered, thereby enriching the concentration of oxygen of the air breathed through the mouth. Patients with nasal obstructions, however, will not benefit much from use of a nasal cannula.

25. **c.** A child or infant mask may be placed over the stoma of a laryngectomy patient to provide supplemental oxygen. The use of a humidifier is recommended because the oxygen bypasses

the normal structures of the nose and throat, which would naturally humidify it.

26. **d.** The proper flow rate when using a nonrebreather mask is 15 lpm in most cases.

27. **b.** The reservoir of a nonrebreather mask allows delivery of high concentrations of oxygen. The reservoir should be filled with oxygen before placing the mask on the patient. If the reservoir deflates completely with each patient breath, the oxygen flow rate to the mask is too low and it should be increased. There are no circumstances under which the reservoir should be removed.

28. **a.** The nasal cannula may be used as an alternative when a patient will not tolerate a nonrebreather mask despite reassurances from the caregiver that adequate oxygen is being delivered.

29. **c.** When using a nasal cannula, flow rates greater than 6 lpm are of little value because they do not improve oxygen delivery and high flow rates can cause discomfort to the patient.

30. **b.** To administer oxygen to a conscious child who will not tolerate a mask, use a blow-by technique. This may be accomplished through various methods. Oxygen tubing can be held about 2 inches from the patient's face, or it may be inserted into a paper cup held near the child's face. Or, an oxygen mask may be held near the child's face. The objective is to increase the concentration of oxygen in the surrounding air. A good indication of how badly the child needs oxygen is whether he or she will accept it. Seriously ill or injured infants or children usually do not fight the oxygen mask.

31. **b.** A nasopharyngeal airway, although often overlooked, is better tolerated in a semiconscious patient with a gag reflex. Oral airways, dual lumen airways, and oral endotracheal tubes can only be used when the gag reflex is absent or deeply depressed. Attempts at nasotracheal intubation may be appropriate, but nasotracheal intubation attempts will also stimulate a gag reflex.

32. **c.** If the patient will tolerate it, an adjunctive airway should always be used when ventilating a patient with a flow-restricted, oxygen-powered ventilation device or when a single rescuer is using a bag-valve-mask. Various airways are available for use with patients of all ages.

33. **d.** Measuring from the bottom of the patient's earlobe to the corner of the mouth will provide a useful guide for sizing an oral airway. An alternate method is to measure from the corner of the patient's mouth to the angle of the jaw.

34. **a.** To place an oral airway in an adult, insert it upside down and then rotate it 180 degrees. An alternate method is to use a tongue depressor to manage the tongue while inserting the airway right side up.

35. **b.** To determine the proper size of a nasopharyngeal airway to be inserted, measure from the tip of the nose to the earlobe or to the angle of the jaw.

36. **d.** Before inserting a nasopharyngeal airway, lubricate it with a water-based lubricant. Do not use petroleum jelly. Because the bevel should be toward the septum, most nasopharyngeal airways are designed to be placed in the right nostril, but if resistance is met, the other nostril can be attempted.

37. **a.** As a general rule, if a patient's breathing rate falls below 8 breaths a minute, assist the patient's breathing. Some patients with higher breathing rates may also need assistance. Decisions should be based on the patient's overall condition and the quality of respirations, not simply the breathing rate.

38. **d.** Although a bag-valve-mask (BVM) can be used with room air, supplemental oxygen should be connected to the device whenever it is available. Also, an oxygen reservoir should always be attached. In essence, the bag-valve-mask should be considered a multi-part system, and all its parts (i.e., the bag-valve-mask, oxygen reservoir and tubing) should be stored and used together.

39. **c.** The advantage to using a bag-valve-mask (BVM) over a flow-restricted, oxygen-powered ventilation is that the operator can manually monitor lung compliance. If it gets increasingly difficult to squeeze the bag, the patient should be assessed for the possible development of a tension pneumothorax. Without supplemental oxygen, lower concentrations of oxygen will be delivered by the BVM. Although BVMs are simple to operate, personnel still need to be trained on their proper use.

40. **a.** Flow-restricted, oxygen-powered ventilation devices should not be used on infants or small children (consult local protocols for exact age criteria). They can be used on some trauma patients and in patients without a gag reflex. The devices may be used to support ventilations in a patient who is breathing.

41. **a.** The major problem associated with a bag-valve-mask (BVM), especially when it is used by one rescuer, is an inability to maintain a good seal with the mask to adequately ventilate the patient. This problem can be lessened if two operators use the device, with one maintaining a mask seal and the other squeezing the bag. BVMs are capable of delivering high concentrations of oxygen. Clear facemasks should be used so the user can see if the patient vomits.

42. **b.** If a patient with an oral airway in place develops a gag reflex, remove the airway and suction the patient if necessary. Suction may be needed to prevent aspiration of vomitus.

43. **c.** Suction units should provide no less than 300 mm Hg of negative pressure.

44. **c.** The hard suction catheter (also known as a rigid catheter, tonsil tip, tonsil sucker, or Yankauer) and soft suction catheter (also known as a French catheter) are commonly used by EMS personnel.

45. **a.** When suctioning a patient, insert the catheter without suction. Suction should be applied only while withdrawing the catheter. Rotating the catheter between the fingers with a twirling motion will keep the tip from sticking to the tissue and will cover all areas being suctioned. Always wear gloves while suctioning.

46. **b.** An adult patient should not be suctioned for longer than 15 seconds at a time. The goal of suctioning a patient's airway is to clear the airway. But remember, while suctioning fluids the rescuer is also suctioning oxygen. It may be necessary to suction the patient a number of times to thoroughly clear the airway. Oxygenate the patient between each suctioning period.

47. **d.** A soft suction catheter should not be inserted farther than the base of the patient's tongue.

Generally, a hard suction catheter is preferred when suctioning the oropharynx.

48. b. When performing tracheobronchial suctioning through an endotracheal tube, preoxygenate the patient with 100% oxygen and place the patient on a cardiac monitor to immediately detect bradyarrhythmias. Using a sterile technique, the catheter should be advanced to the desired location, usually about at the level of the carina. It may be necessary to inject 3 to 5 mL of sterile saline down the tube to loosen secretions.

49. c. When suctioning a laryngectomy patient, do not insert the catheter more than 3 to 5 inches into the trachea. Inject 3 mL of sterile saline down the trachea to loosen secretions. Coughing during the procedure is normal and will help to loosen secretions. If the procedure does not induce coughing, the patient should be instructed to exhale while the trachea is suctioned.

Endotracheal Intubation

50. c. The epiglottis is the leaf-shaped, flexible cartilage that hangs over the larynx and keeps liquids and solids from entering the trachea. The pharynx is the area directly posterior to the mouth and nose, the carina is the lower end of the trachea where the right and left mainstem bronchi branch, and the vallecula is a groove-like structure anterior to the epiglottis.

51. a. When intubating a patient, the patient's heart rate may slow (bradycardia). This can result from stimulation of the nerves that regulate the heart rate, as well as from hypoxia.

52. a. The laryngoscope should be held in the left hand regardless of whether the user is left or right handed.

53. b. To raise the epiglottis out of the way, the tip of a curved laryngoscope blade should be inserted into the vallecula. The epiglottis is then indirectly lifted.

54. c. A straight blade is used to directly lift the epiglottis, thereby exposing the glottic opening. A MacIntosh blade is a type of curved blade.

55. c. When immediate placement of an endotracheal tube is required, the most common-

size tube used for an average-sized adult is the 7.5 mm. As a general rule, adult females require a 7.0 to 8.0 and males require an 8.0 to 8.5.

56. b. After placing an endotracheal tube, the cuff is usually filled with 5 to 10 mL of air. More air may cause the bulb to burst and less air may allow leakage around the cuff.

57. d. Although it is more complicated to perform and requires special instruments, the advantage of the endotracheal over an EOA or dual lumen airway is that the endotracheal tube protects the airway from aspiration of gastric contents. Endotracheal intubation should not be performed on a patient with an intact gag reflex.

58. d. Proper placement of an endotracheal tube can be verified by attaching an end-tidal CO_2 detector to the tube. The detector senses the presence of carbon dioxide in the exhaled breath. An esophageal intubation detector device also may be used. Although the numerical markings show how deep the tube is, they do not indicate whether the tube is in the trachea or esophagus. Fluid in the tube is usually an indication of improper tube placement.

59. b. The most critical complication of endotracheal intubation is unrecognized esophageal placement because this will prove fatal. Right mainstem bronchus placement, broken teeth, and tongue injuries are also potential complications but are not usually fatal.

60. d. When intubating a nontrauma patient, place the patient's head in the sniffing position. To accomplish this, flex the neck and extend the head at the base of the skull. A towel may be placed under the supine patient's occiput to help accomplish this.

61. c. When a trauma patient is being intubated, the patient's head should be placed in a neutral, in-line position so as not to potentially damage the spinal cord.

62. a. When properly placed in an endotracheal tube, the tip of the stylet should not protrude from the end of the airway. It is best if it does not extend past the proximal end of the Murphy's eye.

63. b. When inserting the laryngoscope blade into the patient's mouth, insert the blade into the right side of the mouth and displace the tongue to the left to obtain greater visibility of the cord.

64. d. If lung sounds are heard only on the right side, this indicates a right main stem intubation. Remove air from the cuff and pull the tube back slightly. Check breath sounds after repositioning the tube.

65. d. Most adults can be intubated with a size 3 curved or straight blade.

66. d. Uncuffed endotracheal tubes are generally used for children less than 8 years old because the cricoid cartilage is the narrowest part of the airway and serves as a functional cuff.

67. a. A technique for deciding what size endotracheal tube to insert in an infant or child is to match the tube size to the diameter of the patient's little finger or nasal opening.

68. d. While one rescuer attempts to intubate the patient, a second rescuer can perform the Sellick maneuver, that is, provide cricoid pressure. The Sellick maneuver helps to compress the esophagus, thereby reducing the risk of the patient regurgitating. Chest compressions should be discontinued during intubation attempts, and the person performing the intubation should hold both the laryngoscope and the endotracheal tube. The Heimlich maneuver is abdominal compressions used to relieve an obstructed airway and is not performed when attempting intubation.

Questions 69 through 75 deal with rapid sequence intubation (RSI).

69. b. The two types of neuromuscular blocking drugs are depolarizing and nondepolarizing agents. Depolarizing agents substitute themselves into the neuromuscular junction and bind to the receptors for acetylcholine. Nondepolarizing agents bind to the receptors for acetylcholine and block the uptake of acetylcholine at the neuromuscular junction without initiating depolarization of the muscle membrane.

70. d. Succinylcholine is the most common neuromuscular blocking agent initially used in the field to paralyze a patient requiring rapid sequence intubation. Succinylcholine is a depolarizing agent. It is often preferred because it has a rapid onset of action and the briefest duration of action of all neuromuscular blocking drugs.

71. c. Premedicating the head injury patient with lidocaine will blunt a rise in intracranial pressure and prevent laryngospasm.

72. a. Fasciculations are uncontrollable muscle twitching. Fasciculations can be produced by depolarizing agents.

73. d. Before performing rapid sequence intubation on a pediatric patient, premedicate the patient with atropine. This will reduce the possibility of the patient going into a bradycardic rhythm.

74. c. Patients undergoing rapid sequence intubation should be sedated with medications such as etomidate, diazepam, or midazolam. One of the key reasons for administering such medications is that they have an amnestic affect, that is, the patient will not remember the procedure.

75. d. Vecuronium (Norcuron) is an example of a nondepolarizing agent. Although nondepolarizing agents have a longer onset of action, they have a longer duration of action and therefore are better for longer-term paralysis. They are best used after endotracheal tube placement has been verified and the tube has been properly secured.

Questions 76 through 78 deal with performing a cricothyrotomy.

76. c. When performing a needle cricothyrotomy, insert the needle through the midline of the membrane at a 45- to 60-degree angle toward the patient's carina. This reduces the risk of the needle going through the posterior wall of the trachea and directs the flow of oxygen from the catheter toward the lungs.

77. b. Before inserting the needle through the cricothyroid membrane, attach a syringe to the needle. Apply negative pressure to the syringe while inserting the needle through the skin. The entrance of air into the syringe indicates that the needle is in the trachea. The rescuer performing the procedure should stabilize the larynx using the thumb and middle finger of one hand. This is not the same as the Sellick maneuver.

78. a. The correct ratio of inflation to deflation depends on whether an airway obstruction is present. Generally, an inspiratory-to-expiratory ratio of 1 second of inspiration to 4 seconds of expiration is used if no upper airway obstruction is present. Ratios of 1 second of inspiration to 8 seconds of expiration are needed if upper airway obstruction is present to prevent barotraumas.

PATIENT ASSESSMENT

1. Scene size-up:
   a. includes taking appropriate body substance isolation measures
   b. is necessary only when approaching a trauma scene
   c. should be performed immediately after the initial patient assessment
   d. is the responsibility of the senior crew member

2. If a scene is not safe and it cannot be made safe:
   a. enter only if the patient's life is in immediate danger
   b. do not enter
   c. one rescuer should enter while another stands by for assistance to arrive
   d. return to the station until the scene becomes safe

3. Match the following injuries with their likely mechanism of injury: chest injury, head/cervical spine injury, hip injury.

   _____ windshield broken in a "spiderweb" pattern

   _____ broken car dashboard

   _____ accident in the shallow end of a swimming pool

   _____ bent steering wheel or steering column

4. The chief complaint is a:
   a. list of what is currently wrong with the patient
   b. brief, short description of the patient's primary problem
   c. history of the present illness
   d. description of the patient's medical history

5. The initial assessment includes the rescuer's general impression of the patient and evaluation of, in order, the patient's:
   a. level of consciousness, airway, breathing, and circulation
   b. blood pressure, level of consciousness, and pulse
   c. airway, pulse, blood pressure, and responsiveness
   d. pulse, bleeding, airway, and family history

6. When a life-threatening condition is discovered during the initial assessment:
   a. immediately skip to a focused trauma history
   b. note it and correct it during the appropriate part of the detailed exam
   c. manage the problem immediately
   d. note the condition on the run report and let the hospital deal with it

7. Cervical spine stabilization should first be accomplished:
   a. while the secondary survey is being performed
   b. after the patient is log-rolled onto the backboard
   c. when the patient's level of consciousness is being assessed
   d. after the vital signs have been checked

8. When the AVPU scale is used for noting a patient's level of consciousness, *V* would signify that the patient:
   a. is "vocal" and able to speak
   b. responds to "verbal" stimuli
   c. responds to "visual" stimuli
   d. has spontaneous "ventilations"

9. The letter *P* in AVPU refers to whether the patient:
   a. is oriented to "place"
   b. is a "priority" patient
   c. has a "pulse"
   d. responds to "painful" stimuli

10. When assessing and reassessing the mental status of a patient with a possible head injury, note all of the following on the EMS report *EXCEPT:*
    a. any changes for the better or worse
    b. whether the assessor thinks the patient is intoxicated
    c. the patient's exact words when answering questions
    d. Glasgow Coma Scale scores

11. Part of maintaining an adequate airway in a trauma patient involves:
    a. placing the patient in a pneumatic antishock garment (PASG)
    b. placing the patient in the shock position
    c. sealing open chest wounds
    d. sitting the patient upright

12. When a severely injured or unconscious multi-system trauma patient is examined, it is important to:
    a. remove as little of the patient's clothing as possible
    b. remove all the patient's clothing
    c. expose only the areas with obvious injury or pain
    d. not remove any clothing, because this may cause hypothermia

13. A rapid trauma assessment should be performed on:
    a. all unresponsive trauma patients
    b. all trauma patients
    c. any patient complaining of neck pain
    d. any patient with a painful, swollen, deformed extremity

14. A rapid trauma assessment is a:
    a. rapid evaluation of the patient's airway and cervical spine
    b. methodical exam limited to the area of injury
    c. rapid examination of the mechanism of injury and scene
    d. quick head-to-toe exam

15. Ideally, a rapid trauma assessment should be performed in:
    a. 10 to 30 seconds
    b. 30 to 60 seconds
    c. 60 to 90 seconds
    d. 90 to 120 seconds

16. When a multisystem trauma patient is encountered:
    a. deal with life-threatening conditions first
    b. focus on the patient's most painful injury first
    c. focus on the injury that appears to be most serious first
    d. do not manage any injuries until the rapid trauma assessment is complete

17. If a conscious trauma patient is complaining of severe pain in the pelvic region:
    a. do not flex or compress the pelvic girdle
    b. compress the pelvic region to see if compression elicits further pain
    c. log-roll the patient onto his or her side and assess the posterior pelvis
    d. have the patient move his or her legs into a position that relieves the pain

18. Your patient was the driver of a car involved in a motor vehicle crash. A haze is present in the vehicle. Because the air bag has deployed:
    a. there is little chance the patient received significant injury
    b. it is unlikely the patient has any serious injuries if he appears stable after the first 5 to 10 minutes
    c. the patient should be checked for steam burns
    d. the air bag should be lifted and the steering wheel checked for damage

19. Evaluation of the adult patient's extremities involves checking for:
    a. capillary refill, sensation, and circulation
    b. circulation, motor function, and sensation
    c. reflexes, pulses, and color
    d. blood pressure, reflexes, and motor function

20. An often overlooked but important part of the focused history and physical exam of the trauma patient is checking the patient's:
    a. posterior body
    b. airway
    c. reflexes
    d. mental status

21. If only one rescuer is present, the rapid trauma assessment should be performed:
    a. before the initial assessment
    b. after baseline vital signs and history are obtained
    c. before any cervical spine precautions are taken
    d. after an initial assessment is done

22. Your patient was working in his wood shop when he sustained a serious laceration to his forearm as a result of a run-in with his table saw. When performing your examination, begin:
    a. at the head, then work toward the injury
    b. at the site of the injury
    c. with reevaluation of the airway
    d. by performing manual cervical immobilization

23. When an unresponsive medical patient is encountered, the next step after the initial assessment is to complete:
    a. an assessment of the chest to evaluate the lungs and heart
    b. a detailed physical exam
    c. a rapid head-to-toe assessment similar to the rapid trauma assessment
    d. an abbreviated focused history

24. The assessment of a responsive medical patient:
    a. emphasizes the patient's vital signs
    b. is not as critical as that of an unresponsive patient if there is no previous history of medical problems
    c. usually can wait until the patient is moved to the ambulance
    d. is normally based on the patient's chief complaint

25. The most important aspect of the assessment of a child is the:
    a. patient's blood pressure
    b. patient's pulse rate
    c. mother's or father's general reactions
    d. rescuer's general impression of the patient

26. Capillary refill should be checked on:
    a. patients older than 16 years
    b. all patients
    c. any patient in shock
    d. patients younger than 6 years

27. When capillary refill time is checked, color should normally return within:
    a. $1/2$ to 1 second
    b. 2 seconds
    c. 4 seconds
    d. 10 seconds

For questions 28 through 32, refer to the acronym S-A-M-P-L-E.

28. When a patient history is taken, the letter *P* refers to:
    a. location of "pain"
    b. presence of "paralysis"
    c. events "preceding" the injury or illness
    d. "pertinent" past medical history

29. The letter *M* refers to:
    a. present "medications"
    b. ability to "move" all extremities
    c. time of the last "meal"
    d. name of the patient's "MD"

30. The letter *E* refers to:
    a. length of time from onset of problem until "EMS" was called
    b. "events" leading up to the injury or illness
    c. whether the situation should be classified as a true "emergency"
    d. whether there is a need for "extrication"

31. The letter *L* refers to:
    a. the patient's "lifestyle"
    b. things that "led" up to the event
    c. the patient's "last" oral intake
    d. checking the patient's "lung" sounds

32. When routinely questioning a patient about allergies (the *A* in S-A-M-P-L-E), the rescuer is concerned about allergies to:
    a. medications
    b. food
    c. environmental factors
    d. all of the above

33. Given the following list, mark whether each is a sign, symptom, or both.

_____ chest pain

_____ cyanosis

_____ apnea

_____ difficulty breathing

_____ nausea

_____ sweating

_____ cool skin

_____ headache

_____ dizziness

_____ paleness

_____ deformed extremity

_____ vomiting

_____ swelling

_____ double vision

_____ numbness

_____ wheezing

34. When obtaining a history from a female patient between the ages of 10 and 55 who is complaining of abdominal pain, question the patient about all of the following *EXCEPT:*
    a. when was her last menstrual period
    b. if she is sexually active
    c. when she last ate or drank
    d. if she has taken anything to relieve the pain

35. A male patient in his mid-20s appears to be intoxicated. He is acting belligerently, talking in a loud voice, and cursing. While trying to manage the patient, it is best to:
    a. be accepting, not challenging
    b. turn the patient over to police
    c. try to keep the patient in a small area
    d. try to get the patient to lower his voice and stop cursing

36. Given the following list of medical emergencies, note whether you would expect the patient's skin color to be cyanotic, flushed, jaundiced, pale, or pink.

_____ hypoglycemia

_____ heat emergency with dry skin

_____ liver dysfunction

_____ normal skin

_____ late stage carbon monoxide poisoning

_____ insufficient circulation

_____ inadequate oxygenation

_____ hypoperfusion

37. The best part of a patient to check for jaundice is:
    a. the white area of the eye
    b. the lowest areas of the body
    c. the gums
    d. the skin of the thigh

38. When a stethoscope is used, the earpieces should:
    a. face backward
    b. be placed in the most comfortable position
    c. face away from the patient
    d. face forward

39. The diaphragm of the stethoscope is best used for listening to:
    a. high-frequency sounds
    b. low-frequency sounds
    c. heart sounds
    d. gallops

40. The pulse may be defined as:
    a. the number of times the heart contracts each minute
    b. the pressure in an artery
    c. a wave of blood that courses through an artery as the heart contracts
    d. blood flowing through a vein

41. When checking a carotid pulse:
    a. check only one side at a time
    b. check both sides simultaneously
    c. only perform carotid pulse checks on patients older than 65
    d. use the thumb of the hand closest to the head

42. The most common place to check a pulse in a conscious adult patient is the:
    a. brachial artery
    b. radial artery
    c. carotid artery
    d. femoral artery

43. Given the following medical conditions, note whether you would expect the pupils to be dilated, constricted, or unequal.

_____ amphetamine use

_____ post atropine administration

_____ narcotics use

_____ cardiac arrest

_____ head injury

_____ organophosphate poisoning

44. When assessing a pulse, check for:
    a. rate and quality
    b. volume and strength
    c. flow and rate
    d. quality and volume

45. When a patient's pulse is described, the term *quality* refers to its:
   a. strength and regularity
   b. rhythm and rate
   c. rate and regularity
   d. strength and rate

46. Referring to Figure 4-1, match the following key pulse points to their location: brachial, carotid, dorsalis pedis, femoral, posterior tibial, radial.

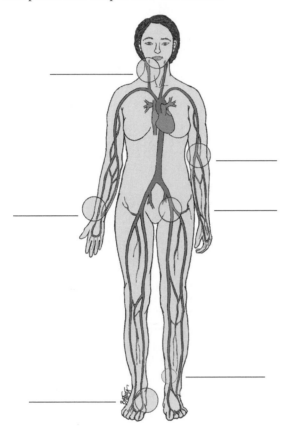

Figure 4-1

47. The normal pulse rate for an adult is:
   a. 50 to 70 beats per minute
   b. 60 to 100 beats per minute
   c. 80 to 120 beats per minute
   d. 110 beats per minute

48. The normal pulse rate for a child is:
   a. 60 to 80 beats per minute
   b. 80 to 100 beats per minute
   c. less than 80 beats per minute
   d. 120 beats per minute

49. The pulse rate of an infant is normally:
   a. 50 to 80 beats per minute
   b. 80 to 100 beats per minute
   c. 100 to 140 beats per minute
   d. 170 to 200 beats per minute

50. Systolic blood pressure can best be defined as:
   a. the pressure blood exerts against the walls of the arteries
   b. the volume of blood in an artery
   c. the pressure exerted by blood against the walls of the veins
   d. the difference between the arterial pressure and venous pressure

51. The first sound noted when taking a blood pressure by auscultation is the:
   a. diastolic pressure
   b. systolic pressure
   c. mean arterial pressure
   d. venous pressure

52. The diastolic pressure corresponds to:
   a. the pressure exerted against the walls of the arteries when the heart is pumping
   b. the difference between the resting pressure and pumping pressure
   c. the pressure exerted against the walls of the arteries when the left ventricle is at rest
   d. half the systolic pressure

53. Systolic blood pressure may indicate a serious problem if it is:
   a. 90 mm Hg
   b. 130 mm Hg
   c. less than 100 mm Hg
   d. less than 140 mm Hg

54. Obtaining a blood pressure by feeling a pulse rather than by listening with a stethoscope is known as:
   a. auscultating a blood pressure
   b. pulsing a blood pressure
   c. tamponading a blood pressure
   d. palpating a blood pressure

55. Normal adult systolic blood pressure is:
   a. 80 to 120 mm Hg
   b. 100 to 140 mm Hg
   c. 120 to 160 mm Hg
   d. 140 to 180 mm Hg

56. Normal adult diastolic blood pressure is:
   a. 40 to 70 mm Hg
   b. 50 to 80 mm Hg
   c. 60 to 90 mm Hg
   d. 70 to 100 mm Hg

57. Vital signs on an unstable patient should be checked:
a. every 5 minutes
b. every 10 minutes
c. every 15 minutes
d. only if a medical intervention is performed

58. To obtain an accurate blood pressure, the sphygmomanometer cuff should:
a. be the length of the forearm
b. cover about two thirds of the patient's upper arm
c. be twice the diameter of the arm
d. be placed even with the bend in the patient's elbow

59. An error in blood pressure measurement may be the result of:
a. incorrect cuff size
b. operator error
c. loud background noise
d. all of the above

60. If it is difficult to hear a blood pressure sound, the sounds may be augmented by:
a. slowly inflating the cuff
b. lowering the arm before inflating the cuff
c. elevating the arm before inflating the cuff
d. rapidly deflating the cuff

61. To obtain an accurate blood pressure, the blood pressure cuff should be deflated at a rate of:
a. 1 to 2 mm Hg per second
b. 2 to 3 mm Hg per second
c. 3 to 4 mm Hg per second
d. 4 to 5 mm Hg per second

62. Referring to Figure 4-2, match the following key thoracic landmarks to their location (*Some answers may be used more than once*): anterior axillary line, midaxillary line, midclavicular line, midsternal line, posterior axillary line, scapular line, vertebral line.

63. When assessing your patient's chest, you note that the chest wall diameter is noticeably increased. You would expect to find this patient has a history of:
a. congestive heart failure
b. previous flail chest
c. chronic obstructive pulmonary disease
d. hypertension

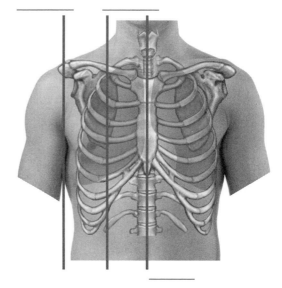

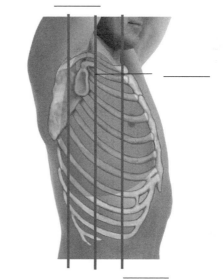

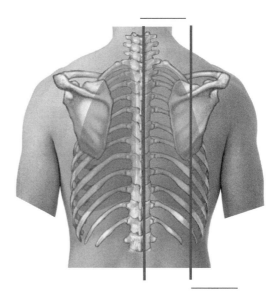

Figure 4-2

64. High-pitched, discontinuous sounds often described as similar to the sound of hair being rubbed between the fingers and heard during the end of inspiration are known as:
    a. rhonchi
    b. crackles
    c. sibilant wheezes
    d. sonorous wheezes

65. Wheezes can be described as a:
    a. harsh, raspy sound created by fluid in the lungs
    b. crowing sound heard on inspiration
    c. fine, crackling sound indicating the presence of fluid in the small airways
    d. high-pitched, whistling sound created as air flows through narrowed airways

66. The most typical causes of crackles are:
    a. pulmonary edema and pneumonia
    b. chronic obstructive pulmonary disease and asthma
    c. congestive heart failure and emphysema
    d. bronchitis and croup

67. Wet, low-pitched breath sounds are:
    a. coarse crackles
    b. fine crackles
    c. sibilant wheezes
    d. sonorous wheezes

68. Continuous, low-pitched rumbling sounds usually heard on expiration are:
    a. discontinuous breath sounds
    b. fine crackles
    c. rhonchi
    d. sibilant wheezes

69. An inspiratory, crowing type sound that can usually be heard without the aid of a stethoscope is:
    a. coarse crackles
    b. fine crackles
    c. sibilant wheezes
    d. stridor

70. Given the following list of medical conditions, note whether you would expect to hear crackles, pleural friction rub, stridor, or wheezes.

    _____ pulmonary edema
    _____ emphysema
    _____ pneumonia in its early stages
    _____ asthma
    _____ viral croup
    _____ pleurisy
    _____ anaphylaxis

71. When assessing the patient's chest:
    a. look for paradoxical movement
    b. check breath sounds
    c. feel for crepitation
    d. all of the above

72. While percussing the chest of a patient with hyperinflation due to pneumothorax, asthma, or other pulmonary disease, you are most likely to hear:
    a. resonance
    b. dullness
    c. hyperresonance
    d. flatness

73. When auscultating heart sounds, ensure that the patient is:
    a. in a right lateral recumbent position or lying flat
    b. sitting up and leaning slightly forward or in a left lateral recumbent position
    c. lying flat or sitting up and leaning slightly backward
    d. in Trendelenburg position or a prone position

74. For maximal effectiveness, heart sounds should be auscultated over the:
    a. xyphoid process
    b. third intercostal space, midaxillary line
    c. left fifth intercostal space near the sternal border
    d. manubrium

75. Heart murmurs normally indicate:
    a. the presence of an aneurysm
    b. a local blood flow obstruction
    c. a narrowing of a coronary artery
    d. the presence of a valvular defect

76. A bruit is a:
    a. fine vibration or tremor that is always benign
    b. sign of a heart valve defect
    c. low-pitched sound that may indicate local obstruction
    d. abnormal breath sound usually heard in pediatric patients

77. Referring to Figure 4-3, label the following organs with the abdominal quadrants in which they are primarily located (*Some organs may be in more than one quadrant*).

_____ appendix

_____ gall bladder

_____ large intestine

_____ left adrenal gland

_____ left kidney

_____ left ovary and salpinx

_____ left ureter

_____ liver

_____ pancreas (body)

_____ pancreas (head)

_____ right adrenal gland

_____ right kidney

_____ right ovary and salpinx

_____ right ureter

_____ small intestine

_____ spleen

_____ stomach

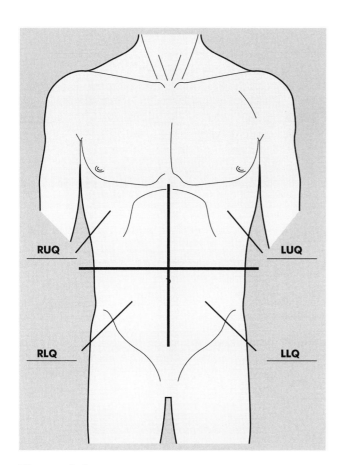

Figure 4-3

78. When you are palpating a patient's abdomen, it is generally considered to be normal if it is:
a. hard
b. soft
c. distended
d. rigid

79. When assessing the abdomen:
a. inform the patient before starting palpation
b. palpate using only one finger
c. palpate only in the area of discomfort
d. press as deeply as possible

80. While examining a patient's abdomen, you note Cullen's sign. The presence of Cullen's sign may indicate:
a. kidney injury
b. bowel obstruction
c. cirrhosis of the liver
d. peritoneal bleeding

81. The "Pronator Drift" test is performed by having the patient:
a. close the eyes and hold both arms out from the body
b. squeeze the rescuer's finger with both hands simultaneously
c. push the soles of the feet against the rescuer's palms
d. touch the finger to the nose, alternating hands

Questions 82 through 87 refer to the acronym O-P-Q-R-S-T.

82. The letter *O* refers to:
a. the patient's last "oral" intake
b. whether the patient is "oriented"
c. the time of "onset" of the problem
d. performing an "ongoing" assessment

83. The letter *P* relates to:
a. severity of "pain"
b. "provocation"
c. what the main "problem" is
d. the "primary" complaint

84. The letter *Q* refers to:
a. how "quickly" the problem started
b. the "quality" of the pain
c. the "quantity" of medications regularly taken by the patient
d. whether the patient "qualifies" as a priority patient

85. The letter *R* component involves asking the patient if:
    a. anything provides "relief" of the pain
    b. this is a "regular" problem
    c. the onset of the problem was "rapid"
    d. the pain "radiates" to other areas

86. The letter *S* is associated with:
    a. "symptoms"
    b. "severity"
    c. "signs"
    d. "sensation"

87. *T* refers to:
    a. "time"
    b. the patient's "temperature"
    c. whether the problem involves "trauma"
    d. the "type" of problem

88. When an unresponsive patient is encountered:
    a. O-P-Q-R-S-T information cannot be obtained
    b. it is not important to gain O-P-Q-R-S-T information
    c. O-P-Q-R-S-T information may be obtained from family, friends, or bystanders
    d. accurate O-P-Q-R-S-T information can only be obtained if the patient regains consciousness

89. The absence of a sign or symptom that may be expected to be present when assessing a patient with a particular medical problem is known as:
    a. a pertinent positive
    b. a nonspecific complaint
    c. a pertinent negative
    d. extraneous information

90. The detailed physical exam is a:
    a. rapid neurological exam
    b. breathing and pulse check
    c. 15-minute thorough exam limited to the injured body system
    d. methodical head-to-toe examination

91. The primary purpose of the detailed physical exam is to:
    a. check for signs of abuse or drug use
    b. find hidden injuries or medical problems
    c. confirm a medical problem exists
    d. help diagnose the patient's problem

92. An example of a patient who would not need a complete and thorough detailed physical exam is:
    a. an unresponsive medical patient
    b. a trauma patient with an altered mental status
    c. a patient with a history of heart problems who is complaining of mild chest pain
    d. a patient who was ejected from a vehicle but is complaining only of shoulder pain

93. When assessing the patient's ears, be alert for the presence of blood mixed with:
    a. vitreous humor
    b. cerebrospinal fluid
    c. synovial fluid
    d. lacrimal fluid

94. Ideally, the detailed physical exam should be performed:
    a. while still in the house
    b. before leaving for the hospital
    c. after Advanced Life Support personnel arrive
    d. while en route to the hospital

95. When performing the ongoing assessment:
    a. ensure adequacy of oxygen delivery and artificial ventilations, and the adequacy of medical interventions
    b. repeat a head-to-toe exam
    c. record the vital signs and S-A-M-P-L-E history every 10 minutes
    d. perform a detailed physical exam

96. A stable patient should receive an ongoing assessment every:
    a. 5 minutes
    b. 10 minutes
    c. 15 minutes
    d. 20 minutes

97. In essence, the ongoing assessment repeats all the components of the:
    a. detailed physical exam
    b. initial assessment
    c. rapid trauma assessment
    d. S-A-M-P-L-E history

98. An important component of patient assessment that must not be neglected is:
    a. providing emotional reassurance to the patient
    b. obtaining insurance information for billing purposes
    c. passing information on to law enforcement officers
    d. assuring the patient everything will be all right

99. When an injured patient is found at a crime scene:
    a. have the police bring the patient to the medical care personnel for them to provide patient care
    b. wait to begin patient care until law enforcement officials have completed their investigation
    c. try to disturb the scene as little as possible while providing patient care
    d. immediately move the patient to the ambulance before providing any care

100. When checking whether a patient is oriented to person, place, time, and purpose, the last thing the patient will normally forget is:
    a. place
    b. person
    c. purpose
    d. time

101. When palpating a patient's neck and upper chest, you note it appears swollen and you feel a crackling sensation similar to popping bubble wrap. This condition is known as:
    a. rales
    b. ischemia
    c. subcutaneous emphysema
    d. parenchyma

Questions 102 through 104 refer to the Glasgow Coma Scale in Box 4-1.

102. Your patient is a 30-year-old male who is lying on the sidewalk. His eyes are closed and he opens them only on voice command. He can speak, but his answers are inaccurate. During the exam, he reacts to pain by attempting to push your hand away from the painful area. His Glasgow Coma Scale score is:
    a. 11
    b. 12
    c. 13
    d. 14

103. A hit-and-run patient is found lying next to the road. She does not open her eyes in response to any stimulus. She does respond to painful stimuli by groaning and moving her arms away from the source of pain. Her Glasgow Coma Scale score is:
    a. 5
    b. 6
    c. 7
    d. 8

104. A Glasgow Coma Scale score that would be considered normal is:
    a. 9 to 10
    b. 11 to 12
    c. 14 to 15
    d. 17 to 18

Box 4-1 Glasgow Coma Scale

1. Eye Opening	Points	
• Spontaneous	4	
• To voice	3	
• To pain	2	
• None	1	_____

2. Verbal Response	Points	
• Oriented	5	
• Confused	4	
• Inappropriate words	3	
• Incomprehensible sounds	2	
• None	1	_____

3. Motor Response	Points	
• Obeys commands	6	
• Localizes pain	5	
• Withdraws (pain)	4	
• Flexion (pain)	3	
• Extension (pain)	2	
• None	1	_____

| Total (1 + 2 + 3) | | _____ |

ANSWERS TO CHAPTER 4: PATIENT ASSESSMENT

1. **a.** Scene size-up includes taking appropriate body substance isolation measures. It should be done on all calls. The rescuer must determine if the scene is safe before assessing the patient. Everyone on the crew is responsible for looking for unsafe situations.

2. **b.** If a scene is not safe and cannot be made safe, do not enter the scene. Remember, dead EMTs don't save lives.

3. Match the following injuries with their likely mechanism of injury: chest injury, head/cervical spine injury, hip injury.

head/cervical spine injury	windshield broken in a "spiderweb" pattern
hip injury	broken car dashboard
head/cervical spine injury	accident in the shallow end of a swimming pool
chest injury	bent steering wheel or steering column

4. **b.** The chief complaint is a brief, short description of the patient's primary problem, such as "chest pain" or "difficulty breathing."

5. **a.** The initial assessment includes the rescuer's general impressions of the patient and assessing the patient's level of consciousness, airway, breathing, and circulation.

6. **c.** All life-threatening conditions discovered during the initial assessment should be managed immediately. If the problem is not managed immediately it may be forgotten, and even if it is not forgotten, a delay in management may lead to death from an otherwise survivable problem.

7. **c.** Cervical spine stabilization should take place while the patient's level of consciousness is being assessed.

8. **b.** The letter *V* signifies that the patient responds to verbal stimuli, *A* corresponds to alert, and *U* means the patient is unresponsive to any stimuli.

9. **d.** The letter *P* refers to whether the patient responds to only painful stimuli.

10. **c.** When assessing and reassessing mental status, note any changes for the better or worse. Changes are important as they act as a baseline for comparison. The Glasgow Coma Scale is a great way to quantify patient trends. The patient's answers do not need to be written verbatim. If a good reason exists to suspect the patient is intoxicated, or if the patient admits to being intoxicated, it may be noted as well. However, a patient who appears to be intoxicated, or even someone who admits to being intoxicated, may have underlying trauma or a medical problem affecting his or her mental status.

11. **c.** Open chest wounds compromise the lungs' ability to function; therefore they must be sealed with an occlusive dressing to maintain adequate oxygenation. Sitting a trauma patient upright is contraindicated because of the possibility of cervical spine injury. Placing the patient in a PASG or the shock position will not ensure a patent airway; however, it may increase the circulation of hemoglobin to vital organs.

12. **b.** It is generally recommended that all clothing be removed from a seriously injured multisystem trauma patient, especially if the patient is unconscious and cannot verbally communicate. In many cases, it is not the injuries you see that will kill the patient, but rather, the injuries you don't see. Discretion should be exercised to keep embarrassment to a minimum. Because it can be avoided by using blankets, hypothermia is not a valid reason to leave clothing in place.

13. **a.** A rapid trauma assessment should be performed on any unresponsive trauma patient as well as any trauma patient who has a significant mechanism of injury.

14. **d.** A rapid trauma assessment is a quick head-to-toe exam.

15. **c.** A rapid trauma assessment should be performed in 60 to 90 seconds.

16. **a.** When a multisystem trauma patient is encountered, deal with life-threatening conditions first. Do not be fooled into focusing on the patient's most painful injury or the worst-appearing injury first.

17. a. If a conscious trauma patient is complaining of severe pain in the pelvic region, do not flex or compress the pelvic girdle because this may cause further injury. If the patient is unconscious, or if the patient is not complaining of pelvic pain but pelvic injury is suspected, checking the stability of the pelvis is warranted. This can be done by pressing downward and outward on each anterior iliac crest and by pressing downward on the symphysis pubis. Do not log-roll or move the legs of a patient with a suspected pelvic injury.

18. d. Although air bags can reduce the incidence of injuries from vehicle crashes, they can be misleading. A patient may sustain an injury yet not show immediate signs of the injury. If an air bag has been deployed, lift the air bag and check the steering wheel for deformity or damage. If either is noted, suspect injury to the patient, especially chest injury. The haze present after a deployment is a nontoxic powder that is used to lubricate the bag.

19. b. Evaluation of the patient's extremities includes checking circulation (distal pulses), motor function, and sensation.

20. a. Many times we forget to check a patient's posterior body during the trauma assessment. But critical life-threatening injuries may be missed if this important part of the patient exam is forgotten. The patient's level of consciousness and airway are checked during the initial assessment. Reflexes usually are not checked in the field by EMS personnel.

21. d. If only one rescuer is present, the rapid trauma assessment should be performed after an initial assessment is done. Vital signs and history are taken after the rapid assessment. Although it may be difficult when only one rescuer is present, cervical spine precautions should still be taken to the best extent possible before the rapid trauma assessment is performed. If two rescuers are present, some procedures can be performed at the same time.

22. b. When managing a patient with single-system trauma, such as a lacerated arm, a focused history and physical examination, which begins at the site of the injury, is indicated. However, if the patient appears confused or a significant mechanism of injury exists, a complete head-to-toe exam is necessary.

23. c. When an unresponsive medical patient is encountered, a rapid head-to-toe assessment similar to the rapid trauma assessment should be done after the initial assessment. This will help identify any life-threatening problems in need of immediate correction.

24. d. The assessment of a responsive medical patient is normally based on the patient's chief complaint. Do not delay assessment until the patient is in the ambulance. If assessment is delayed, then management of the patient, such as assisting with medications, also may be delayed.

25. d. The rescuer's general impression of a sick or injured child is more important than vital signs. Children can maintain what appear to be normal vital signs, but their condition can suddenly deteriorate.

26. d. Capillary refill time should only be checked on patients younger than 6 years. Remember that if the patient's extremities are cold, capillary refill time will not be an accurate indicator. The capillary refill test is not considered to be as reliable an indicator of cardiovascular status in adults.

27. b. When checking capillary refill, you should see the color returning within 2 seconds. Delays can indicate poor peripheral circulation and can be an indicator of shock.

For questions 28 through 32, refer to the acronym S-A-M-P-L-E.

28. d. The letter *P* refers to pertinent past medical history, such as previous illnesses or injuries.

29. a. The letter *M* refers to the patient's present medications. When asking about current medications, also ask about any herbs and other over-the-counter medications the patient is taking.

30. b. The letter *E* relates to the events that led up to or caused the injury or illness.

31. c. The letter *L* refers to the patient's last oral intake, whether solids or liquids.

32. d. All of the above. The allergies EMS personnel are concerned with are allergies to medications, food, or environmental factors, such as pollen or insect stings.

33. A sign is something the rescuer sees, feels, or hears. A symptom is something the patient tells the rescuer. A syndrome is a collection of symptoms. The *S* in S-A-M-P-L-E refers to signs and symptoms.

symptom chest pain

sign cyanosis

sign apnea

both difficulty breathing

symptom nausea

sign sweating

sign cool skin

symptom headache

symptom dizziness

sign paleness

sign deformed extremity

sign vomiting

sign swelling

symptom double vision

symptom numbness

sign wheezes

34. b. A female patient complaining of abdominal pain should be asked when her last menstrual period was. She should also be asked when she last ate and drank and whether she has taken anything to relieve the pain. In most cases, questioning whether she is sexually active is not appropriate. However, she should be asked whether it is possible she is pregnant. Keep in mind that younger females can be pregnant; therefore use your best judgment in deciding which young patients should be asked about the possibility of pregnancy.

35. a. Dealing with an intoxicated patient can be quite challenging. In general, when trying to manage intoxicated patients, be accepting and not challenging. Do not attempt to have them lower their voices or stop cursing as this may aggravate them. Also, avoid trapping them in small areas. Because a medical problem may be present, simply turning the person over to the police is not appropriate. A thorough exam should be performed to ensure no serious medical problems exist that should be treated.

36. Given the following list of medical emergencies, note whether you would expect the patient's skin color to be cyanotic, flushed, jaundiced, pale, or pink.

pale hypoglycemia

flushed heat emergency with dry skin

jaundiced liver dysfunction

pink normal skin

flushed late stage carbon monoxide poisoning

pale insufficient circulation

cyanotic inadequate oxygenation

pale hypoperfusion

37. a. Jaundice manifests early in the white area of the eye. This area is easy to see, and no clothing must be removed to view it.

38. d. The earpieces of a stethoscope should face forward to match the natural direction of the listener's ear canals.

39. a. The diaphragm of the stethoscope best amplifies high-frequency sounds, such as breath sounds. The bell is used to listen to low frequency sounds, such as heart sounds. Gallops are types of heart sounds.

40. c. The pulse may be defined as a wave of blood that courses through an artery as the heart contracts. It is not the number of times the heart contracts each minute. Sometimes, such as when a patient has a rapid heart rate, the heart may not refill completely. It does contract, but no pulse is felt because not enough blood is in the ventricles to push the blood through the circulatory system.

41. a. When checking a carotid pulse, check only one side at a time. Checking both sides simultaneously may obstruct blood flow to the brain. Rubbing the carotid artery may cause vagal stimulation resulting in a drop in pulse rate, especially in the elderly. Never use the thumb to check any pulses; it has its own pulse.

42. b. EMS personnel most commonly check a radial pulse in any patient older than 1 year. If the radial pulse cannot be felt, assess the carotid pulse. For children younger than 1 year, check the brachial pulse.

43. Given the following medical conditions, note whether you would expect the pupils to be dilated, constricted, or unequal.

<u>dilated</u> amphetamine use

<u>dilated</u> post atropine administration

<u>constricted</u> narcotics use

<u>dilated</u> cardiac arrest

<u>unequal</u> head injury

<u>constricted</u> organophosphate poisoning

44. **a.** The pulse should be checked for rate and quality. Quality refers to volume (strong or weak) and regularity. If it is irregular, check for a regular irregularity (i.e., an extra beat every second or third beat) or irregular irregularity (i.e., no pattern to the irregularity).

45. **a.** The quality of a patient's pulse is determined by its strength and regularity.

46. Referring to Figure 4-1, match the following key pulse points to their location: brachial, carotid, dorsalis pedis, femoral, posterior tibial, radial.

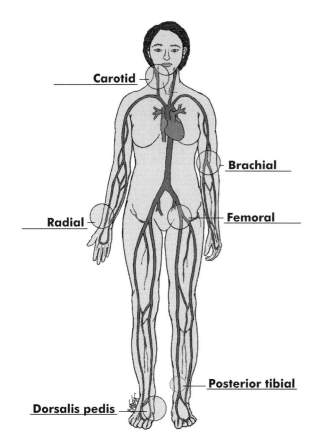

Figure 4-1

47. **b.** The normal adult pulse range is 60 to 100 beats per minute. Remember that the overall patient picture is more important than focusing on the patient's exact pulse rate.

48. **b.** The normal pulse range for a child is 80 to 100 beats per minute. In younger children, the pulse rate normally may be greater than 100.

49. **c.** The pulse rate of an infant is normally 100 to 140 beats per minute. The pulse rate of a newborn may be as high as 150 to 160.

50. **a.** Systolic blood pressure is the pressure blood exerts against the walls of the arteries.

51. **b.** The first sound noted when taking a blood pressure by auscultation is the systolic pressure. The point when the sounds fade or disappear during deflation of the cuff corresponds with the diastolic pressure.

52. **c.** The diastolic reading corresponds to the pressure exerted against the walls of the arteries when the left ventricle is at rest. The systolic reading is the pressure during ventricular contraction.

53. **c.** A systolic blood pressure less than 100 mm Hg may indicate a serious problem, especially if the patient has associated signs and symptoms of trauma or a medical problem.

54. **d.** This is known as palpating a blood pressure. To do this, palpate a pulse below the blood pressure cuff, then inflate the cuff. When the pulse is no longer felt, the cuff is inflated another 30 mm of Hg. The pressure is then released. The first pulse felt as the cuff is deflated is the systolic pressure. Palpated blood pressures should be noted as the systolic pressure over *P* (e.g., 126/P).

55. **b.** Normal adult systolic blood pressure is 100 to 140 mm Hg.

56. **c.** Normal adult diastolic blood pressure is 60 to 90 mm Hg.

57. **a.** Vital signs on an unstable patient should be checked every 5 minutes. If the patient is stable, the patient should be checked every 15 minutes.

58. b. The blood pressure cuff should cover about two thirds of the patient's upper arm. The width of the blood pressure cuff bladder should be at least 20% greater than the diameter of the patient's arm or 40% of the limb circumference. The bottom of the cuff should lie about an inch above the bend of the elbow.

59. d. All of the above. Incorrect cuff size, operator error, and loud background noise all can cause inaccurate blood pressure measurements.

60. c. Elevating the arm before inflating the cuff may reduce venous congestion, which makes it difficult to hear blood pressure sounds. The cuff should be rapidly, not slowly, inflated in 7 seconds or less. The cuff should then be deflated slowly.

61. b. A blood pressure cuff should be deflated at a rate of 2 to 3 mm Hg per second. A faster deflation rate will result in erroneous readings.

62. Referring to Figure 4-2, match the following key thoracic landmarks to their location (*Some answers may be used more than once*): anterior axillary line, midaxillary line, midclavicular line, midsternal line, posterior axillary line, scapular line, vertebral line.

63. c. Patients with chronic obstructive pulmonary disease often have increased chest wall diameter. Their "barrel-shaped" appearance is the result of air trapping.

64. b. High-pitched, discontinuous sounds often described as similar to the sound of hair being rubbed between the fingers and heard during the end of inspiration are known as *crackles.* Crackles may be further classified as coarse crackles or fine crackles.

65. d. Wheezes can be described as a high-pitched whistling or "musical" sound created as air flows through narrowed airways. They are usually louder during expiration.

66. a. The most typical causes of crackles are pulmonary edema and pneumonia in its early stages. Crackles may be difficult to hear and may be overridden by louder respiratory sounds. Asking the patient to cough may clear secretions and make crackles easier to hear.

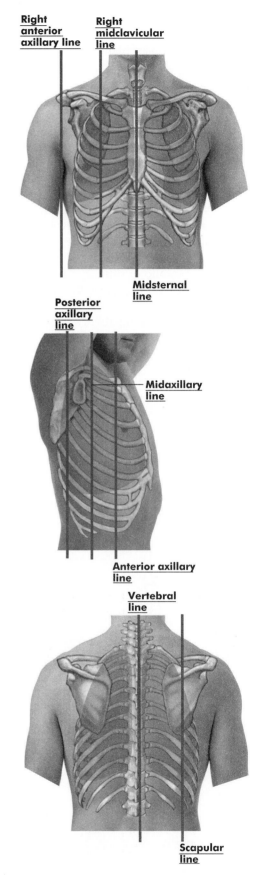

Figure 4-2

67. a. Coarse crackles are wet, low-pitched sounds. Fine crackles are dry, high-pitched sounds.

68. c. Rhonchi are continuous, low-pitched rumbling sounds usually heard on expiration. Rhonchi are categorized as continuous breath sounds and are also known as *sonorous wheezes.*

69. d. Stridor usually is an inspiratory, crowing-type sound and usually can be heard without the aid of a stethoscope. It indicates significant narrowing or obstruction of the larynx or trachea.

70. Given the following list of medical conditions, note whether you would expect to hear crackles, pleural friction rub, stridor, or wheezes.

crackles pulmonary edema

wheezes emphysema

crackles pneumonia in its early stages

wheezes asthma

stridor viral croup

pleural friction rub pleurisy

wheezes anaphylaxis

71. d. All of the above. Check breath sounds when assessing the patient's chest. Note whether they are present or absent, equal or unequal. Note their quality, too. Also, look for paradoxical movement and feel for crepitation.

72. c. While percussing the chest of a patient with hyperinflation resulting from pneumothorax, asthma, or other pulmonary disease, you are most likely to hear hyperresonance. Dullness or flatness suggests the presence of fluid and/or pulmonary congestion. Resonance usually is heard over normal lungs.

73. b. Ideally, when auscultating heart sounds, the patient should be sitting up and leaning slightly forward or in a left lateral recumbent position. These positions bring the heart closer to the left anterior chest wall.

74. c. For maximal effectiveness, heart sounds should be auscultated over the left fifth intercostal space near the sternal border.

75. d. Heart murmurs normally indicate the presence of a valvular defect. They are prolonged extra sounds that are caused by a disruption in the flow of blood into, through, or out of the heart.

76. c. Bruits are low-pitched sounds that may be heard while auscultating the carotid artery or another organ or gland and may indicate local obstruction. Thrills are similar but are fine vibrations or tremors that may indicate blood flow obstruction. They may be serious or benign.

77. Referring to Figure 4-3, label the following organs with the abdominal quadrants in which they are primarily located (*Some organs may be in more than one quadrant*).

RLQ appendix

RUQ gallbladder

RUQ, LUQ, RLQ, LLQ large intestine

LUQ left adrenal gland

LUQ left kidney

LLQ left ovary and salpinx

LLQ left ureter

RUQ liver

LUQ pancreas (body)

RUQ pancreas (head)

RUQ right adrenal gland

RUQ right kidney

RLQ right ovary and salpinx

RLQ right ureter

RLQ, LLQ small intestine

LUQ spleen

LUQ stomach

78. b. When palpating a patient's abdomen, it is generally considered to be normal if it is soft. A hard, rigid, or distended abdomen is indicative of underlying abdominal problems, including internal bleeding.

79. a. When assessing the abdomen, inform the patient before palpating. Otherwise, the patient may be surprised and tighten the abdominal muscles. Do not begin in the immediate area of pain; if any pain exists, save that area for last. There is no need to press deeply to note whether the abdomen is soft, firm, or distended.

80. d. Cullen's sign is discoloration around the umbilicus and may indicate peritoneal bleeding. Grey-Turner's sign is discoloration found in the flank and may indicate possible kidney injury or pancreatic problems.

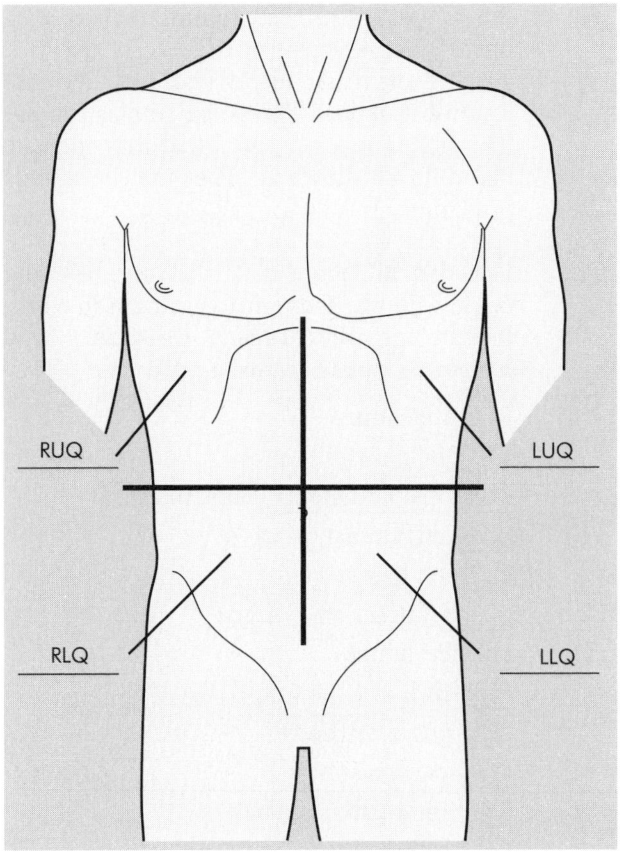

Figure 4-3

81. **a.** The "Pronator Drift" test is performed by having the patient close the eyes and hold both arms out from the body. The test result is considered normal if both arms move the same or both arms do not move at all. It is considered abnormal if one arm does not move in concert with the other, or if one arms drifts down compared with the other.

Questions 82 through 87 refer to the acronym O-P-Q-R-S-T.

82. **c.** The letter *O* refers to the time of onset of the problem. This is when the medical problem first started, and it may be a short or long period prior to when EMS was called.

83. **b.** The letter *P* stands for provocation, that is, what made the pain start or what makes it worse. It also stands for palliation, or what makes the pain lessen or disappear.

84. **b.** The letter *Q* refers to the quality of the pain. This is a description of the characteristics of the discomfort, such as whether the pain is sharp, dull, or stabbing, or whether it is a constant or intermittent pressure.

85. **d.** The *R* involves asking the patient if the pain radiates to or is felt in other areas of the body. However, if the patient is complaining of pain it may not radiate, but just stay in one place.

86. **b.** The letter *S* is associated with severity, or how bad the pain is on a scale of 1 to 10.

87. **a.** The letter *T* refers to time. Time relates primarily to duration of the pain, such as if pain has been going on for some time, or if it has gotten better then worse. It is also important to note if there was a particular time when the problem got worse, prompting the patient to call EMS.

88. **c.** When an unresponsive patient is encountered, O-P-Q-R-S-T information may be obtained from family, friends, bystanders, or anyone familiar with the patient and the problems.

89. **c.** The absence of a sign or symptom that may be expected to be present when assessing a patient is known as a pertinent negative. For example, a patient experiencing chest pain may have no radiation of the pain or no accompanying dyspnea. This is a pertinent negative. Although pertinent negatives do not warrant medical care, noting a pertinent negative is as important as noting a pertinent positive, that is, a positive finding. It also shows the thoroughness of the field assessment.

90. **d.** The detailed physical examination is a methodical head-to-toe examination. Although it covers many items that were checked in the rapid trauma assessment, the detailed exam is slower, methodical, and more comprehensive. It expands upon the assessment steps in the focused history and physical examination.

91. b. The primary purpose of the detailed physical exam is to find hidden injuries or medical problems that may not have been discovered during an earlier exam.

92. c. A patient with a history of heart problems who is complaining of mild chest pain would not need a detailed physical exam because little information is likely to be gained from palpating every body part of this patient. This would also be true of a patient with minor single-system trauma such as a foot laceration. A detailed physical exam should be performed on any unresponsive medical and trauma patient, patients with altered mental status, or patients with a significant mechanism of injury involved.

93. b. Check for cerebrospinal fluid when checking the ears. If blood is also present, place some on a 4 × 4 gauze pad. If cerebrospinal fluid is mixed with the blood, it forms a halolike ring of fluid around the blood in the middle. Vitreous humor is fluid within the eye, synovial fluid lubricates joints, and lacrimal fluid is tears.

94. d. Ideally, the detailed physical exam should be performed in the back of the ambulance while en route to the hospital. This saves precious time and does not delay delivering the patient to definitive care.

95. a. During the ongoing assessment, ensure adequacy of oxygen delivery and artificial ventilations, as well as the adequacy of medical interventions, such as checking dressings and splints.

96. c. A stable patient should receive an ongoing assessment every 15 minutes. An unstable patient should be reassessed every 5 minutes or less.

97. b. In essence, the ongoing assessment repeats all the components of the initial assessment. During the ongoing assessment the patient's response to medical interventions also should be evaluated.

98. a. An important component of patient assessment that must not be neglected is providing emotional reassurance to the patient. Often, patients are distraught and worried about their condition. EMS personnel can help to alleviate some of the anxiety by being compassionate and caring. However, do not tell the patient everything will be all right, because this may not be the case.

99. c. An injured patient at a crime scene still needs medical attention. However, try to disturb the scene as little as possible. Be careful not to be in such a hurry to move the patient that further harm is done.

100. b. Normally the last thing patients forget is "person," that is, who they are. The reason is that this information is stored in long-term memory. Short-term memory, such as where they are (place), what time it is, and what they were doing (purpose) immediately before the event, is forgotten first.

101. c. Subcutaneous emphysema is a collection of air in the soft tissue. This often is associated with some type of disruption of the tracheobronchial tree and is a serious finding. *Rales* refers to an abnormal lung sound, parenchyma is the substance of a gland or solid organ, and ischemia involves inadequate blood flow to a tissue.

```
┌─────────────────────────────────────────────┐
│ Box 4-1   Glasgow Coma Scale                  │
│                                               │
│ 1. Eye Opening              Points            │
│    • Spontaneous              4               │
│    • To voice                 3               │
│    • To pain                  2               │
│    • None                     1      _____    │
│                                               │
│ 2. Verbal Response          Points            │
│    • Oriented                 5               │
│    • Confused                 4               │
│    • Inappropriate words      3               │
│    • Incomprehensible sounds  2               │
│    • None                     1      _____    │
│                                               │
│ 3. Motor Response           Points            │
│    • Obeys commands           6               │
│    • Localizes pain           5               │
│    • Withdraws (pain)         4               │
│    • Flexion (pain)           3               │
│    • Extension (pain)         2               │
│    • None                     1      _____    │
│                                               │
│ Total (1 + 2 + 3)                    _____    │
└─────────────────────────────────────────────┘
```

Questions 102 through 104 refer to the Glasgow Coma Scale in Box 4-1.

102. b. The patient's score is 12: eye opening = 3, verbal response = 4, motor response = 5.

103. c. The patient's score is 7: eye opening = 1, verbal response = 2, motor response = 4.

104. c. A normal total score is 14 to 15. A patient's condition would be considered serious if the score were less than 13.

COMMUNICATIONS AND DOCUMENTATION

1. Communication is vital to the performance of a prehospital provider's duties because:
   a. it is required to facilitate scene control
   b. teamwork is improved by effective communication
   c. it is required to relay accurately patient information and assessment
   d. all of the above

2. Prehospital communication typically does not occur between the:
   a. patient and the 911 dispatcher
   b. nurse and the patient
   c. paramedic in the field and the hospital
   d. on-line medical control physician and the paramedic

3. Place the phases of an EMS event in the proper order:
   a. occurrence, detection, notification and response, EMS arrival/treatment/transport, preparation for next call
   b. detection, occurrence, notification and response, EMS arrival/treatment/transport, preparation for next call
   c. occurrence, detection, EMS arrival/treatment/transport, notification and response, preparation for next call
   d. preparation for next call, detection, occurrence, EMS arrival/treatment/transport, notification and response

4. The use of _____ ensures that EMS communication is brief, accurate, unambiguous, and a common means of communications between medical professionals.
   a. 10 codes
   b. call signs
   c. proper terminology
   d. encrypted signals

5. A paramedic calls in to the hospital stating that the patient is comatose and the on-line medical control physician asks whether the patient responds to painful or verbal stimuli. This is an example of what kind of problem encountered during verbal communication in EMS?
   a. semantic
   b. technical
   c. cultural
   d. professional

6. Proper verbal communication during an EMS event promotes all of the following *EXCEPT*:
   a. exchange of patient information
   b. professionalism
   c. coordination of system resources
   d. raising the esteem of the paramedic

7. An example of a technical problem that impedes verbal communication is:
   a. using incorrect 10 codes
   b. speaking too rapidly
   c. speaking too softly
   d. radios that can't communicate on the same frequency

8. The written communication of a prehospital event is most complete in the:
   a. radio transmission log
   b. bedside report given to the receiving nurse
   c. Patient Care Report (PCR)
   d. run critique by the medical director

9. All of the following are purposes of the Patient Care Report *EXCEPT*:
   a. to prove who is at fault during an accident investigation
   b. legal documentation of care rendered to a patient
   c. billing
   d. quality improvement

10. Information contained in the Patient Care Report is:
    a. not discoverable
    b. confidential
    c. judgmental
    d. not considered part of the patient medical record

11. The medical director uses the information collected by the EMT to:
    a. perform quality improvement and develop prehospital protocols
    b. avoid lawsuits
    c. ensure proper spelling of technical terms
    d. get rid of "frequent flyers" who abuse the system

12. The use of handheld computers, voice recognition software, global positioning systems, and wireless communication devices:
    a. is far-fetched and too expensive to consider
    b. does not allow the performance of diagnostic tests in the field
    c. is an example of how technology is changing the way information is being gathered during an EMS event
    d. guarantees improved patient care

13. As with the written medical record, the most important factor to consider in implementing electronic information gathering is:
    a. deciding on the appropriate computer operating system
    b. ensuring that devices use long-lasting batteries
    c. using competitive bidding to get the best price
    d. maintaining patient confidentiality

14. Patient information gathered electronically:
    a. always results in a written record
    b. has the same legal status as a written record
    c. is less easily modified and corrected
    d. is always more accurate than a written record

15. Communication on a single frequency where only one person can speak at a time is what kind of system?
    a. simplex
    b. duplex
    c. multiplex
    d. trunked

16. For less congestion on radio frequencies, _____ systems receive a transmission and then retransmit it on a specific frequency, thereby "locking out" others from using that frequency until the service has completed its transmissions.
    a. simplex
    b. duplex
    c. multiplex
    d. trunked

17. The ability of two medics to communicate simultaneously to each other over the radio is facilitated by what kind of communication system?
    a. duplex and multiplex
    b. simplex
    c. computerized
    d. repeater

18. A _____ receives a transmission from a low-powered radio and then retransmits it at a higher power.
    a. digital encoder
    b. repeater
    c. multiplexer
    d. trunking station

19. Use of laptop computers, mobile fax machines, and GPS systems are examples of what type of technology?
    a. digital
    b. analog
    c. simplex
    d. duplex

20. One advantage of using cellular phones in prehospital communications is:
    a. secure and encrypted communication
    b. all communications are electronically recorded for later review
    c. on-line medical control physician can speak directly to the patient
    d. universal coverage regardless of geography

21. Licensing, frequency allocation, and enforcement of regulations of equipment used for radio operation are the responsibility of the:
    a. Federal Communications Commission (FCC)
    b. Office of Homeland Security (OHS)
    c. Federal Trade Commission (FTC)
    d. Food and Drug Administration (FDA)

22. Components of the dispatch communication system include all of the following *EXCEPT:*
    a. voice print recognition of callers
    b. predefined access number (911)
    c. emergency medical dispatcher
    d. prearrival instructions

23. Enhanced 911 (E911):
    a. indicates the severity of the call and communicates patient medical history
    b. allows automatic caller identification and displays phone number and address on the dispatcher's console
    c. is universally available
    d. alleviates the need for the dispatcher to ask the location of the emergency

24. The Emergency Medical Dispatcher (EMD) is:
    a. responsible only for dispatching the ambulance
    b. able to provide life-saving information through the use of prearrival instructions
    c. not required to be trained or educated
    d. not required to be CPR certified

25. Appropriate information to be gathered by the Emergency Medical Dispatcher includes all of the following *EXCEPT:*
    a. phone number and address of the caller
    b. nature of the patient's complaint
    c. whether the caller wants the paramedics or just an EMT-Basic
    d. severity of the patient's condition

26. The Emergency Medical Dispatcher is responsible for all of the following *EXCEPT:*
    a. coordination of EMS response
    b. ensuring that all radio frequencies are operational and fully licensed
    c. delivery of prearrival instructions
    d. being the first contact point in the EMS system

27. Prearrival instructions given by the Emergency Medical Dispatcher:
    a. do not include relaying information to the responding ambulance
    b. do not include providing emotional support to the caller
    c. are not required in a fully functional and quality EMS system
    d. provide immediate and potentially life-saving information

28. When providing a radio report to the receiving hospital:
    a. think before you speak, formulate the message, then relay it
    b. use 10-codes to facilitate a shorter transmission
    c. inform the hospital of the patient's name so that they can have the medical records prepared before arrival
    d. repeat each phrase or line to ensure that the listener is able to copy your transmission

29. Items to include in the radio report include all of the following *EXCEPT:*
    a. estimated time of arrival
    b. patient's age, sex, and chief complaint
    c. patient's insurance information
    d. brief history, physical exam, and treatment given

30. The purpose of the radio report is to:
    a. alert the hospital of your impending arrival and convey relevant patient information
    b. document the care rendered to the patient
    c. avoid the need to provide a bedside report
    d. reassure the patient that he or she is being well cared for

31. Put the following components of the prehospital radio report in their proper order (1-6).
    ____ patient complaint
    ____ estimated time of arrival
    ____ patient age and sex
    ____ unit identification
    ____ pertinent history and physical findings
    ____ treatment given so far

32. After receiving instructions from the on-line medical control:
    a. request confirmation that the orders are actually in your protocol manual
    b. immediately perform them
    c. perform them only if the transmission is recorded
    d. use the "echo" procedure by repeating back what was heard and confirming receipt of the message

33. The primary reason for writing a legible, accurate, and complete Patient Care Report is:
   a. it demonstrates professionalism and is the primary means by which a prehospital provider can document the quality of care
   b. policy and protocols dictate that a PCR must be completed prior to the end of the shift
   c. the state EMS oversight agency requires it
   d. the hospital requires it for the medical record

34. You care for a 56-year-old man complaining of chest pain. Documenting the absence of nausea, diaphoresis, and shortness of breath is an example of:
   a. making sure that the patient doesn't need oxygen
   b. listing pertinent negatives
   c. performing a thorough exam
   d. following state-mandated protocol

35. The most appropriate means to document a patient's important statements is to:
   a. make a tape recording of the patient's statement
   b. place the statement within quotation marks
   c. have the patient review and sign the Patient Care Report
   d. paraphrase his or her statements using appropriate medical terminology

36. All of the following are components to a professionally written report *EXCEPT:*
   a. correct spelling
   b. accepted terminology and abbreviations
   c. judgments as to who was at fault in a motor vehicle crash.
   d. legible handwriting

37. Which of the following is an example of an inappropriate and judgmental statement that should not be included in a Patient Care Report?
   a. The patient was drunk when he fell off the bar stool.
   b. The patient stated that he had consumed two beers before our arrival.
   c. The patient stated, "I ran the red light and hit the truck."
   d. The patient's speech was slurred.

38. Patient Care Reports should be completed:
   a. before the billing report is completed
   b. once you have enough time to complete it uninterrupted
   c. after the emergency physician has made the diagnosis and informed you of the patient's final disposition
   d. as soon as possible after the patient interaction

39. Each of the following is an acceptable way to make a correction to a Patient Care Record *EXCEPT:*
   a. mark a line through the entry
   b. complete a supplementary report indicating the need for the correction
   c. ensure the person making the correction is the same person who wrote the initial report
   d. use a black marker to obscure the previous entry

40. When documenting a patient's refusal of care you must include:
   a. your advice to the patient regarding the benefits of treatment and the risks of refusal
   b. the advice rendered by on-line medical control
   c. the signature of reliable witnesses to the event
   d. all of the above

41. Which of the following is not considered a system for writing the narrative component of the Patient Care Report?
   a. SOAP
   b. START
   c. head to toe
   d. chronological

42. The difference between subjective and objective information is:
   a. subjective refers to statements and opinions while objective information comes from observation and measurement
   b. subjective information is more accurate than objective information
   c. subjective information is always in quotes
   d. objective information comes from conclusions as to the cause of the event

43. Documentation during mass casualty situations:
   a. is completed by the receiving hospital
   b. needs to be completed only on patients requiring advanced life support
   c. must wait until all victims have been triaged and transported
   d. cannot be performed while en route to the hospital

44. You are transporting three "walking wounded" or "green" victims with minor injuries from a disaster site. Your radio report should:
   a. consist of all the usual elements of patient information, findings, and interventions
   b. be kept short and precise so as to relieve congestion on the frequency
   c. not be given because they are probably already expecting you
   d. none of the above

45. You are transporting a young boy with an allergic reaction. The on-line medical control physician orders you to administer 100 mg of diphenhydramine while your protocols allow you to administer only 25 mg. You should:
   a. repeat the order to the physician and confirm his order
   b. indicate to the physician that the order is not contained in your protocols and not perform the order
   c. wait until you arrive at the hospital to address the issue with the physician
   d. all of the above

ANSWERS TO CHAPTER 5: COMMUNICATIONS AND DOCUMENTATION

1. **d.** The ability to effectively communicate is a critical component of a prehospital professional. The ability to assume leadership of a scene and coordinate the activities of your team is dependent on your understanding of how to relay information.

2. **b.** Vital information must be communicated between all phases of the EMS response. The dispatcher must be able to convey the seriousness of the patient's condition to the medic. To obtain appropriate orders and prepare the hospital to care for the patient, the medic must effectively communicate the patient's physical findings and medical impression.

3. **a.** The event occurs, it is detected by either the patient or bystander, EMS is notified by 911, and the response occurs. EMS arrives, treats the patient, and transports to the hospital. Finally, the crew prepares for the next call.

4. **c.** Communication in EMS occurs between several agencies and people. The use of proper terminology is vital to ensure effective communication. Proper terminology includes the use of appropriate medical terms and plain English to convey information.

5. **a.** It is vital to use terms that are understood equally when communicating. Semantics refers to how the same word can mean more than one thing depending on its use. *Comatose* is not a standard term for level of consciousness, whereas *AVPU* is.

6. **d.** The primary purpose of communication is to benefit the patient and facilitate the best care possible. Attempting to look knowledgeable by using big words and complicated terminology does not benefit the patient.

7. **d.** Technical difficulties in EMS communication occur when any of the various electronic equipment used does not operate properly. This includes the 911 system, dispatch equipment, and radios.

8. **c.** Although the EMT may write notes in the field and give these to the receiving staff, the formal written communication of what occurred to the patient and the care rendered is contained in the Patient Care Report, sometimes referred to as the *run sheet*.

9. **a.** The Patient Care Report should be objective and nonjudgmental. It becomes a legal part of the patient's medical record, is used to justify billing charges, and is critical for the effective performance of quality assurance.

10. **b.** It is vital to recognize that the Patient Care Report is confidential and cannot be released without permission from the patient. It is part of the patient's medical record and should not contain judgmental language or comments. The fact that it can be obtained by a subpoena means that it is discoverable in a legal action.

11. **a.** The Patient Care Record contains vital information to perform quality improvement, such as skills that were performed and whether proper care was provided. The medical director uses this information to monitor the paramedic and develop protocols for care. The other listed uses are not considered proper uses of this confidential information.

12. **c.** As technology advances, it changes the way information can be obtained, stored, and conveyed. With ongoing development and broad acceptance, technology becomes more affordable. If used properly, advanced technology improves patient care.

13. **d.** As technology makes information gathering easier it also increases the potential for breaches of confidentiality to occur. It is the legal responsibility of the service to ensure appropriate protection of this information regardless of how it is gathered, stored, or conveyed by and between agencies.

14. **b.** The accuracy of an electronic patient record depends on the person entering it and may contain errors if not examined closely, but with the use of technology may be easily corrected. The information contained holds equal legal status to the written report. Although it may be printed out, it may not have to be accompanied by a written record, depending on your local protocols.

15. **a.** The simplex system allows only one person to speak at a time.

16. d. If the same frequency is used simultaneously by two transmissions, one or both of the transmissions may be blocked by interference. This leads to confusion as to who is talking to whom. The trunked system closes the frequency from use by more than one service.

17. a. The duplex system is similar to a telephone, where two transmissions can occur simultaneously and both be heard by each radio.

18. b. A repeater allows the paramedic to use a low-powered handheld radio at the patient bedside to consult with medical control. Repeaters work by receiving a lower-power radio signal and rebroadcasting it at a higher power so that the signal may reach a distant receiver such as a hospital base station.

19. a. Digital technology refers to the use of binary computer language to transmit information rather than modulating radio waves, which are used in analog systems.

20. c. Although the use of cellular phones does allow you to more privately speak to on-line medical control, you must remember that it is not secure from being overheard by certain types of scanners. The ability to have a physician speak directly to a patient can help alleviate issues such as treat and release and against medical advice departures. Unfortunately, the communication might not be recorded, and therefore it is vital that you document accurately the content of your communication in your written record.

21. a. The Federal Communication Commission is responsible for these activities.

22. a. The dispatch communication system must have a clearly recognized and predefined number to make access easy for the caller. The emergency medical dispatcher is trained to interview the caller to determine the severity of the emergency, dispatch the appropriate level of response, and provide important and sometimes lifesaving instructions to the caller before the arrival of EMS. As yet, voice print recognition is merely fantasy.

23. b. Enhanced 911 automatically displays the caller identification on the dispatcher's console. However, the site of the emergency may not be at the location of the caller, and the dispatcher must still verify this as well as ask questions to determine the severity of the emergency.

24. b. The professional Emergency Medical Dispatcher (EMD) has completed a formal course of study and is certified and sometimes licensed. The EMD's responsibilities far exceed that of merely dispatching the ambulance and include providing vital instructions to the caller. Therefore EMDs must be CPR certified to enable them to provide appropriate instructions over the phone.

25. c. The level of EMS response to be dispatched is determined by the answer to a set of predefined questions according to the nature of the patient's complaint. Regardless of whether E911 is used, the location of the caller and the emergency must be verified in the event of technical difficulties.

26. b. The administration of the communication center is responsible for radio frequency maintenance and licensure. The other listed items are critical responsibilities of the professional emergency medical dispatcher.

27. d. The professional emergency medical dispatcher is trained to provide instructions in CPR, bleeding control, childbirth, and the relief of choking. Dispatchers are also trained to calm and reassure the victim or caller while EMS is en route. The role of the emergency medical dispatcher is critical to the quality of any EMS system.

28. a. Regardless of the severity of the situation it is vital that you remain calm while transmitting your report. The receiving hospital must obtain a clear understanding of the patient's condition and your requests. To facilitate this take a few seconds before transmitting to formulate your message. The use of 10 codes does not improve the efficiency of the transmission and the use of the patient's name may breach confidentiality. If you speak clearly and calmly there is no need to repeat your statements unless asked to by the hospital.

29. c. Insurance information has no bearing on the care rendered and should not be part of your report. Your goal is to convey a picture of the patient and their condition. To do this you must include age, sex, chief complaint, a brief history, and pertinent physical findings, as well as any treatment you have given and the response to that treatment. Generally, you should start and end your report with your ETA.

30. a. The most important information you can give the receiving hospital is the severity of the patient's condition and your estimated time of arrival. This helps them to prepare for your patient's needs. You will still need to provide a more comprehensive report at the bedside when handing off the patient to the emergency department staff.

31. Put the following components of the prehospital radio report in their proper order (1-6).

  _3_ Patient complaint

  _6_ Estimated time of arrival

  _2_ Patient age and sex

  _1_ Unit identification

  _4_ Pertinent history and physical findings

  _5_ Treatment given so far

32. d. By repeating any on-line medical control orders, both you and the medical control physician will be sure that the orders were received and understood. Only request confirmation of orders if you believe they are not part of your standard protocols. Perform them only once you have made sure they are correct and appropriate.

33. a. The written report is usually the only legal record of the care you rendered and is best defended against critique if it is written legibly and accurately. You must include all care rendered and assessments performed. If it is not written, it did not happen.

34. b. The absence of particular signs and symptoms is as important as their presence, and documenting them justifies your treatment and diagnostic impression.

35. b. By quoting patients you are documenting statements in their own words rather than making a judgment as to what they are saying. For example, it is better to state, "I was beat up" rather than, "The patient was beaten." Accurate quotation of the patient's statements reduces your liability.

36. c. The professionally written patient record is nonjudgmental and is easy to read and understand. It should be written with this thought in

mind: "Could I present this in a court of law 10 years from now?"

37. a. Any use of slang or judgmental language will taint the record and appear biased and will place you at risk of being accused of altering your care based on personal beliefs rather than professional assessment. The use of quotations further insulates you from liability and increases the accuracy of your report.

38. d. The sooner the report is completed the more accurate it will be. After several calls the facts of the event can become blurred. Waiting until you have learned the patient's diagnosis will taint your perception of the event and lead you to depict your report in an unfair manner. You must report only what you know, saw, and did.

39. d. It must be very apparent that any correction to the Patient Care Report occurred and the original mistake must be visible. Corrections should be made only by the person who completed the record and dated and signed. If substantial corrections are needed, the use of a supplementary report is advised rather than crossing out large sections of the report.

40. d. It is vital that you document the patient's competence to make a decision to refuse care. This includes what assessments you made about whether the patient understood the risks associated with the refusal and whether there was an absence of mental impairment from drugs or alcohol. All of these actions should be witnessed by a reliable individual, and, if possible, medical control should be consulted.

41. b. START is the system of disaster triage. The SOAP format consists of the Subjective, what the patient was complaining of and the history of present illness; Objective, what you observed and assessed; Assessment, your diagnostic impression; Plan, your list of interventions. The head-to-toe narrative lists complaints and assessments of each major organ system and is completed with your impression and plan. The chronological narrative records things in the order in which they occurred. The complete EMS narrative often uses a combination of all three methods.

42. a. Subjective information consists of patient statements and answers to your questions as well as their pertinent medical history. Because it cannot be verified it may be less than accurate. Objective information contains elements that you can verify, such as blood pressure and physical findings. Although some of the subjective information is contained in the patient's quoted statements, items such as medical history are not.

43. c. During a disaster, minimal documentation is required to triage each victim into immediate, delayed, and nontransport categories. Full documentation must be completed to the extent possible after the victims are cared for.

44. c. During a mass casualty incident the transportation officer would be responsible for notifying the receiving hospital of the incoming patients. During disasters, radio communication frequencies easily become congested and should not be used to relay nonemergent information.

45. d. You should never perform an intervention or administer a medication outside your accepted scope of practice. Any disagreement with on-line medical control should be handled off the air and in person in a professional manner. You should record accurately in your written record the receipt of the order and your refusal to carry it out.

TRAUMA I: HEMORRHAGE AND SHOCK

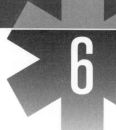

6

1. When managing a patient with severe external blood loss:
   a. control the bleeding before donning gloves
   b. only gloves and eye protection are needed
   c. determine whether the patient has a communicable disease before donning personal protective equipment
   d. use gloves, eye protection, gown, and mask when possible

2. A serious amount of sudden blood loss in an adult is:
   a. 1 unit
   b. 500 cc
   c. 1 L
   d. 2 cups

3. Venous bleeding is best described as:
   a. a slow flow of bright red blood
   b. oozing of blood from a wound
   c. a steady flow of dark-red blood
   d. difficult to control with direct pressure

4. Bleeding from the artery of a normovolemic, oxygenated patient:
   a. is bright-red and spurts with each heartbeat
   b. is not life-threatening
   c. can be easily controlled by direct pressure
   d. can be controlled only with a tourniquet

5. Capillary bleeding is:
   a. associated with long clotting times
   b. slow, oozing, and is dark red
   c. bright red and steady
   d. normally controlled by use of pressure points

6. After personal protective equipment is donned, the first step to control bleeding is:
   a. applying direct pressure
   b. placing the patient in shock position
   c. applying digital pressure to an artery
   d. applying a cold pack

7. All of the following may be used to provide pressure to control bleeding *EXCEPT*:
   a. a gauze bandage
   b. the hand
   c. an air splint
   d. a narrow cravat

8. Along with using direct pressure to control bleeding from an extremity:
   a. immerse the extremity in cold water
   b. lower the extremity
   c. apply ice to the area of the wound
   d. elevate the extremity

9. The pressure point of choice for controlling bleeding from a proximal forearm injury is the:
   a. radial artery
   b. popliteal artery
   c. brachial artery
   d. tibial artery

10. A 26-year-old tree service worker has cut his thigh with a chain saw. There is uncontrolled bleeding from the injury despite the application of direct pressure. The pressure point of choice in this situation is the:
    a. posterior tibial artery
    b. popliteal artery
    c. dorsalis pedis artery
    d. femoral artery

11. A tourniquet should be used:
    a. on all crush injuries involving an extremity
    b. only as a last resort
    c. when direct pressure alone will not control bleeding
    d. whenever an amputation is encountered

12. When a bandage is used as a tourniquet, it should be:
    a. wrapped around an extremity twice
    b. loosened every 20 minutes to resupply the area below with blood
    c. between 1 and 2 inches wide
    d. applied as far from the wound as possible

13. Tighten a tourniquet:
    a. just enough to occlude venous blood flow
    b. enough to occlude arterial blood flow
    c. as much as possible
    d. until pain below the wound is relieved

14. After applying a tourniquet:
    a. document its use and the time it was applied on the EMS report
    b. cover the wound and tourniquet with sterile dressings and bandages
    c. lower the extremity below the level of the heart
    d. apply digital pressure to the appropriate pressure point

15. A potential problem with using a blood pressure cuff as a tourniquet is:
    a. it is not wide enough
    b. it cannot occlude arterial blood flow
    c. there is a greater likelihood of damaging underlying structures
    d. pressure in the cuff gradually may be lost

16. The three primary components of the cardiovascular system are:
    a. blood, heart, and blood vessels
    b. red blood cells, white blood cells, and platelets
    c. water, glucose, and plasma
    d. oxygen, blood, and carbon dioxide

17. Shock is best defined as:
    a. low blood pressure
    b. inadequate tissue perfusion
    c. the body's response to any blood loss
    d. rapid pulse rate associated with dilation of blood vessels

18. The three principal stages of shock, in the proper order, are:
    a. initial, medial, endstage
    b. reversible, irreversible, terminal
    c. compensated, decompensated, irreversible
    d. hypovolemic, compensatory, final

19. Lack of tissue perfusion will eventually lead to:
    a. aerobic metabolism
    b. oxymetabolism
    c. anaerobic metabolism
    d. arteriosclerotic metabolism

20. Most of the water in the body can be found in the form of:
    a. intracellular fluid
    b. extracellular fluid
    c. intravascular fluid
    d. interstitial fluid

21. The extracellular fluid between the cells and outside the vascular bed is:
    a. intravascular fluid
    b. interstitial fluid
    c. intracellular fluid
    d. plasma

22. By-products of anaerobic metabolism include:
    a. glucose and glycogen
    b. pyruvic and lactic acid
    c. epinephrine and norepinephrine
    d. glucagons and insulin

23. An early sign of shock is:
    a. low blood pressure
    b. red, dry skin
    c. rapid heart rate
    d. lethargy

24. Of the various types of shock, the one least likely to present with an increased pulse, sweating, and pallor is:
    a. hypovolemic shock
    b. septic shock
    c. cardiogenic shock
    d. neurogenic shock

25. The types of shock that are associated with systemwide vasodilation are:
    a. cardiogenic, anaphylactic, hypovolemic
    b. neurogenic, septic, hypovolemic
    c. septic, anaphylactic, neurogenic
    d. hypovolemic, cardiogenic, neurogenic

26. The type of shock associated with loss of blood or fluid volume from the body caused by hemorrhage or secondary to dehydration is:
    a. septic
    b. hypernatremic
    c. cardiovascular
    d. hypovolemic

27. The type of shock associated with simple fainting is:
    a. hypotonic
    b. neurogenic
    c. cardiogenic
    d. oligemic

28. A patient who experiences a severe allergic reaction may have:
   a. cardiogenic shock
   b. hypovolemic shock
   c. septic shock
   d. anaphylactic shock

29. In cardiogenic shock, the primary cause of decreased cardiac output is:
   a. vasoconstriction
   b. pump failure
   c. fluid loss
   d. rapid heart rate

30. A patient experiencing neurogenic shock experiences relative hypovolemia as a result of:
   a. antigen release
   b. a severe infection
   c. vasodilation
   d. weakening of the heart muscle

31. Of the patients listed below, the one who is most likely to develop septic shock is a patient with a:
   a. gunshot wound to the abdomen
   b. recent bee sting
   c. history of serious heart problems
   d. urinary tract infection

32. When administering fluids to a patient with an uncontrollable hemorrhage and shock, the goal is to:
   a. administer enough fluid to normalize vital signs
   b. withhold fluids totally to avoid potential for pulmonary edema
   c. administer fluids rapidly to achieve a 3:1 replacement ratio of fluid infused to blood lost
   d. titrate fluids until the patient shows signs of clinical improvement

33. Stagnant capillary blood flow results in:
   a. reduced carbon dioxide levels and improved aerobic metabolism
   b. increased venous return and capillary constriction
   c. reduced delivery of oxygen and increased anaerobic metabolism
   d. hypocoagulability and improved removal of cellular metabolites

34. During the capillary washout phase as it relates to hemorrhagic shock:
   a. cardiac output increases slightly
   b. metabolic acidosis results
   c. perfusion improves as clogged capillaries are cleared
   d. postcapillary sphincters tighten causing blockages

35. Pulse pressure:
   a. is the difference between the patient's systolic blood pressure and pulse
   b. is of less importance when evaluating the shock patient than systolic pressure
   c. reflects the tone of the arterial system
   d. is unaffected by peripheral vascular resistance

36. To check for orthostatic vital sign changes:
   a. have the patient lie flat and check the vital signs 1 minute later
   b. have the patient rise from a recumbent position to a standing position and immediately check vital signs before compensation can occur
   c. have the patient stand for 1 minute, then place the patient in a sitting position and check vital signs 1 minute thereafter
   d. have the patient rise from a recumbent position to a sitting or standing position and check vital signs 1 minute later

37. A patient would be considered to have positive orthostatic vital sign changes if he or she displayed a:
   a. rise in blood pressure of 10 to 15 mm Hg and/or a concurrent rise in pulse rate of 15 to 20 beats per minute
   b. fall in blood pressure of 10 to 15 mm Hg and/or a concurrent rise in pulse rate of 10 to 15 beats per minute
   c. fall in blood pressure of 5 to 10 mm Hg and/or a concurrent fall in pulse rate of 10 to 15 beats per minute
   d. rise in blood pressure of 15 to 20 mm Hg and/or a concurrent fall in pulse rate of 15 to 20 beats per minute

38. Positive orthostatic vital sign changes indicate the patient:
    a. is going into irreversible shock
    b. has significant internal bleeding
    c. has a significant volume depletion of at least 10%
    d. is experiencing widespread vasodilation

39. In compensated shock, the body:
    a. reduces venous capacitance in response to blood loss
    b. is hemodynamically unstable and shows pronounced symptoms of shock
    c. can no longer maintain preload
    d. is incapable of meeting its metabolic needs

40. When assessing a patient in compensated shock, the EMS provider would expect to see:
    a. normal or slightly elevated blood pressure
    b. severe tachycardia
    c. decreased respiratory rate
    d. flushed skin

41. A patient in decompensated shock would be expected to display:
    a. a widening pulse pressure
    b. an increase in cerebral perfusion due to blood shunting
    c. decreased systolic and diastolic pressure
    d. decreased pulse rate

42. Your patient has lost a significant amount of blood because of a severe leg laceration. His blood pressure is 80/62. This blood pressure would be classified as:
    a. normotensive
    b. hypotensive
    c. hypertensive
    d. profoundly hypotensive

43. Of the following patients, the one that would most likely receive and benefit from aggressive fluid therapy is:
    a. an 18-year-old male with multiple gunshot wounds to the chest
    b. a 22-year-old male with multiple stab wounds to the abdomen and whose bleeding appears to be controlled
    c. a 35-year-old male with a large laceration to the thigh caused by a chain saw and whose bleeding is controlled
    d. a 63-year-old female who has been throwing up coffee ground emesis for 3 days and is now also passing bright red blood from the rectum

44. The mechanisms by which it is thought that the pneumatic antishock garment (PASG) helps to manage shock include all of the following *EXCEPT*:
    a. increasing peripheral vascular resistance in the tissues beneath the PASG
    b. arresting hemorrhage by tamponading bleeding vessels in the lower extremities and pelvis
    c. stabilizing pelvic and lower extremity fractures thereby decreasing movement and subsequent blood loss
    d. providing a substantial autotransfusion of blood from the extremities to the body core

45. If signs of shock are present, use of the pneumatic antishock garment (PASG) would be indicated in the event of:
    a. an open wound to the chest with severe external bleeding
    b. a pelvic injury with signs of abdominal bleeding
    c. blunt trauma to the chest with signs of internal bleeding
    d. an isolated open head injury accompanied by severe external bleeding

46. An absolute contraindication for the use of PASG is:
    a. first trimester of pregnancy
    b. pulmonary edema
    c. abdominal evisceration
    d. a knife imbedded in the abdomen

47. When properly placed, the top of the PASG should lie:
    a. below the last pair of ribs
    b. at the nipple line
    c. at the level of the umbilicus
    d. at the level of the sixth rib

48. When applying the PASG, inflate it until the:
    a. patient states he or she feels better
    b. patient's blood pressure reaches 120 systolic
    c. Velcro starts to crackle
    d. pressure gauges reach 90 mm Hg

49. Deflation of the PASG should be accomplished:
    a. in the field after IVs are started
    b. by first deflating the legs, then the abdomen
    c. slowly, stopping deflation after each blood pressure drop of 10 to 15 mm Hg to stabilize the patient with fluids
    d. only by trained personnel in a clinical setting

50. Your patient is a 76-year-old female who is in a nursing home. Upon your arrival, you notice she is semiconscious. Her pulse is 120, her respirations are rapid, and her blood pressure is 88/60. She is slightly warm to the touch. There are no signs of internal bleeding. According to the staff, her only history is that of a recent urinary tract infection. You suspect her low blood pressure to be related to:
    a. hypovolemic shock
    b. septic shock
    c. cardiogenic shock
    d. neurogenic shock

ANSWERS TO CHAPTER 6: TRAUMA I: HEMORRHAGE AND SHOCK

1. d. When managing a patient with obvious external blood loss, wear appropriate personal protective equipment as dictated by the circumstances. For example, if minimal bleeding without the risk of splash is encountered, gloves may be all that are needed. However, in the event of severe bleeding, the risk of splashing or spurting is much greater, and eye protection, gown, and mask should be used. Use of personal protective equipment should never be based on the patient's admission of having a communicable disease. All patients must be assumed to pose a risk to the caregiver.

2. c. The loss of 1 L of blood in an adult patient can cause hypovolemic shock. In children, a loss of 500 cc of blood is serious, as is a loss of 100 to 200 cc of blood in infants.

3. c. Venous bleeding can be recognized as dark-red blood that flows steadily. This type of bleeding often is controlled easily with direct pressure.

4. a. Arterial bleeding from a patient who is normovolemic and well oxygenated is usually bright red, and the blood spurts with each heartbeat. This type of bleeding may not be controlled easily and can be rapidly fatal. If the patient is hypoxic, the blood may be darker in color. If the patient is hypovolemic and hypotensive, the spurting may not be as pronounced.

5. b. Bleeding from the capillaries is characterized by a slow, oozing flow of dark-red blood. Pressure points are not used to control capillary bleeding.

6. a. Application of direct pressure is the first step in bleeding control. The pressure may be concentrated (such as when a fingertip is used to press on the bleeding point) or diffuse (such as when pressure is applied over a larger area of injury). Diffuse pressure occludes the arteries and veins that supply blood to the injured area.

7. d. A gauze bandage, the hand, or an air splint may all be used to apply direct pressure to a wound. A narrow cravat should not be used because it acts like a tourniquet and applies too much pressure to a narrow area and may impair circulation or damage underlying blood vessels and nerves.

8. d. Elevation of an extremity above the level of the heart may supplement direct pressure for bleeding control. Ice should never be placed directly on a wound.

9. c. The brachial artery, located in the upper arm, is the pressure point of choice for controlling bleeding from a forearm injury.

10. d. The femoral artery, located in the groin, is the best pressure point to use to control bleeding from a leg injury.

11. b. Tourniquets should be used *only* as a last resort, after trying all other bleeding control techniques. They are not automatically necessary in cases of amputation or crush injury.

12. a. When a bandage is used as a tourniquet, it should be wrapped twice around an extremity before being tightened. It should be 4 inches wide and 6 to 8 layers deep. The tourniquet is applied proximal to the wound, but as distal on the extremity as possible. It should never be loosened once it is applied, because this may flood the body with acidotic blood.

13. b. Tourniquets must be applied tight enough to occlude arterial blood flow. If only venous blood flow is occluded, bleeding may become worse because the bleeding site is still supplied with blood, but return of venous blood is restricted.

14. a. After applying a tourniquet, document its use and the time it was applied on the EMS report. Some sources advocate writing the letters *TK* and the time the tourniquet was applied on the patient's forehead.

15. d. Blood pressure cuffs may gradually lose pressure. They are wide enough to be used as tourniquets; however, if used as such they must be constantly monitored for pressure loss. Hemostats may be used to clamp the cuff tubes, potentially reducing pressure loss.

16. a. Blood, the heart, and blood vessels are the three primary components of the cardiovascular system.

17. b. Shock can be defined as an abnormal condition of inadequate blood flow to the body's peripheral tissues. It is associated with life-threatening cellular dysfunction.

18. c. The three principal stages of shock are compensated, decompensated (or uncompensated), and irreversible.

19. c. Lack of tissue perfusion will eventually lead to anaerobic metabolism, that is, metabolism that occurs in the absence of oxygen.

20. a. Most of the water in the body can be found in the form of intracellular fluid, fluid within the cell membranes throughout most of the body. Intracellular fluid accounts for 40% of body weight.

21. b. Interstitial fluid is the extracellular fluid between the cells and outside the vascular bed. It accounts for 15% to 16% of body weight and also includes special fluids such as cerebrospinal fluid and intraocular fluid.

22. b. Anaerobic metabolism produces pyruvic acid, which is converted to lactic acid. The buildup of lactic acid and other by-products of anaerobic metabolism creates a cellular and interstitial acidosis. Without the return of oxygen and the subsequent removal of lactic acid and other toxins, the cells will soon die.

23. c. A rapid heart rate is an early sign of shock. The heart rate increases in an attempt to maintain cardiac output. Low blood pressure will come at a much later time.

24. d. Neurogenic shock is the type of shock least likely to present with increased pulse, sweating, and pallor because there is a loss of the sympathetic impulses, which usually produce the tachycardia, diaphoresis, and pallor.

25. c. Septic, anaphylactic, and neurogenic shock are associated with systemwide vasodilation as the cause of hypotension rather than a frank loss of blood or other fluids. This vasodilation causes a relative hypovolemia.

26. d. Hypovolemic shock is associated with loss of blood or fluid volume from the body caused by hemorrhage or secondary to dehydration.

27. b. Simple fainting is a mild, readily reversible neurogenic shock that can occur in the absence of injury.

28. d. A patient who experiences a severe allergic reaction may develop anaphylactic shock, a type of distributive shock.

29. b. Failure of the heart to pump properly, or pump failure, is the primary cause of decreased cardiac output in a patient experiencing cardiogenic shock.

30. c. The relative hypovolemia experienced by a patient in neurogenic shock is the result of widespread vasodilation.

31. d. Septic shock is related to infection. It is thought to be mediated through toxins that either are a part of the microorganism or are released by the organism. These toxins stimulate the release of complex vasoactive agents that compromise the vascular system's ability to control blood vessels and distribute blood.

32. d. When hemorrhage cannot be controlled, such as in cases of internal bleeding caused by trauma, it is best to be cautious with fluid administration. The goal is to stabilize the patient's condition until the patient reaches a trauma center, not to return vital signs to normal. Increasing the blood pressure can have negative effects because it can dislodge clots that are forming and disrupt the normal clotting process.

33. c. Stagnant capillary blood flow results in reduced delivery of oxygen and increased anaerobic metabolism. Perfusion is affected, thereby preventing the removal of cellular metabolites. The effect on the body's clotting mechanisms is hypercoagulability.

34. b. During the capillary washout phase, postcapillary sphincters relax. Cells swell and die and metabolic acidosis results. Additionally, cardiac output drops further.

35. c. Pulse pressure reflects the tone of the arterial system. It is calculated by subtracting the patient's diastolic blood pressure from the systolic blood pressure. It is more sensitive to changes in perfusion than the systolic or diastolic pressure alone. Pulse pressure changes significantly as a result of peripheral vascular resistance.

36. d. To check for orthostatic vital sign changes, have the patient rise from a recumbent position to a sitting or standing position, or from a sitting position to a standing position, and then check vital signs 1 minute later.

37. b. A patient would be considered to have positive orthostatic vital sign changes if he or she displayed a fall in blood pressure of 10 to 15 mm Hg and/or a concurrent rise in pulse rate of 10 to 15 beats per minute.

38. c. Positive orthostatic vital sign changes (postural hypotension) indicate the patient has a significant volume depletion of at least 10% and therefore a decrease in perfusion status.

39. a. Compensated shock is the initial shock state. In this stage, the body reduces venous capacitance by initial vasoconstriction in response to blood loss. Through this and other actions, the body is still capable of meeting its metabolic needs.

40. a. In compensated shock, the body's compensatory responses are sufficient to overcome the decrease in available fluid. Blood pressure is maintained as a result of the compensatory mechanism. Mild tachycardia, increased respiratory rate, and pale skin also would be expected.

41. c. A patient in decompensated shock would be expected to display decreased systolic and diastolic pressure. The pulse pressure is likely to narrow as systolic pressure drops to a greater degree than diastolic pressure. The pulse rate increases, and cerebral perfusion decreases, leading to altered mental status.

42. b. This patient would be considered to be hypotensive. Blood pressure is classified as normotensive if it is normal, hypotensive if the systolic is between 70 and 100 mm Hg, and profoundly hypotensive if it is less than 70 mm Hg.

43. c. If external bleeding can be controlled and there is no reason to suspect serious internal hemorrhage, aggressive fluid resuscitation may be used. If uncontrollable internal bleeding is suspected, fluids should be administered with caution. Always consult local protocols regarding fluid resuscitation guidelines.

44. d. The mechanisms by which it is thought that the pneumatic antishock garment (PASG) helps to manage shock include increasing peripheral vascular resistance in the tissues beneath the PASG, arresting hemorrhage by tamponading bleeding vessels in the lower extremities and pelvis, and stabilizing pelvic and lower extremity fractures, thereby decreasing movement and subsequent blood loss. The PASG does not provide a substantial autotransfusion of blood from the extremities to the body core. Research indicates that only about 250 mL of blood is returned to central circulation.

45. b. A pelvic injury with signs of abdominal bleeding is an indication for the use of the PASG. The PASG should not be used if the patient has chest injuries or an isolated head injury.

46. b. PASG should not be applied if chest auscultation reveals pulmonary edema. Depending on local protocol, PASG may be used even in cases of evisceration or impaled objects in the abdomen. In such cases the abdominal compartment is not inflated.

47. a. The top of the PASG should lie below the last pair of ribs to prevent compression of the thoracic cavity.

48. c. The PASG should be inflated until the Velcro starts to crackle or the pop-off valves release. Gauges tend to be inaccurate and are not often used. If gauges are used, a pressure of 60 mm Hg is recommended. Always follow your local protocols.

49. d. Deflation of the PASG should not be done in the field. It should be accomplished by trained personnel in a clinical setting. Generally, deflations should be stopped after each 5 mm Hg drop in the patient's blood pressure. EMS personnel should be familiar with deflation procedures in the event that instruction needs to be given to hospital personnel who are less familiar with the device. Always follow your local protocols for deflation.

50. b. This patient is most likely in septic shock. Good clues are that the patient has a history of a recent urinary tract infection and that she still may have the infection, as evidenced by the possible fever. Not all patients in septic shock will be febrile, however.

Trauma II: Soft Tissue Trauma and Burns

1. Two main functions of the skin are:
   a. blood cell production and waste disposal
   b. temperature regulation and fluid absorption
   c. protection and temperature regulation
   d. waste disposal and fluid absorption

2. The outermost layer of the skin is known as the:
   a. epidermis
   b. dermis
   c. subcutaneous tissue
   d. hyperdermis

3. The sweat glands and hair follicles are contained in the:
   a. dermis
   b. subcutaneous tissue
   c. pleura
   d. epidermis

4. Directly beneath the dermis lies the:
   a. bone
   b. subcutaneous layer
   c. meninges
   d. subfascia layer

5. Sebacious glands secrete:
   a. acids
   b. sweat
   c. saliva
   d. oils

6. The body's natural ability to stop bleeding, the ability to clot blood, is known as:
   a. platelet aggregation
   b. hemostasis
   c. vasoconstriction
   d. collagen synthesis

7. The three basic steps of the clotting mechanism include all the following *EXCEPT*:
   a. release of platelet factors
   b. formation of thrombin
   c. conversion of fibrinogen into prothrombin
   d. trapping of red blood cells in fibrin to form a clot

8. An example of a closed soft-tissue injury would be:
   a. an incision
   b. a hematoma
   c. a compound fracture
   d. an abrasion

9. When bruising is noted over the area of a vital organ:
   a. a superficial injury should be suspected
   b. direct pressure should be applied to the area
   c. damage to the underlying organ and internal bleeding should be suspected
   d. it is of concern only if it is noted on the abdomen and not the chest

10. Another term for a bruise is:
   a. abrasion
   b. urticaria
   c. hematocrit
   d. contusion

11. A lump at a wound site caused by blood collecting within damaged tissue is a:
   a. hematoma
   b. varicose vein
   c. fistula
   d. melanoma

12. Match the following types of open soft-tissue injuries with their descriptions: abrasion, amputation, avulsion, laceration, puncture.

_____ A break in the skin caused by forceful impact with a sharp object. The wound edges may be regular (linear) or irregular (stellate).

_____ Caused by a simple scraping or scratching of the outer layer of the skin. Examples include "rug-burns" or "friction-burns."

_____ A portion of tissue or skin that is torn loose and left hanging as a flap or is completely pulled from the body

_____ A small opening or perforation of the skin typically caused by pointed sharp objects

_____ The removal of an appendage (such as an arm) from the body

13. A consideration when managing abrasions is that:
a. bleeding may be severe
b. they may become contaminated by foreign matter
c. pain is usually minimal
d. sterile dressings are not needed because the wound is not deep

14. Bleeding from a laceration:
a. is always easy to control
b. usually cannot be controlled using direct pressure
c. may be severe and difficult to control
d. is primarily from the capillaries

15. A gunshot wound with no exit is classified as a:
a. laceration
b. puncture wound
c. perforating wound
d. sterile wound

16. One of the goals of managing open wounds is to:
a. thoroughly clean the wound before dressing it
b. remove any clots that have formed prior to the arrival of EMS
c. immediately apply a bandage
d. prevent further contamination of the wound

17. A dressing should do all of the following _EXCEPT_:
a. hold a bandage in place
b. help control bleeding
c. prevent further contamination and infection
d. protect the wound from further injury or damage

18. When bandaging an extremity:
a. place knots over the wound
b. cover all fingertips and toes to prevent further injury
c. secure any loose bandage ends
d. wrap the bandage tightly enough to occlude venous flow

19. When managing an impaled object:
a. control bleeding by applying pressure on the object
b. stabilize the object with a bulky dressing
c. remove the object and apply direct pressure to the wound to control bleeding
d. never remove the object

20. Examine the patient for an exit wound whenever:
a. a penetration/puncture injury is encountered
b. an avulsion has occurred
c. a partial amputation has occurred
d. a stellate laceration is discovered

21. An impaled object may need to be removed if it:
a. interferes with the airway
b. is lodged in the ear
c. is too small to be x-rayed
d. is lodged in the nose

22. To package an amputated part for transportation to the hospital, the EMS provider should:
a. pack it in ice
b. immerse the part in sterile water
c. wrap it in a sterile dressing and keep it cool
d. wrap it in a wet, sterile dressing and keep it warm

23. When managing a partial avulsion or amputation:
a. leave the part in the position found
b. complete the amputation with sterile scissors
c. apply direct pressure to the skin flap to control bleeding
d. gently straighten and align any skin bridges

24. When managing a patient with an injury to the soft tissue of the neck, always suspect accompanying:
a. rib injuries
b. jaw injuries
c. cervical spine injury
d. chest injuries

25. Injuries that occur as a result of a victim being propelled through space and striking a stationary object or the ground are classified as:
    a. primary blast injuries
    b. secondary blast injuries
    c. tertiary blast injuries
    d. associated blast injuries

26. The most frequent and life-threatening pressure injury associated with explosions is:
    a. intestinal rupture
    b. pulmonary trauma
    c. penetrating wounds
    d. aortic tears

27. When managing a victim of a blast injury, *avoid*:
    a. aggressive positive pressure ventilation
    b. starting an IV
    c. covering the ear canal
    d. removing contaminating material that may be needed as evidence

28. When managing a patient with an impaled object in the eye:
    a. remove the object if it interferes with placement of a metal eye shield
    b. remove the object if transport time to the hospital is greater than 20 minutes
    c. remove the object and apply pressure to the wound
    d. never remove the object

29. When managing a penetrating injury to the eye:
    a. also cover the uninjured eye
    b. leave the uninjured eye uncovered
    c. apply dry gauze pads to the eye
    d. use a compression dressing

30. Early management of an open chest injury includes:
    a. covering the wound with saline-soaked gauze pads
    b. supporting the injured area with sandbags
    c. sealing the wound with an occlusive dressing
    d. placing the patient on a backboard

31. If no spinal injuries are present or suspected, a patient with an open chest injury should be placed:
    a. supine with the legs elevated
    b. in a position of comfort, usually sitting
    c. in a prone position
    d. on the right side with the head lower than the legs

32. Management of an evisceration includes:
    a. replacing the organ within the abdomen
    b. applying a moist, sterile dressing to the area and covering it with an occlusive dressing
    c. applying direct pressure to the evisceration to control bleeding
    d. applying the PASG and inflating the legs and abdominal compartment

33. The position of choice for a patient with an evisceration and no accompanying spinal or leg injuries is on the:
    a. back with the hips and knees flexed
    b. back with the hips and knees straight
    c. left side
    d. right side

34. Management of an open neck injury may include:
    a. placing the patient in a sitting position
    b. applying digital pressure to a brachial artery
    c. covering the wound with a sterile occlusive dressing
    d. applying cold packs to the injury site

35. A major concern after extrication of a crush syndrome patient is that:
    a. patients become alkalotic
    b. patients develop dysrhythmias as a result of becoming hypokalemic
    c. hypophosphatemia may negatively affect the vasculature system
    d. toxic by-products are released into the circulation when entrapped limbs are reperfused

36. Rhabdomyolisis involves:
    a. the destruction of skeletal muscle of the entrapped victim
    b. dehydration and hypothermia, which results from inactivity of the entrapped victim
    c. an accumulation of foreign material in the lungs of the entrapped victim
    d. a progression of cardiac dysrhythmias that results from the prolonged inactivity of the entrapped victim

37. Compartment syndrome involves:
    a. swelling caused by increased circulation to an injured area of tissue
    b. loss of sensation to an injured area caused by increasing pressure on nerves innervating the area
    c. increasing pressure in an enclosed fascial space
    d. internal damage to muscles, blood vessels, and bones caused by compressive forces

38. One of the primary differences between crush injury and other soft tissue injuries is that:
a. hemorrhage is usually easy to control
b. the injury is often a closed injury, so infection is not a major concern
c. the skin remains intact and therefore external bleeding is not present
d. internal damage may be far more extensive than it appears

39. When managing a patient with a crush syndrome:
a. avoid IV fluid administration to prevent development of pulmonary edema
b. aggressively hydrate the patient to manage hypovolemia and maintain urine output
c. consider administering furosemide to help maintain urine output
d. always administer calcium chloride to prevent hyperkalemia

40. Clues that a wound is infected include:
a. inflammation, edema, and dryness
b. itching, dryness, and bleeding
c. pain on palpation, itching, and scar formation
d. purulent drainage, persistent pain, and fever

41. You and your partner are managing a patient with a gunshot wound. The clothing must be removed. When removing clothing:
a. never cut clothing
b. place the clothes in a nonporous plastic bag to reduce the risk of biohazard
c. avoid cutting through any holes in the clothing
d. to reduce the biohazard risk, give the clothing to the family to clean immediately

Burns

42. Burns injuries are typically classified as any of the following *EXCEPT*:
a. chemical
b. steam
c. electrical
d. thermal

43. A burn characterized by reddening, blister formation, and intense pain is a:
a. full-thickness burn
b. superficial burn
c. partial-thickness burn
d. medium-thickness burn

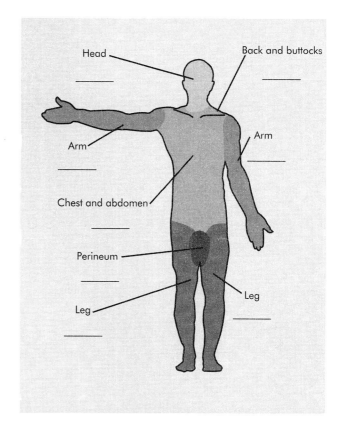

Figure 7-1 Rule of Nines: Adult

44. Using the given list of percentages, label each part of the adult in Figure 7-1 with the proper percentage of body surface area: 1%, 9%, 9%, 9%, 18%, 18%, 18%, 18%.

45. Using the given list of percentages, label each part of the 5-year-old child in Figure 7-2 with the proper percentage of body surface area: 9%, 9%, 14%, 16%, 16%, 18%, 18%.

46. Using the given list of percentages, label each part of the infant in Figure 7-3 with the proper percentage of body surface area: 9%, 9%, 14%, 14%, 18%, 18%, 18%.

For questions 47 through 49, use the Rule of Nines to calculate the approximate percentage of burns.

47. A 48-year-old man has been injured in a gas heater explosion. He has burns covering his entire right arm, entire back, and the back of his head. You estimate the burns to cover a body surface area of about:
   a. 18%
   b. 27%
   c. 31%
   d. 40%

48. A 5-year-old girl has pulled a pot of boiling water off the stove while helping her mother make supper. She has burns on the chest, abdomen, and front of both legs. You estimate the burns to cover a body surface area of about:
   a. 22%
   b. 34%
   c. 48%
   d. 56%

49. An 8-month-old baby has been rescued from a burning house by firefighters. On examination, you find that the infant has partial-thickness burns on the buttocks and back of both legs. You estimate the burns to cover a body surface area of about:
   a. 9%
   b. 14%
   c. 23%
   d. 30%

50. Superficial burns involve:
   a. only the dermis
   b. only the epidermis
   c. the epidermis and dermis
   d. all the layers of the skin

51. Respiratory tract burns should be suspected if a patient:
   a. has singed or sooty nasal hairs, nostrils, or lips
   b. has a hoarse voice
   c. was in a closed room during a fire
   d. all of the above

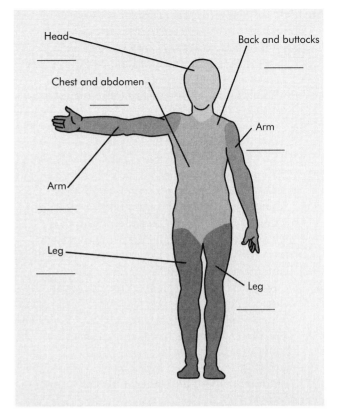

Figure 7-2 Rule of Nines: Child

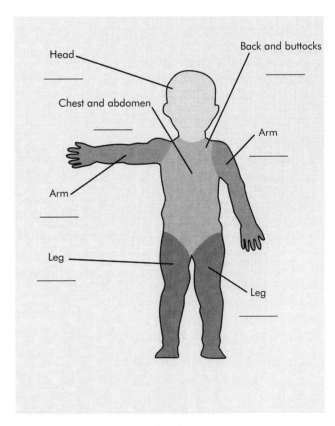

Figure 7-3 Rule of Nines: Infant

52. Patients with suspected inhalation injuries:
    a. should not be given oxygen to avoid drying of the mucous membranes
    b. will display signs of respiratory distress within 1 hour of the injury
    c. should always be transported to the hospital
    d. normally have a cherry-red skin color

53. The palm of a patient's hand may be used as a guide when estimating burn percentages of small areas because it represents an area of approximately:
    a. 0.5% of body surface
    b. 1% of body surface
    c. 2% of body surface
    d. 3% of body surface

54. For adults, moderate burns include:
    a. full-thickness burns covering less than 10% of the body and involving hands, feet, face, or groin
    b. superficial burns covering more than 30% of the body
    c. partial-thickness burns involving 15% to 30% of the body
    d. partial-thickness burns covering more than 40% of the body

55. Mark each of the following burns as minor, moderate, or critical.

    _____ A timer on a tanning bed malfunctions. Superficial burns cover 85% of the patient.

    _____ A weekend mechanic removes the cap from a hot radiator. He manages to protect his face but has partial-thickness burns covering 10% of the front of his chest and abdomen.

    _____ A spark ignites a welder's shirt. Colleagues quickly extinguish the fire but not before it has caused full- and partial-thickness burns to both arms and the chest. Approximately 18% of surface area sustained partial-thickness burns and 5% sustained full-thickness burns.

    _____ A woman cooking supper spills a pot of boiling water on her legs. Partial-thickness burns cover 18% to 20% of body surface area.

    _____ Hot tar is dropped on the body of a roofer wearing shorts and no shirt. Approximately 20% to 24% of the body surface has partial-thickness burns; one arm is completely encompassed.

56. The age of a burn victim is of special concern if the patient:
    a. is between 20 and 45 years
    b. is younger than 5 years or older than 55 years
    c. is younger than 10 years or older than 50 years
    d. is younger than 15 years or older than 65 years

57. A partial-thickness burn in a child is considered moderate if it covers:
    a. 5% to 10% of the body
    b. 10% to 20% of the body
    c. 20% to 30% of the body
    d. 30% to 40% of the body

58. Moderate pain with associated redness but no blistering is characteristic of a:
    a. superficial burn
    b. partial-thickness burn
    c. medium-thickness burn
    d. full-thickness burn

59. A burn associated with a fractured extremity would be considered:
    a. minor
    b. moderate, provided that it only involves a lower extremity
    c. moderate, regardless of the extremity involved
    d. critical

60. The first step in managing a burn patient is to:
    a. estimate the percentage of burns
    b. open the airway and assess breathing
    c. stop the burning process
    d. apply sterile burn dressings

61. A burn characterized by leathery, dry skin that may appear white or charred, and which may be accompanied by little or no pain is a:
    a. superficial burn
    b. partial-thickness burn
    c. medium-thickness burn
    d. full-thickness burn

62. When caring for burns to the hands or feet:
    a. apply burn cream on each individual digit
    b. place nothing between the fingers or toes
    c. separate each digit with sterile gauze
    d. advanced medical care is needed only if full-thickness burns are present

63. Burn management should include:
    a. applying ice directly to the burn
    b. removing jewelry and smoldering clothing
    c. removing charred clothing stuck to a burn
    d. removing hot tar from a burn

64. Ointments or greases should:
    a. be used only on burns if they are sterile
    b. never be used on burns in the field
    c. be applied immediately after the burning process has stopped
    d. be applied only to extremity burns

65. The IV fluid of choice for a burn patient is:
    a. any crystalloid solution
    b. colloid solution
    c. lactated Ringer's solution
    d. plasma

66. When managing a patient with burns caused by a chemical powder:
    a. cover the chemical with a sterile, moist dressing
    b. brush off as much powder as possible
    c. wash the chemical off slowly
    d. cover the chemical with a sterile, dry dressing

67. Irrigate liquid chemical burns to the body:
    a. with only sterile solutions
    b. with a neutralizing solution
    c. for no longer than 15 minutes
    d. with copious amounts of water

68. Chemical burns to the eyes should be irrigated:
    a. with a neutralizing solution
    b. only if it does not interfere with transport
    c. until the patient reaches the hospital
    d. for no longer than 10 minutes

69. When caring for a patient who has suffered an electrical burn:
    a. ground the patient first to discharge any electricity remaining in the patient
    b. check for entrance and exit wounds
    c. pull the patient off energized wires
    d. ascertain the exact voltage that caused the burn

70. Electrical burns differ from other burns in that:
    a. there is no injury from heat
    b. they heal faster than ordinary burns
    c. damage is always limited to the dermis and epidermis
    d. tissue damage may be deeper and more severe than it appears

71. A major problem associated with lightning strikes and electrical shocks is:
    a. respiratory and cardiac arrest
    b. abdominal injury
    c. intracranial bleed
    d. tension pneumothorax

72. You are transporting a patient to a local burn center that is 35 minutes away and are ordered to start an IV while en route to the hospital. An important consideration when starting an IV on a burn patient is:
    a. if a burned area must be used, avoid cleansing the IV site so as not to disturb or remove any tissue
    b. start the IV using a small-bore catheter to minimize additional tissue damage
    c. if an upper extremity is involved, try to find an IV site in the burned area to leave unburned sites for long-term hospital use
    d. use a large-bore catheter

73. An explosion occurred in a local welding shop. One patient is obviously beyond your help. The other patient has second- and third-degree burns over approximately 20% of his body. When assessing the patient, you note that his pulse rate is 126 and his blood pressure is 94/66. The low blood pressure is most likely the result of:
    a. loss of capillary seal with resultant fluid shift
    b. widespread vasodilation
    c. another injury
    d. spinal shock

ANSWERS TO CHAPTER 7: TRAUMA II: SOFT TISSUE TRAUMA AND BURNS

1. c. The skin provides protection to underlying structures and temperature regulation. Because it is rich in nerve endings, it also allows information to be transmitted from the environment to the brain. The skin also senses heat, cold, touch, pressure, and pain.

2. a. The epidermis is the outermost layer of skin. The dermis is the second layer of the skin. Epi- means "upon"; therefore *epidermis* means "upon the dermis."

3. a. The dermis contains sweat glands and hair follicles.

4. b. The subcutaneous layer is a layer of fatty tissue that lies under the dermis.

5. d. Oils are secreted by sebaceous glands. Sweat is secreted by sudoriferous glands.

6. b. Hemostasis is the body's natural ability to stop bleeding, the ability to clot blood. The vascular reaction involves vasoconstriction, formation of a platelet plug, coagulation, and the growth of fibrous tissue into the blood clot to permanently close and seal the injured blood vessel.

7. c. The three basic steps of the clotting mechanism include the release of platelet factors at the injury site, formation of thrombin, and trapping of red blood cells in fibrin to form a clot. In the process, prothrombin is converted to thrombin, and thrombin acts as an enzyme to convert fibrinogen into fibrin threads that entrap platelets, blood cells, and plasma to form the clot.

8. b. A hematoma is an example of a closed soft-tissue injury. Contusions and crush injuries are other examples.

9. c. When bruising is noted over the area of a vital organ, suspect damage to the underlying organ and possible internal bleeding. Direct pressure does not control internal bleeding and can cause further damage. Although the ribs provide some protection, a blow of enough force to bruise the chest wall also can bruise the underlying lung or heart tissue. Although this may not cause internal bleeding as severe as that associated with abdominal organs, the results can be equally as devastating.

10. d. A contusion is a bruise and can be managed with cold application. Urticaria are itchy wheals or hives, and a hematocrit measures the volume of red blood cells in a specimen. An abrasion is an open wound.

11. a. A hematoma is a lump caused by blood collecting within damaged tissue. Varicose veins are distended veins, a fistula is an abnormal passage, and a melanoma is a tumor or growth.

12. Match the following types of open soft-tissue injuries with their descriptions: abrasion, amputation, avulsion, laceration, puncture.

<u>laceration</u> A break in the skin caused by forceful impact with a sharp object. The wound edges may be regular (linear) or irregular (stellate).

<u>abrasion</u> Caused by a simple scraping or scratching of the outer layer of the skin. Examples include "rug-burns" or "friction-burns."

<u>avulsion</u> A portion of tissue or skin that is torn loose and left hanging as a flap or is completely pulled from the body.

<u>puncture</u> A small opening or perforation of the skin typically caused by pointed sharp objects.

<u>amputation</u> The removal of an appendage (such as an arm) from the body.

13. b. Abrasions often are contaminated by foreign matter because they are associated with friction between the skin and another object, such as ground or pavement. As a result, risk of infection is increased. Bleeding is usually minor and from the capillary beds. Abrasions may be very painful because of the large surface area involved.

14. c. Bleeding from a laceration may be severe and difficult to control depending on location and depth. However, in most cases the bleeding can be controlled using direct pressure.

15. b. Gunshot wounds with no exit and stab wounds are classified as puncture wounds. For a gunshot wound to be considered a perforating wound, it must travel through the body and cause an entrance and exit wound. The notion that gunshot wounds are sterile as a result of the heat of the bullet is false; contamination can occur with bits of clothing and dirt carried deep into the wound.

16. **d.** Preventing further contamination of the wound is a goal of wound management. Other goals include bleeding control and immobilizing the injured part. EMS personnel should not attempt thorough cleaning, and clots should not be removed. Although open wounds may be graphic, they should not sidetrack the rescuer from checking for more serious, life-threatening injuries.

17. **a.** Dressings help control bleeding, prevent further contamination and infection, and protect the wound from further injury or damage. Dressings are held in place by bandages.

18. **c.** Loose bandage ends should be secured so that they do not catch on anything. Do not place knots over wounds, over fractures, on the skin, or on the patient's back. Bandages should not be so tight that they restrict circulation. Do not cover fingertips or toes because this will make it difficult to check for signs of impaired circulation.

19. **b.** Impaled objects should be stabilized with bulky dressings. Do not apply pressure to the object. Although the object is usually left in place, there are situations when the object must be removed (follow local protocols). Long objects may be carefully shortened to facilitate transport.

20. **a.** Whenever a penetrating or puncture injury is encountered, check for an exit wound. A stellate laceration has irregular edges.

21. **a.** An impaled object may need to be removed if it interferes with the airway. An object may need to be removed if it interferes with chest compressions or with patient transportation. Objects lodged in the ear or nose should not be removed if the airway is patent.

22. **c.** An amputated part should be wrapped in a sterile dressing and kept cool. It should not be immersed or soaked in water or allowed to freeze. Always follow local protocols.

23. **d.** Any skin bridges should be gently straightened and aligned to maintain circulation in the partially avulsed or amputated part. Skin bridges

may also be used to cover the stump if surgical amputation becomes necessary. Never complete an amputation or apply pressure to the skin bridge.

24. **c.** Always suspect cervical spine injury when an injury to the soft tissue of the neck is encountered because of its anatomical proximity.

25. **c.** Tertiary blast injuries occur as a result of a victim being propelled through space and striking a stationary object or the ground. Primary blast injuries include burn and pressure injuries caused by the heat of the explosion and the overpressure wave. Secondary blast injuries include trauma caused by debris and projectiles being propelled by the blast.

26. **b.** Pulmonary injury is the most common and serious trauma associated with explosions. These injuries may not manifest themselves immediately after the blast, so it is important that patients be carefully monitored for respiratory problems.

27. **a.** Because of the high incidence of pulmonary blast trauma that occurs after an explosion, positive pressure ventilation of the blast injury patient should be performed with caution. Because of the high potential for damage to the alveolar-capillary walls and to other lung tissues, positive pressure ventilations may induce pneumothorax and create air emboli. Injuries to the abdomen may be severe enough to cause shock, which may necessitate fluid resuscitation. Contaminating material should be removed from wounds, but it should not be discarded because it may be needed as evidence. Because ruptured eardrums are common, the ear canals should be protected to keep out contaminants.

28. **d.** Objects impaled in the eye should not be removed. Stabilize the object, if possible, and cover it with a cone to protect the protruding object from being accidentally displaced. Because both eyes move together, cover the uninjured eye to minimize the chances of eye movement.

29. **a.** When managing a penetrating injury to the eye, cover both eyes. If the uninjured eye is not covered, the injured eye will move whenever the uninjured moves. This is known as *sympa-*

thetic movement. Do not cover an exposed part of the eyeball with dry gauze because this can be irritating and the gauze will absorb eye fluids.

30. c. Early management of an open chest injury includes sealing the wound with an occlusive dressing. This should be accomplished the same time as the airway is assessed in the initial assessment.

31. b. If no spinal injuries are suspected, a patient with an open chest injury should be placed in a position of comfort that does not interfere with breathing.

32. b. Eviscerations should be covered with moist, sterile dressings that are then covered with an occlusive dressing. The organs should not be replaced, and direct pressure should not be applied to the area. The abdominal compartment of the PASG should not be inflated over an evisceration.

33. a. If there are no accompanying spinal or leg injuries, transport an evisceration patient on his or her back with the hips and knees flexed to decrease abdominal pressure.

34. c. A neck vein laceration should be covered with an occlusive dressing to reduce chances of air embolism. The patient should not stand or sit up because this increases the chances of air embolism.

35. d. While the patient is trapped, the metabolic by-products are confined to the entrapped part. After extrication, toxic by-products are released into the circulation. The patient may rapidly deteriorate and die. Even if the patient survives, he or she is at a greater risk of developing renal failure. Because of anaerobic metabolism, the patient's blood will be acidotic. Hyperkalemia will also develop, as will hyperphosphatemia, which can lead to abnormal calcifications in the vasculature and nervous system.

36. a. Rhabdomyolisis involves the destruction of skeletal muscle and results in the release of many toxins including myoglobin, a muscle protein. Myoglobin can lodge in the filtering tubules of the kidneys and lead to renal failure, which can result in the death of the crush injury patient.

37. c. Compartment syndrome involves muscle ischemia that results from rising pressures within an anatomical fascial space. The increasing pressure is usually the result of an extremity injury that causes significant edema and swelling in the deep tissues. External swelling may or may not be evident. The swelling also impairs circulation to the area, which causes ischemia. Pain out of proportion to the injury is commonly present.

38. d. Because a crush injury involves the body tissues being subjected to severe compressive forces, muscles, blood vessels, and bones may be affected. Therefore the internal damage may be far more extensive than it appears on the outside. Hemorrhage may be difficult to control because the source of bleeding may be hard to identify and several large blood vessels may be involved. Limited circulation to the affected tissues creates an excellent growth medium for bacteria. Although the skin may remain intact, in some cases the skin may be cut or torn by the compressive forces.

39. b. When managing a patient with a crush syndrome, aggressively hydrate the patient to manage hypovolemia and maintain urine output. Although maintaining urine output is a goal, loop diuretics such as furosemide should be avoided because they can acidify the urine and further dehydrate the patient. The urine should be alkalinized by administering sodium bicarbonate. This helps control hyperkalemia and acidosis and can prevent acute myoglobinuric renal failure. Calcium chloride generally is not indicated to prevent hyperkalemia but rather to treat severe hyperkalemia.

40. d. Signs that a wound is infected include increasing inflammation or edema, purulent drainage, foul odor, persistent pain, delayed healing, and fever.

41. c. The patient's clothing is evidence and should be turned over to law enforcement officials. When cutting clothing that may be considered evidence, avoid cutting through any existing holes in the clothing. Also, do not place the clothes in a plastic bag because mold or mildew may develop on the clothing because of the trapping of moisture within the bag. Place evidence in a paper bag instead.

Burns

42. b. Burns may be classified as thermal, chemical, or electrical. Some sources also add radiation burns as a fourth category. A steam burn is a thermal burn.

43. c. Partial-thickness burns are characterized by reddening, blister formation, and intense pain.

44.

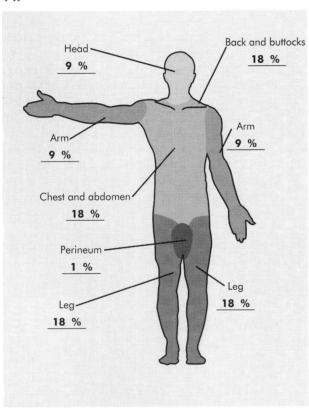

Figure 7-1 Rule of Nines: Adult

45.

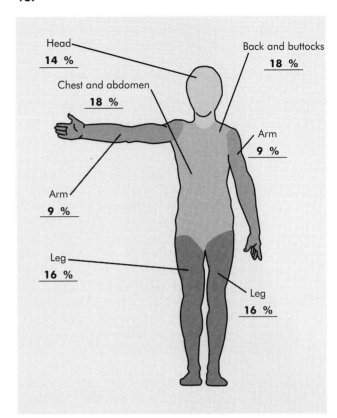

Figure 7-2 Rule of Nines: Child

46.

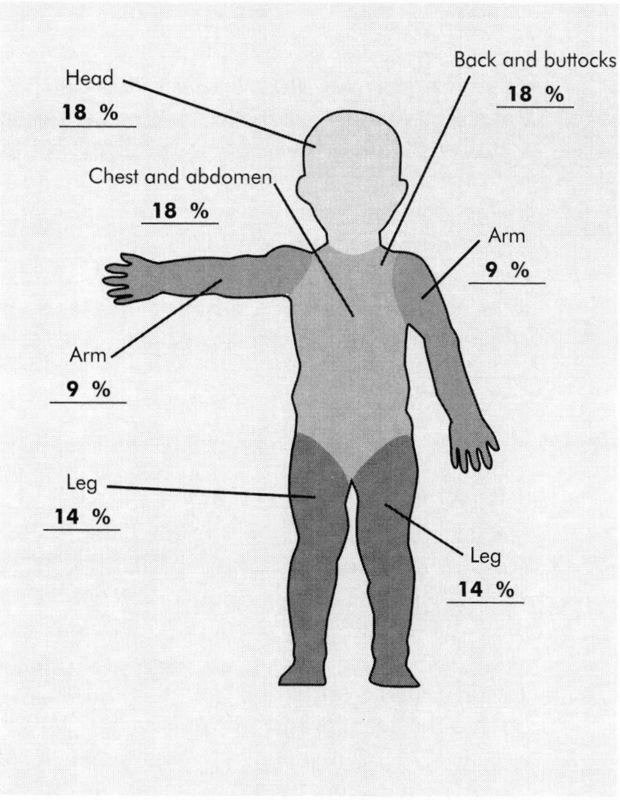

Figure 7-3   Rule of Nines: Infant

For questions 47 through 49, use the Rule of Nines to calculate the approximate percentage of burns.

47. c. The burns cover approximately 31% of body surface area (right arm = 9%, entire back = 18%, back of head = 4%).

48. b. Approximately 34% of body surface area is involved (chest and abdomen = 18%, front of both legs = 16%).

49. c. The infant has burns covering approximately 23% of its body (buttocks = 9%, backs of legs = 14%).

50. b. A superficial burn involves only the epidermis. Partial-thickness burns involve the epidermis and part of the dermis. Full-thickness burns involve the full thickness of the skin and may involve underlying muscles, bones, or other structure.

51. d. All of the above. Singed or sooty nasal hairs, nostrils, or lips or a hoarse voice are signs of possible respiratory tract burns. Also, respiratory tract burns should be suspected if a patient was in a closed room or confined area that was on fire.

52. c. Always transport patients with suspected inhalation injuries to the hospital. The structures of the respiratory tract may swell to a point that the airway becomes occluded. Cherry-red skin color is a sign of carbon monoxide exposure but is usually a late sign of extremely elevated carboxyhemoglobin levels.

53. b. Generally, the palm of the patient's hand equals approximately 1% of body surface area. This can be helpful when estimating burn percentages of small areas.

54. c. For adults, moderate burns include superficial burns covering more than 50% to 75% of the body, partial-thickness burns covering 15% to 30% of the body, or full-thickness burns (not involving face, hands, feet or genitals) covering 2% to 10% of the body.

55. Mark each of the following burns as minor, moderate, or critical.

moderate A timer on a tanning bed malfunctions. Superficial burns cover 85% of the patient.

minor A weekend mechanic removes the cap from a hot radiator. He manages to protect his face but has partial-thickness burns covering 10% of the front of his chest and abdomen.

critical A spark ignites a welder's shirt. Colleagues quickly extinguish the fire but not before it has caused full- and partial-thickness burns to both arms and the chest. Approximately 18% of surface area sustained partial-thickness burns and 5% sustained full-thickness burns.

moderate A woman cooking supper spills a pot of boiling water on her legs. Partial-thickness burns cover 18% to 20% of body surface area.

critical A roofer wearing shorts and no shirt has hot tar dropped on his body. Approximately 20% to 24% of the body surface has partial-thickness burns; one arm is completely encompassed.

56. b. The age of a burn patient is of special concern if the patient is younger than 5 years or older than 55 years because of anatomical and physiological differences in young children and older adults.

57. b. In a child, any partial-thickness burn covering 10% to 20% of the body is considered moderate. Any full-thickness or partial-thickness burn covering more than 20% of the body is considered critical.

58. a. Superficial burns are characterized by redness, moderate pain, and no blister formation.

59. d. Burns associated with a fracture or that involve the respiratory tract are considered critical. They are considered a high-priority injury.

60. c. The burning process must be stopped first or the injury process will continue. An open airway and artificial ventilations will do little good if a patient's tissues are still burning.

61. d. Full-thickness burns are accompanied by little or no pain due to destruction of nerve endings. The skin may be white or charred, and dry and leathery.

62. c. When burns of the hands or feet are being dressed, each finger or toe should be separated with a sterile dressing to keep them from sticking together.

63. b. Jewelry and smoldering clothing should be removed from the burn area. Clothing that is sticking to the burn should be cooled and left in place to avoid removing any burned skin. Attempting to remove tar also may cause further tissue injury, but the tar should be cooled to stop the burning process.

64. b. Never use ointments or grease on burns, even if sterile, because they will trap heat in the tissues. Gelled water may be applied if it is sterile.

65. c. In most cases, lactated Ringer's solution is the fluid of choice for burn patients (always follow local protocols). Normal saline may be used short term, but because it does not contain potassium large amounts can cause hypokalemia. Although D_5W is also a crystalloid solution, it is not preferred because it does not remain in the vascular space as long as Ringer's.

66. b. Powdered chemicals should be brushed off as much as possible, after which the remaining residue may be washed off with copious amounts of water. A special problem associated with some chemicals is that they react with water and may worsen the injury.

67. d. Liquid chemical burns should be flushed with copious amounts of water. A small amount or trickle may do more harm than good in some cases. The water does not have to be sterile. Neutralizing solutions should be avoided, because these often produce heat as the neutralizing takes place. Continue to flush during transportation to the hospital.

68. c. Chemical burns to the eyes should be flushed until the patient reaches the hospital. A sterile solution should be used if possible. Eyes should be flushed from the corner closest to the nose to the outside corner to avoid contaminating the uninjured with the runoff. Flushing of both eyes can be accomplished with a nasal cannula attached to intravenous tubing if available or with commercially available devices designed for eye irrigation.

69. b. Once it is safe to do so, patients who have contacted electrical wires or equipment must be checked for entrance and exit wounds. Electricity does not remain in the patient after removal from the source. If a patient is still in contact with the electrical source, do not touch the patient. Attempt to turn the power off.

70. d. Tissue damage caused by electrical burns may be much deeper and more severe than it appears. Electricity readily travels along nerves, blood vessels, and muscles and is capable of causing severe damage throughout its course of travel.

71. a. Lightning strikes and electrical shocks may cause respiratory and cardiac arrest. As the current passes through the body, it can cause the patient to go into ventricular fibrillation. Even as little as 100 milliamperes can cause ventricular fibrillation. However, these patients have a high survival rate if prehospital intervention is prompt. Although it is not high voltage, 110-volt house current causes most electrocutions because wires and equipment using this current are accessible to most people.

72. d. When starting an IV on a burn patient, use a large-bore IV catheter in a peripheral vein in an unburned extremity. When a catheter must be inserted through burned tissue the risk of subsequent infection is greater, so good aseptic technique is still important. Because tape may not adhere very well to the skin if fluid leak occurs, bandages may be used as well to secure the IV.

73. c. Generally, shock directly associated with burns takes time to develop. If a burn patient presents with signs of shock in the acute phase, look for other potentially life-threatening injuries.

Trauma III: Head, Facial, and Spinal Trauma

8

1. The most frequent cause of death from trauma is:
   a. open chest wound
   b. severe head trauma
   c. aortic dissection
   d. multisystem trauma

2. Approximately what percent of gunshot wounds to the cranium result in death?
   a. 35% to 40%
   b. 40% to 50%
   c. 75% to 80%
   d. 100%

3. The use of helmets reduces the likelihood of death from motorcycle accidents by what percentage?
   a. 20%
   b. 40%
   c. 50%
   d. 70%

4. Intracranial hemorrhage can result in:
   a. hypoxia
   b. increased intracranial pressure
   c. permanent damage
   d. all of the above

5. The severity of head and neck injuries is often difficult to recognize in the prehospital setting.
   a. true
   b. false

6. Which of the following are critical factors that can decrease the death and disability from head and neck trauma?
   a. rapid transport to the closest appropriate facility
   b. early recognition of signs and symptoms of head and neck injury
   c. maintaining a clear airway and providing appropriate ventilation
   d. all of the above

7. Circulation for the face is provided by the:
   a. external carotid artery
   b. internal carotid artery
   c. subclavian artery
   d. vertebral artery

8. The cranial nerve that innervates the facial region, teeth/gums, and palate and controls chewing is the:
   a. optic or second cranial nerve
   b. hypoglossal or twelfth cranial nerve
   c. trigeminal or fifth cranial nerve
   d. vagus or tenth cranial nerve

9. Facial expression is controlled by which cranial nerve?
   a. olfactory or first cranial nerve
   b. facial or seventh cranial nerve
   c. oculomotor or third cranial nerve
   d. glossopharyngeal or ninth cranial nerve

10. The prominent bone of the cheek is the:
    a. zygoma
    b. frontal
    c. maxilla
    d. mandible

11. The largest opening of the skull is the:
    a. mastoid process
    b. optic foramen
    c. foramen magnum
    d. jugular foramen

12. The lowest layer of the true scalp, which is composed of a dense tendinous sheet of connective tissue, is called the:
    a. occipitalis muscle
    b. cancellous bone
    c. periosteum
    d. galea aponeurotica

13. Which bone forms the posterior and inferior aspect of the cranium?
a. occipital
b. parietal
c. temporal
d. frontal

14. Any expanding lesion within the cranium can result in:
a. tentorium cerebelli
b. increased intracranial pressure
c. decreased intracranial pressure
d. none of the above

15. The dura mater, pia mater, and arachnoid membrane make up the:
a. periosteum
b. meninges
c. cranial cavity
d. layers of the cranial fossa

16. Cerebrospinal fluid is a solution of nutrients and waste products that circulates through and around:
a. the spinal cord
b. the cerebral ventricles
c. the subarachnoid space and dural sinuses
d. all of the above

17. The majority of the cranial cavity is occupied by the:
a. cerebellum
b. spinal cord
c. cerebrum
d. brain stem

18. The outer layer of the cerebral cortex is known as the:
a. white matter
b. falx cerebri
c. tentorium
d. gray matter

19. Conscious thought, personality, voluntary motor control, and tactile perception are the function of the:
a. brain stem
b. medulla oblongata
c. cerebellum
d. cerebral hemispheres

20. The anterior cerebral lobe that controls personality is the:
a. parietal lobe
b. frontal lobe
c. occipital lobe
d. temporal lobe

21. The posterior chamber of the eye contains a clear fluid called:
a. vitreous humor
b. aqueous humor
c. cerebrospinal fluid
d. lacrimal fluid

22. The structure of the eye most responsible for focusing light and images is the:
a. iris
b. retina
c. lens
d. sclera

23. Dilation of the pupil seen in severe head injuries is due to:
a. hypoxia
b. hypotension
c. compression of the third cranial nerve
d. hypertension

24. The primary function of the blood-brain barrier is:
a. to prevent infection
b. to block certain substances from entering the cerebrospinal fluid
c. to limit the spread of bleeding from an injury
d. to protect the neurosurgeon during procedures

25. All of the following are true regarding spinal cord injury (SCI) *EXCEPT*:
a. SCI caused by prehospital care is the most common cause of lawsuits
b. it is more common in men than in women
c. approximately 40% will have permanent disability
d. approximately 25% of these injuries may be caused by improper prehospital handling

26. The most important criterion to consider when assessing a patient with possible spinal injury is the:
a. presence of unconsciousness
b. lack of pain
c. evidence of intoxication
d. mechanism of injury

27. Which of the following is true regarding the bony skeleton of the spine?
a. Lumbar vertebrae are the smallest.
b. The first cervical vertebra is called the axis and the second is called the atlas.
c. The eleventh and twelfth thoracic vertebrae have floating ribs.
d. The sacral and coccygeal vertebrae are very flexible.

28. All of the following are parts of a vertebra *EXCEPT* the:
   a. transverse process
   b. spinous process
   c. intervertebral disk
   d. vertebral foramen

29. Match the nerve root with the motor function it controls.
   a. C 4-5   1. wrist extension
   b. C7   2. anal sphincter tone
   c. L5   3. diaphragm
   d. S1-S2   4. foot dorsiflexion
   e. S4   5. foot plantar flexion

30. Match the sensory level with the nerve root involved.
   a. top of the shoulder   1. T4
   b. middle finger   2. S4
   c. nipple   3. L5
   d. lateral calf   4. C3-C4
   e. perianal area   5. C7

31. Signs and symptoms of spinal cord injury include all the following *EXCEPT*:
   a. paralysis
   b. paresthesias
   c. altered mental status
   d. pain/tenderness

Questions 32 through 34 refer to the following scenario:

A 59-year-old man falls 25 feet from a tree hitting his head on a branch. He denies LOC, pain, paresthesias, or paralysis.

32. Which of the following criteria will determine whether cervical spine immobilization is indicated?
   a. presence of a positive mechanism of injury
   b. presence of a negative mechanism of injury
   c. presence of an uncertain mechanism of injury with clinical criteria
   d. written protocol

33. Which of the following is essential to clinically determine that spinal immobilization is not needed for this patient?
   a. He must have more pain in the neck than in the extremity injury.
   b. He must have pain over the spinous process of the injury.
   c. He must have only a temporary loss of consciousness.
   d. He must be sober, calm, and cooperative.

34. Spinal immobilization for this patient:
   a. may consist of cervical spine alone in the absence of back pain or neurological symptoms
   b. is designed to prevent further injury
   c. should be initiated once all airway maneuvers are completed
   d. is not necessary

35. A 40-year-old man is found hanging by his neck. After being cut down, he is found to be alive but quadriplegic. What type of spinal cord injury is this called?
   a. distraction
   b. flexion/extension
   c. rotational
   d. compression

36. A 19-year-old dives head first into 3 feet of water. Initially he is moving all extremities but begins to develop paralysis. The most likely cause is:
   a. primary injury from impingement of a bone fragment into the cord
   b. secondary injury as a result of swelling and ischemia of the spinal cord
   c. spinal cord transsection
   d. spinal shock

37. After sustaining a knife wound to the back, your patient is found to have paralysis on only the left side of his body and loss of pain sensation on his right. This is an example of:
   a. central cord syndrome
   b. Brown-Séquard syndrome
   c. anterior cord syndrome
   d. spinal cord contusion

38. A 25-year-old is hit by a train and sustains a C2 fracture/dislocation resulting in quadriplegia. His blood pressure is 60/P with a pulse of 52. Your understanding of neurogenic shock is that it is:
    a. usually temporary and the result of the loss of sympathetic vascular tone
    b. common and always should be suspected in multiple trauma patients
    c. exhibited by pale, clammy skin associated with hypotension and tachycardia
    d. treated differently than hypovolemic shock with the use of vasopressor agents only

39. Brain injury is classified as a direct or indirect injury to:
    a. the cerebrum
    b. the cerebellum
    c. the brain stem
    d. any of the above

40. Contrecoup injury to the brain occurs on the same side as the impact.
    a. true
    b. false

41. Bleeding between the dura mater and the skull is called:
    a. a subdural hematoma
    b. an intracerebral hematoma
    c. an epidural hematoma
    d. a subarachnoid hematoma

42. The most severe type of injury to the brain occurs from:
    a. diffuse axonal injury
    b. subdural hematoma
    c. epidural hematoma
    d. cerebral contusion

43. Retroauricular ecchymosis or Battle's sign is an early indication of a basilar skull fracture.
    a. true
    b. false

44. The "halo sign" is most reliable:
    a. with fluid from the ear or nose
    b. with any bloody drainage from the head
    c. when imminent death is obvious
    d. in none of the above

45. A concussion can result in:
    a. immediate unconsciousness
    b. transient episodes of neuronal dysfunction
    c. deteriorating level of consciousness
    d. all of the above

46. A comatose state resulting from diffuse axonal injury is associated with:
    a. long periods of unconsciousness
    b. signs of increased cranial pressure
    c. decerebrate or decorticate posturing
    d. all of the above

47. An adult patient with a serious head injury and signs of increased intracranial pressure should be hyperventilated at a rate of 24 breaths/min and 100% oxygen until the time of surgical intervention.
    a. true
    b. false

48. Displacement of brain tissue causing herniation of the brain stem presents with:
    a. vomiting
    b. decreased level of consciousness
    c. fixed and dilated pupils
    d. all of the above

49. Inability to remember events that occurred before the traumatic event is known as:
    a. delirium
    b. retrograde amnesia
    c. antegrade amnesia
    d. dementia

50. Which of the following is true regarding nontraumatic back pain?
    a. It is an uncommon reason for prehospital transport.
    b. Men are twice as likely to be affected as women.
    c. The most common cause is idiopathic and difficult to diagnose.
    d. Lack of numbness or weakness indicates drug-seeking behavior.

51. The difference between sciatica and a herniated intervertebral disk is that:
    a. symptoms from a herniated disk can occur at any level of the spinal cord, whereas sciatica occurs in the lumbar region
    b. a herniated disk is more common in obese patients
    c. sciatica is caused by a tear in the nucleus pulposus
    d. only sciatica is treated with surgical intervention

52. You respond to a 52-year-old male construction worker who awoke with severe back pain and is unable to get out of bed. He is healthy and complains of "fire" in his back radiating into his left leg, which is worse with coughing and movement. Which of the following is the most correct statement regarding this patient?
    a. Large-bore IVs should be placed as a precaution against a dissecting aortic aneurysm.
    b. Administration of an analgesic such as morphine may be required to facilitate transport to the hospital.
    c. A complete neurological exam is not necessary because he is awake and alert with no history of trauma.
    d. His pain is consistent with renal colic.

53. You are intubating an unconscious motorcycle crash victim who has suffered blunt facial trauma. You notice that the upper jaw and nose seem to move freely from the rest of the head and there is profuse bleeding into the mouth. This represents what kind of facial fracture?
    a. zygoma
    b. basilar skull
    c. Le Fort
    d. nasal

54. Your patient has sustained blunt trauma to the left orbit. On exam you are unable to visualize the pupil because the cornea appears black and fluid filled. This is called a:
    a. hyphema
    b. blowout fracture
    c. ruptured globe
    d. traumatic third nerve palsy

55. The appropriate management of an eye injury may include each of the following *EXCEPT*:
    a. administration of a topical anesthetic such as tetracaine
    b. copious irrigation for chemical burns
    c. stabilizing impaled objects in place
    d. leaving one eye open so that the patient can look around

56. Control of severe bleeding from a scalp wound can be controlled by all of the following *EXCEPT*:
    a. direct pressure on the wound
    b. pressure point control at the temporal artery
    c. clamping the bleeding artery with a hemostat
    d. raising the head of the stretcher

57. As intracranial pressure rises, respirations are affected. The pattern of respirations characterized by alternating cycles of deep and shallow breaths is called:
    a. central neurogenic hyperventilation
    b. ataxic respirations
    c. apnea
    d. Cheyne-Stokes respirations

58. The cerebral perfusion pressure can be calculated by:
    a. the difference between systolic and diastolic blood pressure
    b. diastolic blood pressure plus one third of the pulse pressure
    c. intracranial pressure minus diastolic blood pressure
    d. mean arterial blood pressure minus intracranial pressure

59. A 39-year-old man was mowing the lawn when he felt something sharp hit him in the eye. Each of the following is required during evaluation of the eye injury *EXCEPT*:
    a. visual acuity
    b. pupillary reaction
    c. extraocular eye movement
    d. corneal reflex

60. A 40-year-old man has been stabbed in the neck. Injuries to the neck are divided into three zones. Which of the following is true regarding these zones?
    a. Zone I extends from the angle of the mandible upward to the ear.
    b. Zone II extends from the cricoid membrane to the angle of the mandible and represents the least common site of injury.
    c. Zone I injuries have the highest mortality.
    d. Zone III extends from the base of the neck at the sternal notch to the cricoid cartilage.

61. A 16-year-old girl is riding the family four-wheeler at night when she runs into the clothesline, which strikes her across the neck knocking her to the ground. On examination she is awake and alert. Her voice is hoarse and she has pain with swallowing. All of the following are true *EXCEPT*:
    a. the presence of subcutaneous emphysema indicates tracheal disruption
    b. fracture of the trachea can result in airway obstruction requiring surgical intervention
    c. cervical spine precautions should be taken
    d. emergent intubation should be considered to preclude the possibility of airway obstruction from swelling

62. Basilar skull fractures will compress cranial nerves exiting the base of the skull. The cranial nerves involved in basilar skull fractures include all the following *EXCEPT* the:
a. olfactory nerve (CN I)
b. oculomotor nerve (CN III)
c. facial nerve (CN VII)
d. auditory nerve (CN VIII)

Questions 63 through 65 refer to the Glasgow Coma Scale in Box 8-1.

63. The Glasgow Coma Scale is used to evaluate head injury victims. If your patient opens his eyes to voice command only, localizes pain when you pinch his arm, and is awake but confused his Glasgow Coma Scale is:
a. 3
b. 8
c. 12
d. 15

64. A severe head injury is typically associated with a Glasgow Coma Scale of:
a. 13 to 15
b. 8 to 12
c. less than 8
d. none of the above

65. If the patient's Glasgow Coma Scale is 8 or less:
a. total neurological recovery is impossible
b. intubation is probably indicated
c. manitol is indicated
d. surgery is always indicated

Box 8-1   Glasgow Coma Scale

1. **Eye Opening**	Points	
• Spontaneous	4	
• To voice	3	
• To pain	2	
• None	1	_____

2. **Verbal Response**	Points	
• Oriented	5	
• Confused	4	
• Inappropriate words	3	
• Incomprehensible sounds	2	
• None	1	_____

3. **Motor Response**	Points	
• Obeys commands	6	
• Localizes pain	5	
• Withdraws (pain)	4	
• Flexion (pain)	3	
• Extension (pain)	2	
• None	1	_____

Total (1 + 2 + 3)   _____

ANSWERS TO CHAPTER 8: TRAUMA III: HEAD, FACIAL, AND SPINAL TRAUMA

1. **b.** Head trauma is the major cause of death in multiple trauma because of two facts. First, 60% of major trauma victims have a head injury. Second, severe injury to the brain results in cardiorespiratory arrest.

2. **c.** There is a very high mortality rate associated with gunshot wounds to the head primarily because the bullet usually passes through several vital areas and is associated with greater tissue disruption than blunt head trauma.

3. **c.** Head injuries from motorcycle crashes have been cut in half in states where mandatory helmet use has been legislated.

4. **d.** When bleeding occurs in the brain, it takes up space leading to an increased intracranial pressure. The increased pressure results in decreased perfusion of the brain parenchyma leading to hypoxia and permanent damage if not relieved.

5. **a.** The only information available for evaluation in the prehospital setting is the mechanism of injury and gross neurological findings and complaints. The true severity of the injuries cannot be determined until the head injury victim has been evaluated by a physician and diagnostic studies such as x-rays and CAT scans have been performed.

6. **d.** Because the severity of the injuries cannot be completely determined without specialized diagnostic tests, it is vital that the trauma patient be rapidly transported to the nearest facility capable of performing them. Keeping a high index of suspicion will enable you to recognize those patients who require rapid transport. Because altered levels of consciousness result in hypoventilation and hypoxia, it is critical that the airway be properly maintained and appropriate ventilation be provided.

7. **a.** The aorta branches into the left and right brachiocephalic arteries. The common carotid artery then branches off and divides into the internal and external carotid arteries. The internal carotid supplies the anterior circulation to the brain and the external carotid supplies the circulation to the scalp. The vertebral arteries branch off the aorta to supply the posterior circulation of the brain.

8. **c.** The trigeminal nerve controls chewing and sensation from the face. The optic nerve involves vision in the retina. The hypoglossal nerve controls motor function of the tongue. The vagus nerve controls the muscles involved in swallowing.

9. **b.** The facial nerve innervates the muscles of facial expression and taste from the front two thirds of the tongue. The olfactory nerve is for the sense of smell. The oculomotor nerve allows the eye to look up, down, and medially. The glossopharyngeal nerve is involved in swallowing and taste from the posterior one third of the tongue.

10. **a.** The zygoma is the bone of the cheek and bridges between the temporal bone and the maxilla. The frontal bone is under the forehead. The maxilla forms the upper jaw and contains the upper teeth and base of the nose. The mandible forms the lower jaw.

11. **c.** The foramen magnum is the largest opening in the base of the skull through which the spinal cord exits the cranium. The mastoid process is the bony prominence behind and below the ear and is part of the temporal bone. The optic foramen is the opening in the sphenoid bone in the middle of the cranium through which the optic nerves exit. The jugular foramen is an opening between the occipital and temporal bones, through which the jugular veins exit.

12. **d.** The scalp consists of five layers and can be remembered with the letters of the word *SCALP*: Skin, Connective tissue, Aponeurosis, Loose connective tissue, Pericranium. The first three layers make up the true scalp, and the aponeurosis allows free movement of the scalp over the cranium.

13. **a.** The occipital bone is the posterior and inferior portion of the cranium. The parietal bone comprises the majority of the lateral skull. The temporal bone is lateral but inferior to the parietal bone. The frontal bone makes up the anterior and superior portion of the skull.

14. **b.** As bleeding takes up space within the cranium it exerts pressure on surrounding structures leading to an overall increase in intracranial pressure. Brain tumors can also result in increased pressure, though their effects are more gradual. The tentorium cerebelli is the

sheet of connective tissue that separates the cerebrum from the cerebellum.

15. b. The cranial meninges are internal to the skull and overlie the brain. They protect the brain, form the supporting framework for arteries and veins, and enclose a fluid-filled cavity called the subarachnoid space, which is vital to normal brain function. The outer layer is the dura mater, which is a dense fibrous membrane. Next is the arachnoid mater, which is a more delicate membrane overlying the pia mater, which is a highly vascular and delicate membrane. The subarachnoid space is the area between the arachnoid and pia mater.

16. d. Cerebrospinal fluid provides nutrients to the entire central nervous system by circulating around and through the brain and spinal cord. It also provides a means for the removal of metabolic waste products.

17. c. The cerebrum consists of the frontal, temporal, parietal, and occipital lobes and occupies the majority of the cranial cavity. The brain stem consists of the midbrain, pons, and medulla oblongata at the base of the cranial cavity. The cerebellum occupies the posterior portion of the cranial cavity. The spinal cord begins at the exit of the medulla oblongata from the foramen magnum.

18. d. The cerebral cortex is divided into two layers. The outer or gray matter is the location of all of the interconnections of the central nervous system neurons. The inner or white matter appears lighter because of the axon sheaths. The falx cerebri is the membrane dividing the two cerebral hemispheres and the tentorium is the membrane that divides the cerebrum from the cerebellum.

19. d. The neural interconnections that control the listed actions occur in the cerebral cortex in both the left and right cerebral hemispheres. The cerebellum controls balance; the brain stem and medulla oblongata control survival functions such as heart rate and breathing.

20. b. Injury to the frontal lobe is demonstrated by emotional findings such as irritability, tearfulness, and agitation. The parietal lobe houses memory and pain perception. The temporal lobe controls motor function and speech. The occipital lobe perceives vision.

21. a. The vitreous humor is a gelatinous material in the posterior chamber of the eye behind the iris and gives the eye most of its shape. The aqueous humor circulates in the anterior chamber. Lacrimal fluid is secreted by the lacrimal gland and is commonly known as tears.

22. c. The lens stretches and contracts to focus light on the retina. The iris dilates and constricts to allow light to pass. The sclera of the eye is the white portion of the globe and is not involved in sight.

23. c. As intracranial pressure rises in severe head injuries, compression of the third or oculomotor nerve occurs causing it to lose control of the pupillary muscles. As they relax the pupil dilates.

24. b. The blood-brain barrier protects the brain by controlling what substances can pass from the blood into the cerebrospinal fluid. It influences the effects of medications and may inhibit the body's ability to ward off infection.

25. a. Although it is true that spinal cord injuries do occur from improper handling of patients, it is not the most common cause of lawsuits. Most patients with SCI have already suffered the injury before EMS arrival, and a significant number of them will have permanent disability. Men, primarily because of their increased activity in high-risk activities, suffer the greater share of spinal cord injuries.

26. d. Because the severity of spinal cord injury is difficult to detect in the prehospital setting, the mechanism of injury is the most important criterion that determines the likelihood of injury.

27. c. Each of the thoracic vertebrae has an attached rib. However, the eleventh and twelfth ribs are called *floating ribs* because they do not attach to the sternum anteriorly. The first cervical vertebra is the atlas upon which the cranium rests. The atlas articulates with the axis or second cervical vertebra. The largest vertebrae are the lumbar, and the sacral and coccygeal vertebrae are fused into one solid mass of inflexible bone.

28. c. The intervertebral disk rests between the vertebrae and is not actually part of the vertebra. The transverse and spinous processes attach to ligaments and muscles that support the spine, and the vertebral foramen is the opening through which the vertebral artery traverses up and down the lateral aspect of the spine.

29.   a. diaphragm; b. wrist extension; c. foot dorsiflexion; d. foot plantar flexion; e. anal sphincter tone

30.   a. C3-C4; b. C7; c. T4; d. L5; e. S4

31. c.   Spinal cord injury will present with peripheral nervous system signs such as pain, weakness, tingling, and numbness. Altered mental status is a central nervous system sign and not related to the spinal cord. However, the unconscious trauma patient should be assumed to have a spinal cord injury until proven otherwise.

32. a.   This scenario represents a positive mechanism, one in which you should have a high degree of suspicion that a spinal injury may have occurred. An uncertain mechanism with clinical criteria would be present if he could not remember falling and had not hit his head but was complaining of severe neck pain with tingling in his hands.

33. d.   In your determination of whether spinal immobilization may be withheld, it is vital that patients be able to communicate clearly to you whether they have pain or neurological symptoms. They must not have other injuries that would distract them from perceiving their neck pain, and they must be fully awake and sober.

34. b.   Spinal immobilization is designed to prevent further injury and is the first step taken when assessing the trauma victim. It must be maintained throughout all airway activities. It is vital that the spinal cord be treated as one whole entity by immobilizing the cervical spine and the entire spine on a longboard.

35. a.   Distraction injuries occur when the vertebrae are pulled apart. Flexion/extension injuries occur with sudden stops moving either forward or backward. Rotational injuries occur when the head is turned forcibly to the right or left as would occur when being hit from the side in a T-bone collision. Compression injuries occur from deceleration in the long axis of the spine as would occur from falling from a height and landing on the feet or buttocks.

36. b.   If the spinal cord is contused it will begin to swell, which will gradually impair nerve func-

tion. This is secondary injury. Primary injury to the cord occurs when impingement of a bone fragment or transsection of the cord results in immediate loss of nerve impulses. Spinal shock refers to the loss of vascular tone that can occur with spinal cord injuries.

37. b.   Pain fibers enter the spinal cord and cross to the opposite side and travel up to the brain. Motor fibers enter and travel up the same side of the cord as they enter and cross in the midbrain. Because of this, a wound that cuts through only the right or left half of the spinal cord will result in loss of motor function of that side and loss of pain perception on the opposite side. A central cord syndrome occurs from flexion injuries, where the outer layer of the cord is injured, resulting in greater weakness of the upper extremities than the lower extremities. An anterior cord syndrome occurs from a ruptured intervertebral disk, which results in decreased sensation to pain and temperature below the lesion.

38. a.   Spinal shock is uncommon but is due to loss of sympathetic tone to the vasculature and is temporary. The skin will appear normal to flushed in color and dry. Normal to slow heart rates are encountered. Shock in the trauma patient should always be assumed to be from hypovolemia and treated with fluid administration, which is also the same treatment for spinal shock.

39. d.   Direct injury occurs when the force of trauma is directly on the area of injury. Indirect injury occurs from secondary swelling and hypoxia. Both are causes of brain injury and can occur at all levels of the central nervous system.

40. b.   During blunt head trauma the brain impacts the inner surface of the cranium on the side of injury (coup). Blood vessels are injured as it stretches away from the opposite side (contrecoup). The brain then rebounds against the opposite side and suffers further injury from a secondary impact against the cranium.

41. c.   Blood (hematoma) can collect between any portion of the meninges as well as within the brain tissue itself. A hematoma between the dura mater and the skull is epidural and is usually caused by skull fractures and bleeding from the middle meningeal artery. Blood between the dura and the brain is subdural and is caused by rupture of veins in the subdural

space. Blood between the arachnoid membrane and the brain is within the CSF and is called *subarachnoid*. Intracerebral hemorrhage is within the brain tissue and is usually the result of penetrating trauma or rupture of an aneurysm.

42. a. Diffuse axonal injury is the most severe form of brain injury. It results from brain movement within the skull secondary to both acceleration and deceleration forces. These forces cause shearing of the nerve fibers and subsequent damage to the entire nerve. The other listed injuries, although significant, generally result in localized injury, which if treated quickly results in less brain injury.

43. b. Battle's sign does not appear until several hours after suffering a basilar skull fracture; therefore its absence on exam does not mean the patient has not suffered such an injury.

44. a. The halo sign refers to the effect of placing fluid on a piece of clean white paper such as a coffee filter and observing a "halo" of clear fluid staining the paper outward from the droplet. CSF leakage from either the ear or nose, as may occur in a basilar skull fracture, is most useful, but overall the test is highly unreliable and clinical judgment along with other diagnostic tests should be used to diagnose a basilar skull fracture.

45. d. A concussion of the brain is similar to a bruise or contusion. It can result in immediate loss of consciousness or transient changes in mental status as the tissue swells.

46. d. Diffuse axonal injury, the most severe brain injury, presents with all the signs of increased cranial pressure such as decerebrate and decorticate posturing and usually results in prolonged unconsciousness.

47. b. Ventilation of the head-injured patient should be maintained at a normal rate and depth. Studies indicate that hyperventilation results in worsening of cerebral hypoxia and significant acid-base shifts, which can adversely affect the brain.

48. d. Herniation of the brain stem will present with signs and symptoms of increased intracranial pressure. Early signs include decreased level of consciousness, vomiting, and headache. This is

followed by increased systolic blood pressure, widened pulse pressure, and bradycardia (Cushing's triad). Finally, as pressure results in herniation the patient begins to posture and the pupils become fixed and dilated. Survival is unlikely.

49. b. Inability to remember the events before injury is retrograde amnesia, whereas antegrade amnesia is the inability to remember events after the injury. Both are symptoms of head injury. Delirium is a state of agitation often caused by intoxication or drug use as well as various psychiatric conditions. Dementia is a deterioration of cognitive skills such as math and short-term memory, which is slowly progressive and not associated with head injury.

50. c. Nontraumatic back pain can occur without any obvious cause and is very difficult to diagnose. It represents a common reason for EMS transport. The absence of neurological symptoms does not mean they do not have real pain.

51. a. Herniation can occur at any level of the spinal cord and will give symptoms consistent with that level. Sciatica refers to impingement or irritation of the sacral nerve roots and often occurs from muscular irritation and spasm. Herniation occurs when the nucleus pulposus of the intervertebral disk ruptures and exerts pressure on the spinal cord. Generally, sciatica is treated with nonsurgical modalities. Obesity does not predispose patients to disk herniation.

52. b. Any patient with neurological complaints should undergo a full exam including the testing of reflexes, motor function, and sensation. The pain of an aortic aneurysm rupture is usually not associated with neurological symptoms and is not relieved with rest. Renal colic is usually localized to the flank with radiation into the groin but not the leg and is not affected by movement. Administration of analgesics in the prehospital setting is appropriate and should be guided by medical direction.

53. c. The Le Fort fractures involve the midface structures and are categorized into three types depending on what facial bones are involved. Simple nasal and zygoma fractures would not result in gross instability of the face. A basilar skull fracture occurs at the junction of the anterior and middle fossa in the base of the skull and is associated with severe head injury.

54. a. A hyphema is a collection of blood in the anterior chamber often associated with trauma but can occur spontaneously in persons taking anticoagulants. A blowout fracture of the orbit will be demonstrated by the inability to look upward with the affected eye. A ruptured globe may have a hyphema associated with it but also is recognized by a sunken appearance of the globe and an irregularly shaped pupil. Blunt trauma to the eye can bruise the oculomotor nerve resulting in a fixed and dilated pupil; however, it will not affect the patient's level of consciousness.

55. d. It is important to keep the injured eye at rest. Because both eyes move in concert both eyes should be patched. Tetracaine can be administered for pain in the absence of a globe rupture.

56. c. Never use a hemostat to control bleeding without proper surgical training. Direct pressure on the wound along with compression of the temporal artery on the side of the injury will diminish arterial bleeding. Raising the head will diminish venous bleeding.

57. d. Cheyne-Stokes occurs from early ICP increases and is characterized by alternating cycles of deep and shallow breaths. Central neurogenic hyperventilation occurs as pressure rises in the midbrain and is characterized by rapid but shallow breaths. Increased pressure in the medulla results in erratic or ataxic breaths with no recognizable pattern, which usually ends in apnea.

58. d. Systolic blood pressure minus diastolic blood pressure is the pulse pressure. Mean arterial blood pressure is calculated by adding one third of the pulse pressure to the diastolic blood pressure. Cerebral perfusion pressure is the mean arterial pressure minus the intracranial pressure and can be measured only by surgical implantation of a monitor.

59. d. Visual acuity is usually the first thing checked along with a history of eye conditions. Lack of papillary reaction indicates the possibility of a traumatic third nerve palsy, which is associated with high-impact forces. Inability to look upward without pain and double vision is indicative of a blow out fracture of the inferior orbital wall. The corneal reflex is performed when testing cranial nerve function in the comatose patient.

60. c. Zone I neck injuries extend from the base of the neck to the cricoid cartilage. Zone II extends from the cricoid cartilage to the angle of the mandible. Zone II extends from the angle of the mandible upward. Zone II injuries are more common because of their relatively larger size; however, Zone I injuries have the highest mortality because of risk of injury to the major vascular and thoracic structures.

61. d. Emergency airway management in laryngeal and tracheal trauma is controversial. Endotracheal intubation attempts may precipitate laryngospasm resulting in total airway obstruction. Conservative observation and BVM ventilation is usually preferred over early surgical intervention. Cervical spine and thoracic injuries must be considered, and full spinal immobilization is indicated. Subcutaneous emphysema from tracheal disruption is palpable under the skin and feels like Rice Krispies being compressed.

62. b. Injury to the olfactory nerve is the hallmark of a basilar skull fracture and associated with the loss of smell. Facial nerve injury with facial paralysis and auditory nerve injury with deafness are also associated with basilar skull fractures. Compression of the temporal lobe leads to compression of the third cranial nerve causing a fixed and dilated pupil.

63. c. The Glasgow Coma Scale for the patient is 12: 3 points for opening eyes to verbal stimulus, 5 points for localizing pain, and 4 points for speaking clearly but with confused thought processes.

64. c. Glasgow Coma Scale of 13 to 15 is associated with mild head injury; 8 to 12, moderate injury; and less than 8 indicates a severe head injury.

65. b. The old adage "GCS of 8, Intubate" refers to the fact that as LOC decreases the airway becomes less protected and early intubation is indicated. Mannitol is generally indicated only when an acute rise in intracranial pressure is witnessed. Neurological recovery may occur with any head injury, and surgery is indicated only when space-occupying injuries are discovered.

Trauma IV: Thoracic and Abdominal Trauma

9

Thoracic Injuries

1. The mechanism of injury that causes thoracic injury is usually classified as:
   a. sharp or dull
   b. high velocity or low velocity
   c. crushing or tearing
   d. blunt or penetrating

2. Thoracic injury patterns are generally classified as:
   a. sharp or dull
   b. open or closed
   c. crushing or tearing
   d. external or internal

3. The ribs most often fractured are:
   a. 1 to 5
   b. 4 to 9
   c. 6 to 10
   d. 8 to 12

4. Flail chest is defined as:
   a. three or more fractured ribs on the same side of the chest
   b. rib fractures associated with a sternal fracture
   c. two or more adjacent ribs fractured in two or more places
   d. three or more fractured ribs on both sides of the chest

5. The unusual, opposite motion of a flail segment seen during respirations is commonly referred to as:
   a. paroxysmal movement
   b. paradoxical movement
   c. oppositional movement
   d. inordinate movement

6. Management of a patient with a flail chest may include:
   a. applying PASG
   b. transporting the patient without lights and siren
   c. assisting the patient's ventilations with positive pressure
   d. avoiding any contact with the flail segment

7. When air escapes into the soft tissue of the chest wall or neck, the condition is known as:
   a. rhonchi
   b. subcutaneous emphysema
   c. ischemia
   d. parenchyma

8. A critical injury associated with rapid deceleration, such as occurs when a car suddenly stops after hitting an immovable object, is:
   a. spontaneous pneumothorax
   b. myocardial infarction
   c. aortic tear
   d. pulsus paradoxus

9. Sternal fractures often are accompanied by:
   a. myocardial contusion and pulmonary contusion
   b. liver and spleen lacerations
   c. lacerated ventricles and lacerated aorta
   d. diaphragm rupture and migration of abdominal organs to the thoracic cavity

10. An open pneumothorax develops when:
   a. pressure increases within the thoracic cavity because of air exiting the lungs and being unable to escape
   b. air rushes into the chest cavity through a wound when internal thoracic pressure increases
   c. there is a free passage of air between the atmosphere and the pleural space
   d. there is a tear in the tracheobronchial tree allowing air to escape into the soft tissue of the chest

11. A simple pneumothorax occurs when:
   a. air is sucked into the thoracic cavity during expiration
   b. lung tissue is disrupted and air leaks into the pleural space
   c. intrathoracic pressure is greater than atmospheric pressure
   d. air leaks into the pleural space and cannot escape

12. Tension pneumothorax is best described as:
   a. free movement of air between the atmosphere and the pleural space
   b. a disruption of lung tissue that allows air to leak into the pleural space
   c. an open wound that allows air to enter the thoracic cavity
   d. increasing intrapleural pressure that occurs when air can enter the pleural space but cannot escape

13. Signs and symptoms of a tension pneumothorax include:
   a. narrowing pulse pressure, muffled heart sounds, and distended neck veins
   b. dyspnea, bradycardia, and diminished breath sounds on the uninjured side caused by compression
   c. tachycardia, dyspnea, and diminished breath sounds on affected side
   d. decreasing respiratory rate, increasing blood pressure, and bradycardia

14. When a patient develops tracheal deviation caused by a tension pneumothorax:
   a. the trachea deviates away from the injured side
   b. tracheal displacement always occurs immediately
   c. the trachea deviates toward the injured side
   d. the deviation is easily detectable

15. The neck veins of a patient with a tension pneumothorax will most likely be:
   a. normal
   b. flat
   c. unaffected
   d. distended

16. Death from tension pneumothorax is primarily the result of:
   a. rapid development of hypoxia resulting from inability of the lungs to expand
   b. a decrease in venous return to the heart due to compression of the vena cava
   c. profound hypovolemia cause by bleeding into the chest cavity
   d. mediastinal shift, which kinks the trachea, thereby producing suffocation

17. An accumulation of blood in the pleural space is called:
   a. hemothorax
   b. pneumothorax
   c. hemoptysis
   d. pnemococcus

18. The amount of blood each side of the chest cavity of an adult can hold is:
   a. 500 to 1000 mL of blood
   b. 1000 to 2000 mL of blood
   c. 2000 to 3000 mL of blood
   d. 4000 to 5000 mL of blood

19. A hemopneumothorax is characterized by:
   a. a gradual buildup of pressure in one side of the chest because of blood being trapped in the chest cavity and unable to escape
   b. the development of muffled heart sounds and an increased diastolic blood pressure
   c. an accumulation of blood and air in the pleural space
   d. increasing intrapleural pressure accompanied by mediastinal shift toward the injured side

20. Pulmonary contusion is most often associated with:
   a. blunt trauma to the chest
   b. penetrating trauma to the chest
   c. high-energy shock waves from an explosion
   d. tension pneumothorax

21. When managing a patient with a pulmonary contusion, special care must be taken not to:
   a. lay the patient flat
   b. intubate the patient
   c. administer too much oxygen, which may affect the patient's hypoxic drive
   d. overload the patient with IV fluids

22. Early management of an open chest injury includes:
    a. covering the wound with saline-soaked gauze pads
    b. supporting the injured area with sandbags
    c. sealing the wound with an occlusive dressing
    d. pleural decompression

23. If no spinal injuries are present, a patient with an open chest injury should be placed:
    a. supine with the legs elevated
    b. in a position of comfort, usually sitting
    c. in a prone position
    d. on the right side with the head lower than the legs

24. When performing pleural decompression, the proper location for inserting the needle is the:
    a. second or third intercostal space, midclavicular line
    b. second or third intercostal space, midaxillary line
    c. sixth or seventh intercostal space, midclavicular line
    d. ninth or tenth intercostal space, midaxillary line

25. When inserting a needle to decompress the chest, the needle should be inserted:
    a. directly through the rib
    b. below the lower aspect of the rib
    c. above the upper aspect of the rib
    d. either above or below the rib depending on wound location

26. Pericardial tamponade occurs when:
    a. blood or other fluid builds up in the pericardial sac, thereby restricting cardiac filling
    b. the right ventricle becomes too weak to pump and blood backs up in the body's venous system
    c. penetrating trauma to the heart allows the ventricles to pump blood directly into the thoracic cavity resulting in severe hypovolemia
    d. a blockage occurs in coronary arteries significantly limiting perfusion to a large area of myocardium

27. The components of Beck's triad are:
    a. diminished breath sounds, diminished heart sounds, and diminished blood pressure
    b. tachycardia, dyspnea, and a bluish or purple discoloration of the face, neck, and upper shoulders
    c. chest pain radiating down the left arm, dyspnea, and diaphoresis
    d. systolic hypotension (narrow pulse pressure), elevated central venous pressure (jugular vein distention), muffled heart tones

28. Definitive care for pericardial tamponade includes:
    a. pleural decompression
    b. carefully limiting IV fluids
    c. cardioversion
    d. needle pericardiocentesis

29. Myocardial contusion should be suspected if a patient with blunt trauma to the chest presents with:
    a. increased dyspnea
    b. diminished breath sounds on the left side
    c. ECG abnormalities
    d. jugular vein distention associated with hypotension

30. Emergency care in the field for myocardial contusion may include:
    a. prophylactic atropine to reduce vagal tone and prevent bradycardia
    b. pericardiocentesis
    c. pharmacological therapy for dysrhythmias
    d. needle decompression of the chest to reduce intrapleural pressure

31. Traumatic aortic rupture is most often associated with:
    a. low-speed motor vehicle accidents involving rear-end collisions
    b. blunt trauma to the back
    c. pelvic trauma
    d. rapid deceleration

32. High-pressure blunt abdominal trauma is the most common cause of:
    a. retroperitoneal injuries
    b. diaphragmatic rupture
    c. kidney contusion
    d. myocardial contusion

33. The most common cause of esophageal injuries is:
    a. blunt trauma to the throat
    b. rapid compression of the abdomen
    c. penetrating trauma
    d. falls from great heights

34. A common sign of tracheobronchial disruption is:
a. elevated blood pressure
b. bradycardia
c. Battle's sign
d. subcutaneous emphysema

35. A narrowing pulse pressure difference is indicative of:
a. myocardial rupture
b. pericardial tamponade
c. traumatic asphyxia
d. spontaneous pneumothorax

36. Jugular vein distention would most likely be expected in patients with all of the following medical problems *EXCEPT*:
a. severe hemothorax
b. tension pneumothorax
c. pericardial tamponade
d. right ventricular failure

Abdominal Injuries

37. A patient who had a recent injury or blow to the left upper quadrant of the abdomen and who is experiencing pain in the left shoulder should be suspected of having a:
a. retroperitoneal bleed
b. ruptured appendix
c. ruptured spleen
d. pericardial tamponade

38. At an auto accident scene, abdominal injuries would especially be suspected if:
a. the steering wheel is bent
b. the dashboard is broken
c. the front windshield is cracked
d. a passenger is wearing a lap belt but not a shoulder belt

39. When managing a male patient with a genital injury:
a. use a moist sterile dressing for open wounds
b. avoid direct pressure when treating lacerations
c. do not expose the area; leave any physical exam for hospital personnel
d. avoid applying cold packs to the injury

40. Retroperitoneal structures include the:
a. kidneys
b. spleen
c. liver
d. bladder

41. The morbidity and mortality associated with abdominal structure injury are primarily results of:
a. infection causing septic shock
b. abdominal distention causing respiratory compromise
c. hemorrhage causing hypovolemic shock
d. spilling of gastric contents into the abdomen causing metabolic imbalances leading to dysrhythmias

42. Peritonitis is a result of:
a. acute blood loss into the peritoneal cavity
b. chemical irritation to the peritoneum
c. spasms of the abdominal muscles
d. irritation of abdominal contents causing referred pain

43. Peritonitis is most commonly associated with injury to:
a. solid organs
b. retroperitoneal organs
c. vascular organs
d. hollow organs

44. The primary objective when managing serious abdominal injuries accompanied by suspected internal bleeding is to:
a. transport to the hospital closest to the scene
b. provide rapid transport to a hospital capable of surgical intervention
c. provide early IV access and aggressive fluid resuscitation
d. place the patient in PASG to tamponade abdominal bleeding

45. The two most frequently injured solid organs are the:
a. spleen and liver
b. liver and gallbladder
c. pancreas and kidneys
d. kidneys and spleen

46. Use of the pneumatic antishock garment (PASG) for abdominal injuries would be indicated primarily for a patient with:
a. a gunshot wound to the lower abdomen
b. a pelvic fracture
c. a stab wound to the right upper quadrant
d. significant blunt trauma to the left upper quadrant of the abdomen

47. Management of an evisceration includes:
    a. replacing the organ within the abdomen
    b. applying a moist, sterile dressing to the area and covering it with an occlusive dressing
    c. applying direct pressure to the evisceration to control bleeding
    d. applying the PASG and inflating the legs and abdominal compartment

48. The position of choice for a patient with an evisceration and no accompanying spinal or leg injuries is on the:
    a. back with the hips and knees flexed
    b. back with the hips and knees straight
    c. left side
    d. right side

49. Physical signs of acute abdomen include all of the following *EXCEPT*:
    a. rigidity
    b. guarding
    c. distention
    d. bruising

50. You respond to the scene of a multiple-victim shooting. Although one patient is beyond help, the second patient is still alive, although in obvious distress. The patient is having severe difficulty breathing and appears cyanotic. Neck veins are distended and breath sounds are absent on the right side. Your major concern at this point is that the patient may have a:
    a. pericardial tamponade
    b. myocardial contusion
    c. pulmonary contusion
    d. tension pneumothorax

51. Management of this patient is likely to include:
    a. inserting a needle to decompress the chest
    b. performing pericardiocentesis
    c. early IV access and aggressive fluid resuscitation
    d. nebulized albuterol and IV access

52. Upon arriving at the scene of a single-vehicle crash, you notice that a small sports car has tried to take the space occupied by a large tree. There is significant front-end damage to the car. The restrained driver is alert but looks pale and diaphoretic. Further exam shows clear breath sounds but a weak, rapid pulse. His abdomen is soft and there is no pelvic pain on examination. Vital signs reveal a pulse of 136, a blood pressure of 88/60, and respirations of 32. Witnesses state the driver "was flying and passing every car in sight." Based on the mechanism of injury, you suspect the patient has suffered:
    a. a pelvic fracture
    b. a significant liver laceration
    c. an aortic tear
    d. a hemopneumothorax

53. The intervention that will make the greatest difference for this patient is:
    a. starting two large-bore IVs and flowing them wide open
    b. intubating and hyperventilating him
    c. placing him in PASG and inflating all three compartments
    d. rapid transport to a hospital capable of surgical intervention

54. You and your partner respond to a call to assess a patient who was assaulted yesterday. He states he was kicked "in the stomach" and now has increased abdominal pain and that his "left shoulder hurts." Physical examination reveals a bruise over the left upper quadrant and abdominal rigidity. His pulse rate is 126 and his blood pressure is 104/72. Breath sounds are clear bilaterally and present in all fields. You suspect this patient may have:
    a. a lacerated liver
    b. a spleen injury
    c. peritonitis
    d. a ruptured diaphragm

55. A 24-year-old male was working under his car when the jack suddenly slipped. Just before you arrive, family members and neighbors lift the car enough to pull the patient out from under it. As you approach the patient, you immediately see that the skin of his head, neck, and upper chest have an unusual deep red or purple color, and his eyes appear to be bulging. The patient is having severe dyspnea and further examination reveals signs of shock. You suspect this patient is suffering from:
a. traumatic asphyxia
b. spontaneous pneumothorax
c. myocardial contusion
d. pericardial tamponade

56. You and your partner respond to a call for a 22-year-old experiencing chest pain. Upon arrival, you encounter a tall, thin young man who is in mild to moderate respiratory distress. He tells you he suddenly developed sharp chest pain on the right side and then felt short of breath. Vitals reveal a pulse of 118, blood pressure of 122/76, respiratory rate of 28, and oxygen saturation of 92%. You suspect this patient is suffering from:
a. a myocardial infarction
b. an asthma attack
c. a spontaneous pneumothorax
d. pericardial tamponade

57. A 21-year-old female driver of a small, older model sports car has sustained significant injuries as the result of slamming head-on into a tree. There is major deformity to the steering wheel, and the patient is presenting with jugular vein distention, chest pain, and severe dyspnea. Breath sounds are present bilaterally, but pulmonary edema is noted. You suspect this patient may have a:
a. spontaneous pneumothorax
b. myocardial rupture
c. severe hemothorax
d. tracheobronchial disruption

ANSWERS TO CHAPTER 9: TRAUMA IV: THORACIC AND ABDOMINAL TRAUMA

Thoracic Injuries

1. d. The mechanism of injury that causes thoracic injury usually is classified as blunt or penetrating.

2. b. Thoracic injury patterns generally are classified as open or closed.

3. b. The ribs most often fractured are ribs 4 to 9. The reason is that they are thin and poorly protected. Although fractures to ribs 8 through 12 are not as common, fractures to these ribs may be associated with spleen, kidney, or liver injuries.

4. c. Flail chest is defined as two or more adjacent ribs fractured in two or more places. Flail chest is not easily detected in the field because the muscle spasms that often accompany the injury usually keep the flail segment from being discovered.

5. b. Paradoxical movement is the unusual, opposite motion of a flail segment seen during respirations. Because muscle spasms often accompany the injury and keep the flail segment stabilized, paradoxical movement may not be seen when the patient is assessed in the field.

6. c. Management of a flail chest may include assisting the patient's ventilations with positive pressure. A bag-valve-mask should be used to allow the ventilator to monitor lung compliance. Stabilizing the flail segment also may be indicated depending on local protocols. If done, this should be accomplished gently. A pillow can be used to stabilize the segment. Use of PASG should be avoided in these patients because they are at high risk of developing pulmonary edema. Sand bags also should be avoided because they may worsen the injury.

7. b. Subcutaneous emphysema is a collection of air in the soft tissue. This often is associated with some type of disruption of the tracheobronchial tree and is a serious finding. Rhonchi is an abnormal lung sound, parenchyma is the substance of a gland or solid organ, and ischemia involves inadequate blood flow to a tissue.

8. c. Rapid deceleration may cause aortic tear or disruption, which results in rapid and serious blood loss. This is the most common cause of sudden death related to rapid deceleration often associated with high-speed vehicle crashes.

9. a. Sternal fractures are often accompanied by myocardial contusion, pericardial tamponade, and pulmonary contusion. Vascular disruption of thoracic vessels is rare, and seldom is the fracture displaced enough posteriorly to directly impinge on the heart or vessels.

10. c. An open pneumothorax develops when there is a free passage of air between the atmosphere and the pleural space as the result of an open wound to the chest. As internal thoracic pressure decreases, air rushes through the wound into the chest cavity. These wounds are often referred to as "sucking chest wounds" because a "sucking" sound is heard as air moves into and out of the chest through the opening. As air moves in, it displaces the lung tissue and permits collapse of the lung, resulting in a large functional dead space. Also, when internal thoracic pressure decreases there is an inability to ventilate the affected lung.

11. b. A simple pneumothorax, also known as a *closed pneumothorax*, occurs when lung tissue is disrupted and air leaks into the pleural space. A small simple pneumothorax may be difficult to detect in the field and present with only minor to moderate signs and symptoms.

12. d. Tension pneumothorax can be described as increasing intrapleural pressure that occurs when air can enter the pleural space but cannot escape. It can cause a rapid deterioration in the patient's clinical status.

13. c. Common signs and symptoms of tension pneumothorax include increasing dyspnea, tachycardia, diminished or absent breath sounds on the injured side, tracheal deviation, and unequal expansion of the chest.

14. a. In a tension pneumothorax, the trachea deviates away from the injured side and toward the uninjured side. Death is due to a kinking of the superior vena cava caused by deviation of the mediastinum. However, tracheal deviation is a late sign of tension pneumothorax and may be difficult to detect.

15. d. Jugular vein distention is a sign of tension pneumothorax. The distention is caused by the increase in intrathoracic pressure, which slows jugular emptying. However, if the patient is also hypovolemic, distention may not be as notable.

16. b. Although a tension pneumothorax is thought of as respiratory in nature, the usual cause of death is cardiovascular in nature. As pressure increases and mediastinal shift occurs, the vena cava is compressed. Venous return to heart is decreased to the point that cardiac output is not sufficient to sustain life.

17. a. A hemothorax is an accumulation of blood in the pleural space. It is caused by bleeding from the lung parenchyma or damaged blood vessels.

18. c. Each side of the adult chest cavity has the capacity to hold between 2000 and 3000 mL of blood. The potential is therefore great that a patient with bleeding into the chest can develop profound shock and death.

19. c. A hemopneumothorax is characterized by an accumulation of blood and air in the pleural space.

20. a. Pulmonary contusion is most commonly associated with blunt trauma to the chest or rapid deceleration forces that cause the lung to contact the chest wall. The underlying area of lung bruising is usually directly proportional to the area of injury. It is less frequently associated with penetrating trauma or high-energy shock waves from an explosion. Aggressive CPR may also cause pulmonary contusion.

21. d. Because pulmonary contusion involves bruising of the lung tissue, EMS personnel must be especially careful not to fluid overload patients because this can quickly lead to the development of pulmonary edema. The patient should be given high flow oxygen and may need to be intubated to provide ventilatory support. If spinal injury is suspected, the patient will need to be immobilized on a backboard and the head of the board may need to be slightly elevated to improve respiratory effort.

22. c. Early management of an open chest injury includes sealing the wound with an occlusive dressing. This should be accomplished at the same time as the initial assessment of the airway.

23. b. If no spinal injuries are suspected, a patient with an open chest injury should be placed in a position of comfort that does not interfere with breathing.

24. a. When pleural decompression is performed, the proper location for inserting a needle is the second or third intercostal space, midclavicular line. An alternate site is the fifth or sixth intercostal space, midaxillary line.

25. c. The needle should be inserted over the rib to avoid the nerve, artery, and vein that lie just beneath each rib. To ensure correct insertion, insert the needle in such a way that the upper part of the rib is struck, and then the needle is "walked" up and over the rib.

26. a. Pericardial tamponade occurs when blood or other fluid builds up in the pericardial sac, thereby restricting cardiac filling and reducing cardiac output. Although rare, pericardial tamponade has a high mortality rate.

27. d. The presence of Beck's triad is a good indicator that pericardial tamponade exists. The three components of the triad are systolic hypotension (and more specifically a narrowing pulse pressure), elevated central venous pressure (evidenced by jugular vein distention), and muffled heart tones. Although it is a good indicator of pericardial tamponade, Beck's triad is seen in only about 30% of patients and generally in advanced stages of tamponade. Therefore EMS personnel should be alert to the possibility of pericardial tamponade based on the mechanism of injury.

28. d. Definitive care for pericardial tamponade involves removing some of the fluid that has accumulated in the pericardial sac, a procedure that is not usually performed in the field. Therefore rapid transportation to a hospital is needed. Administration of some IV fluids to maximize venous return may be helpful. Always consult medical direction for specific guidance.

29. c. The clinical findings in myocardial contusion are often subtle and may therefore be easily overlooked especially if there are other more obvious injuries or little evidence of thoracic injury. The patient may have no symptoms or may complain of chest pain similar to that of a myocardial infarction. ECG abnormalities may be the best clue that myocardial contusion has occurred.

30. c. Because myocardial contusion may produce lethal ECG dysrhythmias, pharmacological therapy may be indicated. The patient is often tachycardic, not bradycardic. Also, interventions that increase myocardial oxygen consumption should be avoided.

31. d. Traumatic aortic rupture is thought to be a result of shearing forces that develop between tissues that decelerate at different rates. Rapid deceleration in high-speed motor vehicle crashes and falls from great heights are common mechanisms of injury that can cause traumatic aortic rupture.

32. b. High-pressure blunt abdominal trauma is the most common cause of diaphragmatic rupture. When traumatic diaphragmatic rupture occurs, abdominal organs may herniate into the thoracic cavity. Signs and symptoms may be similar to that seen in tension pneumothorax, with the patient complaining of dyspnea and with signs of hypoxia, hypotension, and JVD present. Breath sounds may be absent below a certain point on the chest because the abdominal organ does not allow the lung to expand into that area. Additionally, bowel sounds may be heard in the chest, most commonly on the left side.

33. c. The most common cause of esophageal injuries is penetrating trauma, such as from knife or missile wounds.

34. d. Subcutaneous emphysema is a common sign of tracheobronchial disruption. This is due to air leaking out of the tracheobronchial tree and into the surrounding soft tissue. Battle's sign is ecchymosis over the mastoid that indicates basilar skull fracture.

35. b. A narrowing pulse pressure difference is indicative of pericardial tamponade. As blood enters the pericardial space, there is an increase in pericardial pressure. The increase in pericardial pressure does not allow the heart to expand and refill with blood, resulting in a decrease in stroke volume and cardiac output.

36. a. EMS providers would expect to see jugular vein distention in patients with tension pneumothorax, pericardial tamponade, or right ventricular failure. Its presence would not be expected in cases of severe hemothorax because there is not enough blood volume to allow the jugular veins to become engorged.

Abdominal Injuries

37. c. A patient who had a recent injury or blow to the left upper quadrant of the abdomen and who is experiencing pain in the left shoulder should be suspected of having a ruptured spleen. The pain in the left shoulder is referred pain, caused by aggravation of the phrenic nerve.

38. d. If a passenger in a vehicle was wearing a lap belt but no shoulder belt, suspect abdominal injuries. Also, even in situations when the patient is wearing a shoulder belt, if the lap belt is worn too loosely, the patient can "submarine" under the lap belt and sustain abdominal injuries.

39. a. A moist sterile dressing should be applied to open wounds of the male genitalia. Direct pressure may be used to control bleeding, and cold packs may be applied to blunt injuries. If a genital injury is suspected, expose the area and do a physical exam to be sure no tissue has been avulsed.

40. a. The kidneys and pancreas are both retroperitoneal structures. The spleen and liver are intraperitoneal and the bladder is a pelvic organ.

41. c. The morbidity and mortality associated with abdominal structure injury are primarily the results of hemorrhage. Hemorrhage may result from injury to both solid and hollow organs and from damage to intraabdominal vascular structures.

42. b. Peritonitis is related to chemical irritation of the peritoneum, usually the result of spillage of gastric contents. Blood is not a chemical irritant to the peritoneum. Muscular spasm is a result of peritonitis, not a cause.

43. d. Injury to hollow organs often results in rupture and spillage of their contents. This results in peritonitis.

44. b. Surgical intervention often is the only effective therapy when managing a serious abdominal injury accompanied by suspected internal bleeding. The closest hospital is not necessarily the best choice, because if the hospital does not have readily available surgical services the patient may have to be transported elsewhere, adding to the delay in definitive care. Use of PASG and aggressive fluid resuscitation are controversial. Pouring in IV fluids or placing PASG on the patient will do little good if the site of the bleeding cannot be controlled. These interventions may actually increase the rate of bleeding by raising blood pressure and/or dislodging blood clots. Always follow local protocols on PASG use and fluid resuscitation.

45. a. The spleen and liver are the two most commonly injured solid organs. Both organs are large and relatively unprotected. Injury to either organ may produce serious blood loss.

46. b. Although guidelines for use of the pneumatic antishock garment (PASG) vary, its primary value appears to be in cases of pelvic fracture, especially if hypotension is present.

47. b. Eviscerations should be covered with moist, sterile dressings that are then covered with an occlusive dressing. The organs should not be replaced, and direct pressure should not be applied to the area. The abdominal compartment of the PASG should not be inflated over an evisceration.

48. a. If there are no accompanying spinal or leg injuries, transport an evisceration patient on his or her back with the hips and knees flexed to decrease abdominal pressure.

49. d. Rigidity, guarding, and distention are all signs of acute abdomen. Although bruising may indicate the presence of an underlying abdominal injury, it is not a sign of acute abdomen.

50. d. The severe dyspnea, distended neck veins, and, most important, absence of breath sounds on one side indicate that this patient most likely has a tension pneumothorax. It is critical EMS personnel recognize tension pneumothorax because it is a condition that will become rapidly fatal if left untreated.

51. a. This patient needs needle decompression to relieve the pressure that has built up in his thoracic cavity.

52. c. Because of the rapid deceleration that has occurred, this patient likely has an aortic tear. Pelvic fracture is unlikely with the absence of pain, and the abdomen would likely be rigid with a liver laceration.

53. d. Aortic tears are associated with rapid exsanguination and result in a very high mortality rate. If there is any chance of saving the patient, he must arrive as quickly as possible at a hospital capable of surgical intervention. Pouring in IV fluids or placing PASG on the patient will do little good because the site of the bleeding cannot be controlled. These interventions may actually increase the rate of bleeding by raising blood pressure and/or dislodging blood clots.

54. b. The blunt trauma to the left upper quadrant, referred pain in the left shoulder, and signs of developing hypovolemic shock should make EMS personnel highly suspicious of splenic injury. Signs of peritonitis, or generalized irritation, are not present. Also, clearly heard breath sounds in all fields help to rule out the possibility of ruptured diaphragm with associated movement of abdominal contents into the thoracic cavity.

55. a. The patient is displaying classic signs of traumatic asphyxia, which is to be expected considering the mechanism of injury. An increase in intrathoracic pressure forces blood from the right side of the heart into the veins of the upper thorax, neck, and face, causing the hallmark discoloration of the face, neck, and upper chest.

56. c. Your patient has most likely experienced a spontaneous pneumothorax. Spontaneous pneumothorax occurs when a subpleural bleb (a cystic lesion on a lobe of the lung) ruptures and allows air to enter the pleural space. This type of pneumothorax often occurs in apparently healthy young, tall, and thin males. Signs and symptoms include a sudden onset of chest pain and dyspnea, tachycardia, decreased breath sounds on the affected side, and in more serious cases, cyanosis and altered mental status. Spontaneous pneumothoraces are often well tolerated by the patient.

57. b. Myocardial rupture occurs when blood-filled chambers of the ventricles are compressed with sufficient force to rupture the chamber wall, septum, or valves. These patients often present with a significant mechanism of injury and signs and symptoms of congestive heart failure or pericardial tamponade.

TRAUMA V: MUSCULOSKELETAL TRAUMA

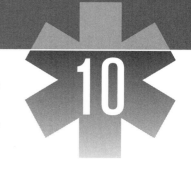

10

1. Which of the following is true about musculoskeletal trauma?
   a. lower extremity injuries generally bleed less than upper extremity injuries
   b. lower extremity injuries are associated with milder mechanisms of injury than upper extremity injuries
   c. upper extremity injuries are rarely life threatening
   d. pelvic injuries are simple to diagnose in the field

2. The axial skeleton consists of how many movable vertebrae?
   a. 21
   b. 24
   c. 26
   d. 29

3. Match the bone with its associated artery, which can be injured by a fracture.
   a. humerus   1. popliteal
   b. radius/ulna   2. tibialis anterior
   c. rib   3. brachial
   d. femur   4. intercostal
   e. tibia/fibula   5. radial

4. The portion of a long bone that contains the marrow is the:
   a. metaphysis
   b. epiphysis
   c. diaphysis
   d. periosteum

5. As we age, all of the following are true *EXCEPT:*
   a. the degree of osteoporosis is related to the incidence of fractures
   b. the costal cartilage ossifies, making the thorax more rigid
   c. wrist fractures are the most common
   d. water content of the intervertebral disks decreases

6. A 16-year-old football player is tackled, landing on his shoulder. He is able to move the upper arm freely but complains of pain over the top of the shoulder. On palpation you find tenderness and swelling at the distal end of the clavicle. He most likely has:
   a. an anterior shoulder dislocation
   b. a shoulder separation
   c. a humerus fracture
   d. a posterior shoulder dislocation

7. _____ connect bone to bone across any joint.
   a. Ligaments
   b. Tendons
   c. Synovial bursae
   d. Cartilage

8. The function and purpose of bones include:
   a. protecting vital organs
   b. acting as attachment points for tendons, cartilage, and ligaments
   c. producing red blood cells
   d. all of the above

9. The types of joints that allow the greatest degree of movement are:
   a. synovial joints
   b. cartilaginous joints
   c. fibrous joints
   d. sutured joints

10. A young boy has fallen on his hand. There is a deformity of the second joint in his third finger, and you suspect a dislocation. This joint is called the:
    a. proximal interphalangeal joint
    b. distal interphalangeal joint
    c. metacarpal-phalangeal joint
    d. metatarsal-phalangeal joint

11. The serious complications associated with musculoskeletal injuries include all the following *EXCEPT:*
    a. hemorrhage
    b. disruption of nerve and arterial supply
    c. fat embolism
    d. unsightly scars

12. While examining a patient who twisted her ankle you check for pulses. Which is correct?
    a. The tibialis anterior pulse is behind the lateral malleolus.
    b. The dorsalis pedis is on the dorsum of the foot proximal to the second and third toes.
    c. The tibialis anterior pulse is anterior to the medial malleolus.
    d. None of the above are correct.

13. A long bone fracture that involves several breaks in the bone with multiple fragments is called a:
    a. greenstick fracture
    b. comminuted fracture
    c. transverse fracture
    d. spiral fracture

14. An injury to the tendons, muscles, or ligaments around a joint, marked by pain, swelling, and discoloration of the overlying skin is called a:
    a. sprain
    b. strain
    c. dislocation
    d. fracture

15. Your patient has an obvious deformity to his forearm and you notice the end of the bone protruding through a large laceration. This is referred to as a(n):
    a. open fracture
    b. contaminated fracture
    c. comminuted fracture
    d. dislocated fracture

16. The difference between a subluxation and a dislocation is:
    a. subluxations are worse than dislocations
    b. dislocations are more easily reduced
    c. dislocations result in greater displacement between the bones
    d. there is no difference

17. Typical blood loss in an uncomplicated femur fracture is approximately:
    a. less than 500 mL
    b. 500 to 1000 mL
    c. 1000 to 2000 mL
    d. 2000 to 3000 mL

18. Tendonitis is:
    a. caused by cartilage damage in the joint
    b. a rupture of the tendon
    c. an inflammation of the bursa surrounding the joint
    d. an inflammation of the tendon

19. All of the following are degenerative conditions *EXCEPT:*
    a. osteoarthritis
    b. bursitis
    c. rheumatoid arthritis
    d. gouty arthritis

20. The most important factor to determine when evaluating patients with serious musculoskeletal trauma is:
    a. whether there is vascular compromise in the injured extremity
    b. whether they have any life-threatening conditions
    c. whether there is a fracture or merely a simple sprain
    d. whether they can bear weight on the injured extremity

21. Which of the following is not considered one of the six Ps of musculoskeletal trauma?
    a. pain
    b. paresthesias
    c. pulses
    d. purple

22. When assessing musculoskeletal injuries the mnemonic *DCAP-BTLS* is used. Complete the following:

    D _____
    C _____
    A _____
    P _____
    B _____
    T _____
    L _____
    S _____

23. The treatment of fractures includes all of the following *EXCEPT:*
    a. apply warm compresses to reduce spasm
    b. splint in position of comfort unless neurovascular compromise is present
    c. elevate injury to reduce swelling
    d. administer analgesics per protocol for the control of pain

24. When applying a splint to an injured extremity:
    a. leave open fractures uncovered so that bleeding can be assessed
    b. check pulses twice only if not present before splint is applied
    c. elevate above heart to improve circulation
    d. splint both the joint above and below the injury site

25. Limb-threatening injuries are due to neurovascular compromise and are associated with each of the following injuries *EXCEPT*:
    a. knee dislocation/fractures
    b. mid-shaft radius fractures
    c. ankle dislocation/fractures
    d. subcondylar fractures of the elbow

26. Reduction of hip, knee, and ankle dislocations:
    a. should be attempted only once if there is neurovascular compromise
    b. is easier the longer the dislocation is left alone
    c. should be attempted before attending to other injuries
    d. should be performed without analgesics, which may cause respiratory depression

27. A pelvic fracture results in severe bleeding from disruption of:
    a. the periosteum, which is rich in blood vessels
    b. the symphysis pubis, causing a rupture of the urethra
    c. the sacroiliac joint, causing rupture of the iliac arteries
    d. the posterior attachment of the aorta, resulting in aortic rupture

28. A patient has had a seizure, and upon arousal, he finds he is unable to move his right shoulder because of pain. He presents holding his arm over his head with the elbow bent and hand resting on his head. He is requesting something for pain. Which of the following is true?
    a. He has suffered an anterior shoulder dislocation.
    b. Having his arm over his head means he has not injured his shoulder and is probably seeking drugs.
    c. He has suffered a posterior shoulder dislocation.
    d. He has suffered a rotator cuff injury from the force of the muscle contractions during the seizure.

29. You respond to the victim of a motorcycle crash. He complains of severe pain in the midthigh of his left leg, and you note a deformity there with marked swelling. Bleeding from a femur fracture can be severe because the popliteal artery is disrupted.
    a. true
    b. false

30. A man reports a sudden pain in his right calf after going up for a rebound while playing basketball. He complains of pain with weight bearing, and on examination you feel a depression at the back of his ankle distal to the calf muscle. You suspect what condition?
    a. ankle fracture
    b. deep venous thrombosis
    c. rupture of the Achilles tendon
    d. fracture of the talus of the foot

31. Appropriate treatment for suspected pelvic fractures includes all of the following *EXCEPT*:
    a. aggressive preparation for shock by establishing large-bore intravenous lines
    b. application of PASG for stabilization of the fractures
    c. forceful manual compression of the pelvis to determine whether an unstable fracture exists
    d. immobilization on a long spine board

32. At the scene of a motor vehicle accident you find that the driver was hit from his side and appears to have a broken humerus. He is complaining of neck pain, and you apply a cervical collar. Which of the following is true about splinting the humerus fracture?
    a. Once the cervical collar is applied the arm may be placed in an arm sling secured around the neck.
    b. The fracture may be difficult to stabilize.
    c. Always immobilize the long bone fracture before securing the patient to the long board.
    d. None of the above are true.

33. All of the following are important points about splinting injuries *EXCEPT*:
    a. the splint should stabilize the joint above and below the injury
    b. only commercially available splints should be used by professional prehospital services to avoid potential claims of negligence
    c. the splint should be appropriately padded over the bony prominences
    d. the splint should allow for assessment of neurovascular status

34. A hockey player falls twisting his ankle. On examination you find it dislocated, and the foot is angulated laterally. The foot is cold and pulseless. Before splinting it you decide to attempt to reduce the dislocation. This is best accomplished by:
a. gentle and steady longitudinal traction in-line with the lower leg
b. administration of analgesics and sedatives such as morphine and midazolam
c. checking the pulse before and after reduction
d. all of the above

35. A Colles' fracture involves:
a. the distal radius of the wrist
b. the mid portion of the forearm resulting in a volar angulation
c. a dislocation of the wrist
d. an impaction of the head of the humerus

ANSWERS TO CHAPTER 10: TRAUMA V: MUSCULOSKELETAL TRAUMA

1. c. Both lower and upper extremity injuries occur from similar mechanisms of injury. Bleeding from a femoral fracture can be severe and is worse than that of the humerus. Upper extremity injuries alone rarely are life threatening. Signs of a pelvic injury usually are limited to pain on palpation and their severity cannot be determined accurately without x-rays.

2. b. The axial skeleton consists of 24 movable (7 cervical, 12 thoracic, and 5 lumbar) and 8 nonmovable vertebrae (5 fused vertebrae in the sacrum and 3 fused vertebrae in the coccyx).

3. a. brachial; b. radial; c. intercostal; d. popliteal; e. tibialis anterior

4. c. Long bones such as the humerus and femur are composed of four components. The diaphysis is the shaft made of dense, compact bone, which contains the bone marrow. The epiphysis is at the ends of the bone, where it articulates with other bones and is the major site of growth. The metaphysis is the portion between the diaphysis and epiphysis. The fourth component, the periosteum, is the outer covering containing vasculature and nerves.

5. c. The most common fractures associated with aging are compression fractures of the vertebra. As we age, loss of calcium results in osteoporosis, which weakens the bones and makes them prone to fractures. Cartilage ossifies and the vertebral disks lose their water content, resulting in loss of height and stiffening of the spine.

6. b. The distal end of the clavicle is joined to the acromion process of the scapula by a ligament. Landing on the top of the shoulder results in a strain or separation of this ligament and is called a *shoulder separation*. A shoulder dislocation would restrict the free movement of the upper arm, and a humerus fracture would be demonstrated by pain and deformity over the upper arm.

7. a. Ligaments connect bone to bone across a joint and give the joint lateral stability. Tendons connect muscle to bone and transfer the force of muscle contraction into motion. Cartilage covers the ends of bones where they articulate and reduces friction. Large joints contain a fluid-filled sac called the *synovial bursa*, which reduces friction between the tendon and the joint it crosses.

8. d. The bony chest wall protects the heart, lung, and upper abdominal organs such as the liver, kidneys, and spleen. They serve as the integral part of joints and provide the structural attachments of tendons, cartilage, and ligaments. The bone marrow is the site of red blood cell production and is vital to our survival.

9. a. There are three classifications of joints. Synovial joints are fluid filled and contain the articulation of two or more bones. The joints involved in movement such as the shoulder, elbow, hip, knee, and ankle are synovial joints. Cartilaginous joints occur where two nonarticulating bones meet. The symphysis pubis is an example of a cartilaginous joint. Fibrous joints occur where two bones grow together as is seen in the skull where they are called *sutures*.

10. a. The fingers, or phalanges, are joined to the hand by the metacarpal-phalangeal joint. Each of the four fingers is composed of three phalanges connected by interphalangeal joints. The proximal and middle phalanxes are connected by the proximal interphalangeal joint and the middle and distal phalanx by the distal interphalangeal joint. The thumb has only two phalanxes. The metatarsal-phalangeal joints are in the foot.

11. d. Although open fractures can result in wounds that scar, this is not a serious physiological complication. Fracture of bones and disruption of muscle and tendons can lead to rupture and injury to arterial and nerve supply, which can result in long-term disability. Hemorrhage from a fracture can be severe and life threatening, and fractures to long bones can result in embolization of bone marrow fat into the bloodstream.

12. b. The tibialis anterior artery runs posterior to the medial malleolus of the ankle, and the dorsalis pedis artery runs across the top (dorsum) of the foot and is usually palpable proximal to the second and third toes.

13. b. When a fracture is described, the direction and number of breaks are used. A greenstick fracture occurs when only one side of the bone is broken and the bone is bent. This occurs in young children whose bones are less calcified and more pliable. The comminuted fracture refers to one in which multiple bony fragments exist. The transverse fracture occurs when the fracture line extends straight across the long axis of the bone as is seen when a blunt object strikes the upper arm. A spiral fracture occurs when the mechanism of injury involves rotation around the long axis of the bone.

14. **a.** Sprains occur when the tissue is torn leading to swelling and discoloration resulting from bleeding. Strains are less severe forms of sprains and do not result in discoloration. They can be limited to muscles. Dislocations occur when the normal articulation of two or more bones is disrupted. Fractures occur only to bones.

15. **a.** Any time the skin is open over a fracture you must consider it an open fracture whether bone was ever seen protruding from the wound. The wound should be protected from further contamination. With the advent of stronger antibiotics, the risk of infection has been reduced dramatically.

16. **c.** The normal articulation is disrupted in both subluxations and dislocations. However, subluxations result in only a portion of the articulation being displaced, whereas dislocations affect the entire articulation. Although both injuries can be reduced with traction, the dislocation requires greater effort and is associated with greater injury to the joint.

17. **c.** The femur fracture can bleed profusely and one fifth or more of the body's blood volume can be lost. For this reason, aggressive treatment for shock should always be initiated when caring for patients with this injury.

18. **d.** When the tendon becomes inflamed a condition called *tendonitis* occurs. The bursa surrounding a joint also can become inflamed, resulting in bursitis.

19. **b.** Bursitis is an acute inflammation of the fluid-filled sack surrounding a joint. Arthritis occurs over time from chronic inflammation and the slow deterioration of age.

20. **b.** Isolated musculoskeletal injuries are rarely life threatening alone. Any patient with trauma should be evaluated for a more serious condition such as impaired airway, breathing, or circulation. The ability to bear weight on an injured extremity does not eliminate the possibility that a fracture or significant injury has occurred.

21. **d.** When assessing a musculoskeletal injury, you can look for six *P*s: Pain, on movement or palpation; Pallor, or pale skin indicating poor capillary refill; Paresthesias, a pins-and-needles sensation from compression on nerves; Pulses, either diminished or absent; Paralysis from total nerve transaction; Pressure, from swelling.

22. DCAP-BTLS is Deformity, Contusions, Abrasions, Punctures, Burns, Tenderness, Lacerations, Swelling.

23. **a.** The application of warm compresses results in more swelling and pain and should not be part of the treatment of fractures. Splinting in a position of comfort or the anatomical position will result in the best blood flow and pain control. Elevation reduces swelling and pain. Analgesics such as morphine are a useful adjunct in the care of fractures.

24. **d.** Proper splinting of a fracture requires the immobilization of the joints above and below the injury as any movement by these joints may cause the fracture site to move. Pulses should be checked both before and after splinting and open fractures should be covered with a dry sterile dressing. Although elevation is helpful, it is not part of the splinting process.

25. **b.** The knee fracture/dislocation can result in disruption of the popliteal artery leading to loss of the lower leg. Similar limb-threatening injuries can occur with ankle fractures involving the tibialis anterior and posterior arteries and the elbow fracture involving the brachial artery. Radius fractures are not typically associated with neurovascular compromise.

26. **a.** Reduction of joint dislocations becomes more difficult as the swelling worsens with time and should be performed only in an attempt to reestablish blood flow to the affected limb. A thorough survey for other injuries should always be performed before attending to any injury. The reduction of a dislocation is best facilitated with the administration of narcotic analgesics.

27. **c.** The iliac arteries bridge and are tightly adhered to the sacroiliac joints. A pelvic fracture

that spreads this joint apart causes them to rupture, resulting in potentially life-threatening hemorrhage.

28. c. Dislocation of the shoulder joint occurs when the humerus pops out of its normal position against the glenoid fossa of the scapula and moves either anterior or posterior to the glenoid. Anterior dislocations result in a boxlike deformity, in which the shoulder loses its normal rounded appearance and the arm is held tightly to the chest. The posterior shoulder dislocation locks the humerus behind the glenoid, inhibiting it from being lowered. The patient will carry the arm over the head for comfort. The posterior shoulder dislocation occurs in seizures because of the forceful contraction of the back and upper arm muscles. Rotator cuff injuries occur from excessive pulling on the shoulder and are not associated with seizures.

29. b. False. The source of bleeding from a femur fracture is from the periosteum of the femur, which is rich in blood vessels. The popliteal artery is rarely injured in the simple femur fracture.

30. c. The Achilles tendon attaches the calf muscles with the heel. It ruptures during forceful plantar flexion as occurs in sprinting or jumping. Usually the rupture can be felt under the skin on the posterior of the ankle. Ankle fractures usually are associated with swelling and deformity to the entire ankle joint.

31. c. Hemorrhage from pelvic fractures can be severe and life threatening and should be treated aggressively by being prepared for it with large-bore IVs. The application of PASG and placement on a long spine board stabilize the fractures and minimize bleeding. It is not necessary to actually feel instability of the pelvis to have a suspicion that a serious injury has occurred. In fact, excessive movement of the pelvis during such a maneuver could result in greater bleeding.

32. b. In the presence of a possible cervical spine injury never affix a splint around the neck and always secure the patient to the long board before splinting the extremity. Because the shoulder joint is difficult to stabilize, it makes stabilization of the humerus fracture difficult.

33. b. Any suitable material may be used to splint a musculoskeletal injury as long as the other listed issues are addressed.

34. d. The reduction of a joint dislocation is most easily performed with in-line traction and a gentle steady pull. It is followed by a palpable rotation into normal position. Pulses should be checked before and after the reduction.

35. a. A Colles' fracture is one of the most common fractures to the wrist and involves a fracture of the distal radius resulting in a "silver-fork" deformity with dorsal angulation.

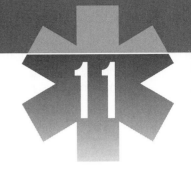

1. Understanding respiratory diseases and how to assess and manage them is vital because:
   a. most of the medications in the drug box are for the treatment of respiratory emergencies
   b. they usually present with minimal signs and symptoms
   c. they represent a significant percentage of EMS calls and often can be life threatening
   d. they rarely lead to death

2. Intrinsic risk factors that increase the chance of developing respiratory disease include all of the following *EXCEPT*:
   a. cigarette smoking
   b. genetic predisposition
   c. cardiac disease
   d. physical and emotional stress

3. The most important intrinsic risk factor that increases the risk of developing respiratory disease is:
   a. cigarette smoking
   b. genetic predisposition
   c. history of cancer
   d. stress

4. Cigarette smoking and environmental pollutants are examples of what _____ factors, which increase the risk of developing respiratory disease?
   a. extrinsic
   b. genetic
   c. inherent
   d. intrinsic

5. The primary function of the respiratory system is:
   a. to buffer the metabolic acids
   b. removal of mucus from the lungs
   c. to filter dust from the air
   d. gas exchange

6. The process of air movement in and out of the lungs is called:
   a. respiration
   b. ventilation
   c. diffusion
   d. perfusion

7. For ventilation to occur all of the following must be present *EXCEPT*:
   a. diaphragm and intercostal muscles must be functional
   b. oxygen must be present in the air
   c. upper and lower airway must be patent
   d. the alveoli must be intact and not collapsed

8. The process by which gas exchange occurs between the air-filled alveoli and the pulmonary capillary bed is called:
   a. osmosis
   b. perfusion
   c. diffusion
   d. dispersion

9. The space between the alveoli and capillary bed is called the:
   a. interstitial space
   b. potential space
   c. inner space
   d. pleural space

10. Enlargement of the interstitial space with fluid or the thickening of the alveoli wall results in:
    a. increased diffusion leading to hypoxia and hypercarbia
    b. decreased perfusion leading to hypoxia and hypocarbia
    c. increased perfusion leading to hypoxia and hypercarbia
    d. decreased diffusion leading to hypoxia and hypercarbia

11. When problems with diffusion cause respiratory emergencies, the treatment initially consists of:
    a. improving perfusion by increasing blood pressure
    b. provision of high-flow oxygen and measures to remove the fluid in the interstitial space
    c. assisting ventilation with a bag-valve-mask
    d. intubation

12. The primary function of the upper airway is to:
    a. filter and humidify the air
    b. facilitate oxygen exchange
    c. generate mucus containing histamine to fight allergies
    d. create the sound of speech

13. The upper airway consists of all of the following *EXCEPT*:
    a. nares
    b. bronchioles
    c. larynx
    d. pharynx

14. The removal of foreign material from the lower airways is the role of the:
    a. alveoli
    b. cilia
    c. bronchi
    d. trachea

15. The lower airway consists of the following *EXCEPT*:
    a. bronchi
    b. alveoli
    c. trachea
    d. bronchioles

16. Carbon dioxide diffuses from the pulmonary capillaries into the alveoli because:
    a. the hemoglobin in the capillaries has very little oxygen
    b. the hydrostatic pressure is greater in the capillaries
    c. the oxygen concentration is higher in the alveoli
    d. the partial pressure of carbon dioxide is higher in the capillaries

17. Protecting the lungs, facilitating ventilation, and supporting the anatomical structures of the respiratory system is the function of the:
    a. abdominal muscles
    b. chest wall
    c. spinal column
    d. vagus nerve

18. During inspiration the:
    a. diaphragm relaxes and the intercostal muscles contract
    b. diaphragm and the intercostal muscles contract
    c. diaphragm contracts and the intercostal muscles relax
    d. diaphragm and intercostal muscles relax

19. The diaphragm is controlled by the _____ nerve
    a. vagus
    b. cranial
    c. phrenic
    d. intercostal

20. Elevation of $PaCO_2$ in the blood results in:
    a. lowering of cerebrospinal fluid pH
    b. elevation of blood pH
    c. elevation of cerebrospinal fluid pH
    d. decreased respiratory rate

21. What part of the brain controls respiration?
    a. medulla
    b. cerebellum
    c. cerebrum
    d. cranial nerves

22. All of the following innervate the structures of the respiratory system *EXCEPT*:
    a. thoracic spinal nerves
    b. Hering-Breuer reflex
    c. vagus nerve
    d. phrenic nerve

23. The last reflex to stimulate respiration occurs:
    a. when the concentration of oxygen in the alveoli decreases to a critical level
    b. when the peripheral chemoreceptors in the aortic arch and carotid artery sense a decrease in the arterial oxygen level
    c. when the pH decreases to a critical level
    d. when the pH increases to a critical level

24. Which of the following statements most accurately describes the difference between ventilation and respiration?
    a. Respiration is the process of breathing, whereas ventilation concerns only the alveoli.
    b. Ventilation is affected by fluid in the interstitial space, whereas respiration is affected by spasm of the bronchioles.
    c. Ventilation and respiration are the same thing.
    d. Ventilation affects removal of carbon dioxide, and respiration concerns the ability to oxygenate the blood.

25. While assessing a patient with a respiratory complaint, you note an alteration in mental status, stridor, diaphoresis, and tachycardia. These are signs of:
   a. cerebral vascular accident
   b. life-threatening respiratory distress
   c. acute myocardial infarction
   d. typical asthma attack

26. Use of accessory muscles, presence of cyanosis, and two-word dyspnea indicate?
   a. need for intubation
   b. indication for intravenous epinephrine
   c. impending respiratory failure
   d. likelihood of aspiration

27. If your patient indicates that during her last respiratory attack she required intubation, this indicates:
   a. increased likelihood that intubation will be required again
   b. she waited too long to seek help
   c. she has moderate disease
   d. she can be treated and released at the scene

28. Common pulmonary medications include all of the following *EXCEPT:*
   a. prednisone
   b. propranolol
   c. albuterol
   d. theophylline

29. The respiratory rate is an excellent indicator of the severity of respiratory distress.
   a. true
   b. false

30. Bradycardia and slowing respiratory rate during a respiratory emergency indicate:
   a. resolution of respiratory distress
   b. exhaustion, hypoxia, and imminent cardiac arrest
   c. expected effects of the medication given to treat the attack
   d. the effects of anxiety and stress

31. Barrel chest deformity, clubbing of the fingernails, and peripheral cyanosis indicate:
   a. acute respiratory distress
   b. hypercarbia
   c. tobacco abuse
   d. long-standing chronic lung disease

32. In which of the following conditions is pulse oximetry completely unreliable?
   a. carbon monoxide poisoning
   b. chlorine inhalation
   c. congestive heart failure
   d. severe asthma attack

33. Albuterol, terbutaline, and epinephrine improve ventilation through what mechanism?
   a. parasympathomimetic
   b. sympathomimetic
   c. anticholinergic
   d. muscarinic

34. The most important medication to administer to someone in severe respiratory distress is:
   a. subcutaneous epinephrine
   b. oxygen
   c. inhaled albuterol
   d. intravenous steroids

35. While a patient in respiratory distress is treated, which of the following is true regarding intravenous steroid administration?
   a. It is indicated in respiratory distress from congestive heart failure.
   b. It decreases the likelihood of the patient requiring prehospital intubation.
   c. It improves oxygenation by reducing mucus production.
   d. It has a delayed onset but may lessen the severity of the attack.

36. Acute respiratory distress syndrome (ARDS) is:
   a. unlikely to result from pneumonia or sepsis
   b. often associated with stridor and signs of airway obstruction
   c. fluid accumulation in the pulmonary interstitial space resulting from increased permeability of the alveoli capillary membranes
   d. the result of repeated asthma attacks leading to scarring of the alveoli walls and the development of blebs

37. Asthma, emphysema, and chronic bronchitis are examples of:
   a. disorders of pulmonary gas diffusion
   b. disorders of pulmonary perfusion
   c. obstructive airway diseases
   d. inherited medical conditions

38. The most common preventable factor that exacerbates obstructive airway disease is:
a. smoking
b. upper respiratory infection
c. exercise
d. allergen exposure

39. Obstructive airway disease is characterized by smooth muscle spasm and mucus secretion in the:
a. trachea
b. alveoli
c. bronchioles
d. posterior pharynx

40. A prolonged asthma attack that does not respond to therapy is called:
a. status asthmaticus
b. acute respiratory distress syndrome
c. unremitting asthma
d. chronic asthma

41. Emphysema, unlike asthma and chronic bronchitis, is:
a. defined as a productive cough for at least 3 months per year for 2 or more consecutive years
b. exacerbated by extrinsic factors in children and intrinsic factors in adults
c. characterized by accumulation of fluid in the interstitial space
d. almost always associated with cigarette smoking and has irreversible airway obstruction leading to blebs and the need to breathe through pursed lips

42. Wheezing is commonly heard during an acute exacerbation of:
a. asthma
b. chronic bronchitis
c. emphysema
d. all of the above

43. Chronic obstructive pulmonary disease (COPD) consists of:
a. asthma, chronic bronchitis, and emphysema
b. chronic bronchitis and emphysema
c. emphysema and upper respiratory infections
d. asthma and anaphylaxis

44. Pharmacological therapy for all of the obstructive airway diseases is aimed at:
a. providing positive airway support
b. increasing oxygenation by decreasing interstitial fluid
c. reversal of bronchiole spasm and reduction of mucus production
d. removing the offending agent that precipitated the event

45. Each of the following medications acts directly on the bronchiole leading to dilation *EXCEPT*:
a. atropine
b. albuterol
c. metaproterenol
d. epinephrine

46. Your patient complains of a productive cough, fever, and malaise. This is most likely:
a. exacerbation of chronic bronchitis
b. pneumonia
c. upper respiratory infection
d. sepsis

47. Pneumonia is most often caused by:
a. bacteria
b. virus
c. fungus
d. yeast

48. Patients with pneumonia may be hypoxic because:
a. infection scars the alveoli, inhibiting oxygenation
b. bronchospasm decreases ventilation
c. mucus and pus accumulate in the alveoli
d. hypotension from sepsis leads to poor lung perfusion

49. The primary difference between cardiogenic and noncardiogenic pulmonary edema is:
a. cardiogenic is seen in high-altitude exposure
b. cardiogenic is a result of elevated vascular pressures, whereas noncardiogenic is caused by increased permeability of the pulmonary vasculature
c. noncardiogenic is seen in acute myocardial infarctions
d. cardiogenic presents with wheezing and noncardiogenic does not

50. Pharmacological treatment and interventions for pulmonary edema consist of diuretics, nitrates, and positive pressure ventilatory support, which result in:
    a. increased oxygen delivery to the lung
    b. decreased blood pressure
    c. increased oxygen to the heart resulting in more efficient contractions
    d. maintenance of alveoli patency and reduction in interstitial fluid

51. A pulmonary embolus is caused by a:
    a. blood clot forming in the lung
    b. large air bubble lodging in the pulmonary artery
    c. globule of fat traveling from a broken bone into the pulmonary artery
    d. all of the above

52. The most common cause of a pulmonary embolus is:
    a. a clot breaking off a deep venous thrombosis in the lower extremity
    b. the sheared tip of a central venous catheter
    c. introduction of air into the vascular tree during diving-related barotraumas
    d. foreign material injected by intravenous drug users

53. The most common presenting symptom of a pulmonary embolus is:
    a. hypoxia
    b. dyspnea
    c. chest pain
    d. hypotension

54. When auscultating the lungs of a patient with a pulmonary embolus, you will most often hear:
    a. wheezes
    b. rhonchi
    c. clear and normal breath sounds
    d. rales

55. Prehospital treatment of pulmonary embolus may include all of the following *EXCEPT:*
    a. high-flow oxygen
    b. administration of heparin to dissolve the clot
    c. positive pressure ventilation
    d. transport to the nearest most appropriate facility

56. Which of the following preventions would result in the greatest decrease in the incidence of lung cancer?
    a. never start smoking
    b. cancer screening programs
    c. avoidance of hazardous material such as asbestos
    d. smoking cessation in smokers

57. The emergency presentation of patients with lung cancer is:
    a. usually associated with hemoptysis
    b. easily distinguished from other causes of respiratory distress
    c. dependent on the type and aggressiveness of the tumor
    d. accompanied by altered level of mentation

58. Sore throat, fever, chills, nonproductive cough, and runny nose, which are usually self-limited and caused by a virus, are known as:
    a. strep throat
    b. upper respiratory infection
    c. mononucleosis
    d. pneumonia

59. A thin, healthy male teenager presents with acute onset of pleuritic right-sided chest pain and shortness of breath. The patient denies recent trauma. Auscultation of the chest reveals no obvious differences between the left and right sides. These findings are most consistent with:
    a. pulmonary embolus
    b. spontaneous pneumothorax
    c. pericarditis
    d. rib fracture

60. A spontaneous pneumothorax:
    a. usually requires prehospital chest needle decompression
    b. often progresses to tension pneumothorax
    c. rarely recurs
    d. is usually partial rather than complete and is well tolerated

61. The presence of hyperventilation in the absence of a clear etiology should be considered to be anxiety induced until proven otherwise.
    a. true
    b. false

62. The presence of carpopedal spasm indicates that hyperventilation has resulted in:
a. respiratory alkalosis
b. respiratory acidosis
c. metabolic alkalosis
d. hypoxia of the nerves

63. The most appropriate treatment of the hyperventilating patient is:
a. have patient breathe into a paper bag
b. assist ventilations with a bag-valve-mask
c. look for any possible cause of respiratory distress and treat appropriately
d. apply a nonrebreather mask but do not attach to oxygen

64. You are treating a 24-year-old woman with asthma. Hearing wheezes both during inspiration and expiration indicates a less severe attack because it takes more air movement to make noise during both phases of breathing.
a. true
b. false

65. You respond to a near drowning. The patient is barely breathing and you hear rales on auscultation. The use of continuous positive airway pressure (CPAP) is indicated in this condition for all of the following reasons *EXCEPT:*
a. it keeps the patient breathing
b. it forces fluid out of the alveoli
c. it improves ventilation by preventing the alveoli from collapsing
d. it improves oxygenation

66. Your COPD patient has quit breathing, and you have intubated the trachea. When you compress the bag, you feel significant resistance and hear wheezes on auscultation. The most effective and immediate treatment would include:
a. administering IV solumedrol
b. administering an in-line nebulized albuterol treatment
c. titrating the oxygen concentration to the patient's pulse oximeter reading
d. none of the above

Questions 67 through 70 refer to the following scenario:

An 87-year-old man is found in severe respiratory distress, breathing slowly through pursed lips and unable to answer your questions regarding his medical history. Auscultation of his lungs reveals diminished but clear breath sounds.

67. Which physical finding would be most compatible with COPD?
a. pedal edema
b. morbid obesity
c. clubbing of his fingernails
d. cyanosis

68. All of the following physical findings would provide evidence of the severity of his condition *EXCEPT:*
a. use of accessory muscles to breathe
b. cyanosis
c. tachycardia
d. absence of tachypnea

69. You establish an IV and administer an albuterol updraft. Which of the following is most likely to result in an exacerbation of his disease?
a. pneumonia
b. upper respiratory infection
c. tapering of his prednisone
d. smoking cessation

70. During transport to the hospital the patient's breathing becomes more labored. Which of the following is most likely to predict the need for intubation?
a. recent hospitalization
b. high-dose prednisone use
c. history of intubation
d. history of lung cancer

Questions 71 through 75 refer to the following scenario:

A 65-year-old woman has suffered a cardiac arrest. CPR is in progress and your partner has delivered a series of stacked shocks. The monitor reveals ventricular fibrillation.

71. You begin to ventilate the patient with the bag-valve-mask attached to oxygen. Which of the following will most accurately reflect the adequacy of your ventilations?
a. rise and fall of the chest wall with minimal resistance
b. pulse oximetry reading
c. absence of vomit
d. absence of gastric distention

72. All of the following maneuvers improve artificial ventilation *EXCEPT:*
    a. placement of an oral-pharyngeal airway
    b. performance of the Sellick maneuver
    c. having a partner maintain mask seal while you compress the bag
    d. hyperextension of the neck

73. You begin to assemble your equipment in preparation for endotracheal intubation. Which of the following will most likely affect your ability to successfully intubate the patient?
    a. morbid obesity
    b. clenching of the jaw
    c. presence of vomit
    d. use of a straight rather than a curved blade

74. After passing the endotracheal tube through the cords and inflating the balloon, you begin to assess the proper placement of the tube. Which of the following is the most reliable indication of proper tube placement?
    a. obtaining a high end-tidal CO_2 reading
    b. obtaining a low end-tidal CO_2 reading
    c. seeing the tube pass the vocal cords
    d. bilateral breath sounds with absent gastric sounds

75. Your first attempt at intubation is unsuccessful, with the tube in the esophagus, and you are preparing to try again. Which of the following would NOT improve the likelihood of success?
    a. leaving the first tube in the esophagus
    b. decompressing the stomach with a nasogastric tube
    c. repositioning the patient's head
    d. choosing a tube smaller than the first one

ANSWERS TO CHAPTER 11: MEDICAL EMERGENCIES I: RESPIRATORY

1. c. Respiratory complaints are one of the most common EMS requests. The complications associated with them can be life threatening and can present dramatically.

2. a. Cigarette smoking along with air pollution and toxic exposures represent extrinsic risk factors. Intrinsic risk factors are those that are inherited or acquired by the body.

3. b. Genetics plays the most important role in defining who is predisposed to respiratory illness and compounds the effects of all extrinsic risk factors. Asthma can be inherited as with any other condition of allergic response. Body type and immunological status also play an important role as risk factors.

4. a. Extrinsic risk factors are those that are external to the body and involve various exposures and activities. Both genetic and inherent are forms of intrinsic risk factors.

5. d. Although the respiratory system is involved in the removal of metabolic acids, it accomplishes this through gas exchange. The movement of mucus and the filtering of dust are secondary functions.

6. b. It is vital to understand the various processes that occur during breathing. Respiration is the process of oxygenating the tissues. Ventilation is the movement of air containing both oxygen and carbon dioxide in and out of the lungs. Diffusion occurs at the alveoli, where oxygen and carbon dioxide move across the epithelial membranes. Perfusion is the function of the heart to move blood through the lung and other organs.

7. b. An open and unobstructed airway, along with a working diaphragm and chest wall, is all that is required for ventilation to occur. Because ventilation refers only to the movement of gases, it is not dependent on the presence of oxygen.

8. c. Oxygen and carbon dioxide move across the alveoli-capillary interface from an area of high to lower concentration. This is the process of diffusion. Perfusion refers to circulation of molecules. Dispersion occurs within a solution and not across a membrane. Osmosis refers to the movement of fluid and not gases across cell membranes.

9. a. Between the cells of the alveoli and the pulmonary capillary bed is the interstitial space composed of fluid and connective tissue. Increases in the amount of fluid and/or scarring of the connective tissue inhibit diffusion of gases. The pleural space is the potential space between the visceral and parietal pleura and becomes an actual space with a pneumothorax.

10. d. Because diffusion relies on the short distance across the interstitial space, oxygen and carbon dioxide diffusion will be diminished. This results in lowered cellular oxygen delivery, hypoxia, and elevated levels of carbon dioxide, hypercarbia.

11. b. Diffusion is diminished by the interstitial fluid resulting in hypoxia. Therefore administration of supplemental oxygen is required. Diuretics and nitrates reduce the interstitial fluid, thus improving oxygen diffusion. Diffusion is not dependent on blood pressure and advanced airway interventions are performed only once inadequate ventilation is determined.

12. a. The upper airway filters dust and humidifies the air to improve the lungs' ability to absorb oxygen. It is not directly involved with diffusion. The mucus secreted by the lung is to moisturize the mucosa and aid in humidification and the removal of dust.

13. b. The upper airway is defined as extending from the opening of the nose and mouth to the vocal cords. All structures below the vocal cords such as the trachea and bronchioles are part of the lower airway.

14. b. Small hairlike structures on the mucosal surface of the trachea and bronchioles are called *cilia* and move in a wavelike pattern up the airway to transport dust and mucus out of the lung.

15. b. Although many consider the alveoli to reside in the lower airway it is more accurate to consider the alveoli, interstitial space, and pulmonary capillary bed as the gas exchange interface. The upper and lower airways are involved primarily in the movement of air.

16. d. The term *partial pressure* refers to the amount of a gas dissolved in a liquid. Because carbon dioxide is dissolved in the serum of the blood and is in higher concentration there than in the alveoli, it will move across the capillary wall into the alveoli.

17. b. The chest wall performs all three functions and any mechanical injury to it will inhibit its function. The vagus nerve innervates the heart. The intercostal muscles are used to expand and contract the chest with no assistance from the abdominal muscles.

18. b. Inspiration occurs when the interior volume of the chest increases, creating a negative pressure gradient facilitating movement of air into the lungs. When the diaphragm contracts, it flattens and expands the chest volume. When the intercostal muscles contract, they spread the ribs apart, further increasing chest volume.

19. c. The phrenic nerve innervates the diaphragm, causing it to contract.

20. a. As the partial pressure of carbon dioxide rises in the blood, it dissolves and becomes carbonic acid lowering the blood pH. This acid moves easily across the blood-brain barrier into the cerebrospinal fluid, thus lowering its pH. It is sensed by the brain stem, resulting in an increased respiratory rate to eliminate it from the system.

21. a. The medulla, which is part of the brain stem, is the primary control center for breathing.

22. c. The vagus nerve innervates the heart. The thoracic spinal nerves control the contraction of the intercostal muscles, whereas the phrenic nerve contracts the diaphragm. The Hering-Breuer reflex refers to the nervous stimulation of the spiral muscles around the terminal bronchials and is responsible for terminating inspiration. It becomes hyperactive with bronchospasm.

23. b. Breathing is stimulated primarily by the rise and fall of carbon dioxide in the system. The oxygen or "hypoxic drive" is stimulated last as a survival reflex and becomes clinically important in the care of COPD patients.

24. d. Ventilation refers to the movement of air, affecting primarily the removal of carbon dioxide, whereas respiration refers to the movement of oxygen into the blood and is more affected by the alveoli-interstitial space-capillary bed interface.

25. b. Any alteration in mental status combined with a respiratory complaint is indicative of hypoxia and hypercarbia. Stridor indicates decreased ventilation, whereas diaphoresis and tachycardia are a result of increased work of breathing. Any one of these findings should alert you to the likelihood of a potentially life-threatening emergency.

26. c. As the work of breathing increases, the accessory muscles are used to further increase the chest volume. Cyanosis and severe dyspnea indicate that these reflexive mechanisms are failing.

27. a. Any person with respiratory disease who has required ventilatory support in the past has a severe condition that can deteriorate quickly. Aggressive treatment is indicated and vigilance in assessing the work of breathing required.

28. b. Beta-blockers, used to treat hypertension, are generally not indicated in patients with reactive airway because they can precipitate bronchospasm. Prednisone is used to reduce inflammation, albuterol is a bronchodilator, and theophylline causes smooth muscle relaxation in the terminal bronchioles.

29. b. In the early stages of respiratory distress the rate will increase. As the work of breathing increases and the patient fatigues, the rate will slow, indicating the onset of respiratory failure.

30. b. Increases in the respiratory and heart rate are seen initially during a respiratory emergency. Bradycardia is an ominous sign and indicative of impending cardiorespiratory arrest. It is imperative to examine the entire combination of vital signs and patient mental status along with apparent work of breathing to determine whether or not the patient is responding to therapy.

31. d. With COPD, the chronic hypoxia results in a deformity of the finger, which gives the appearance of flat rounded clubs. Peripheral cyanosis is due to poor peripheral vascular supply. Over time the chest becomes rounded with an increased total volume. There are no long-term physical findings associated with hypercarbia.

32. **a.** The pulse oximeter measures the percentage of saturated hemoglobin. Because hemoglobin binds to carbon monoxide in a similar manner to oxygen, it will appear the same to the oximeter. Therefore a victim of carbon monoxide poisoning may have a pulse oximeter reading of 100% on room air.

33. **b.** The alpha- and beta-agonist effects of these drugs mimic the sympathetic nervous system, resulting in relief of bronchospasm and increasing ventilatory rate.

34. **b.** Regardless of the cause, the most vital medication to administer is oxygen. All other treatments are to improve the delivery of the oxygen and to improve ventilation.

35. **d.** Intravenous steroids are beneficial in severe exacerbations of asthma and COPD. However, their effect takes 8 to 12 hours and will not affect the need for intubation in the field. Steroids improve these conditions by reducing the overall reactivity of the lungs to bronchospasm.

36. **c.** ARDS occurs when the lung is exposed to irritant fumes or as a result of infection resulting in accumulation of fluid in the interstitial space. It is not related to the congestive heart failure where the primary problem is secondary to fluid accumulation from poor perfusion. It presents with rales, wheezes, and hypoxia.

37. **c.** Asthma, emphysema, and chronic bronchitis constitute the three conditions known as obstructive pulmonary diseases. They each present with decreased ventilation from bronchospasm and mucus plugging. Although asthma does have a genetic predisposition, all three are generally acquired and chronic.

38. **a.** An exacerbation of COPD can be caused by respiratory infections, exercise, and exposure to allergens leading to bronchospasm. However, each of these is difficult to prevent, whereas avoidance of smoking is a conscious and preventable activity that causes the most damage.

39. **c.** The smooth spiral muscles of the Herring-Breuer complex reside in the bronchioles,

which are responsible for bronchospasm and wheezing. The lining of the bronchioles contains mucus-producing cells, which along with the cilia assist in the movement of foreign material from the lung. When these cells become inflamed, they produce an increased amount of mucus, leading to small airway obstruction.

40. **a.** When bronchospasm cannot be stopped with the administration of the usual arsenal of alpha- and beta-agonist agents, the condition is termed *status asthmaticus* and is indicative of a poor outcome. Endotracheal intubation and the use of smooth muscle relaxants including paralytics may be required.

41. **d.** Asthma is caused by bronchospasm from exposure to allergens or other extrinsic factors. Although chronic bronchitis and emphysema are most often caused by smoking, chronic bronchitis is a condition of increased mucus production resulting in a chronic productive cough. Over time, scarring of the alveoli from emphysema results in the development of blebs.

42. **d.** All three conditions will result in wheezing because of narrowing of the airway from bronchospasm, excessive mucus production, or a combination of both.

43. **b.** Although asthma is an obstructive lung disease, it does not result in the chronic changes seen in chronic bronchitis and emphysema. It is more accurately referred to as reactive airway disease because the bronchospasm is reactive to some extrinsic factor.

44. **c.** Nebulized medications such as albuterol, atrovent, and the administration of epinephrine and terbutaline exert their effect by relieving bronchospasm and mucus production.

45. **a.** Atropine is a parasympathetic medication that reduces mucus production through its muscarinic action, which allows the effect of the sympathetic innervation to produce more bronchodilation. It does not act directly on the bronchioles. Albuterol, metaproterenol, and epinephrine exert their effects through alpha- and beta-agonist actions.

46. **b.** Pulmonary infections will result in a productive cough of the pus that accumulates in the

alveoli and bronchi. Fever and malaise is the systemic body response to the infection. Upper respiratory infections usually have a dry, non-productive cough and minimal systemic symptoms. Sepsis can occur from pneumonia but also has many other causes. An acute exacerbation of chronic bronchitis usually is not associated with fever and malaise.

47. a. Although each of the listed agents can cause pulmonary infections, bacteria are the most common. Viral lung infections usually cause an upper airway infection without the production of pus in the alveoli. Fungus and yeast can result in pneumonia but are uncommon.

48. c. As mucus accumulates in the alveoli, it interferes with oxygen delivery to the pulmonary capillary bed. Chronic infections, particularly fungal, can result in scarring of the alveoli but are not characteristic of typical pneumonias.

49. b. Pulmonary edema can result from two separate processes. Exposure of the alveoli-capillary bed to irritants can cause inflammation resulting in increased capillary permeability and fluid accumulation in the interstitial space. This is noncardiogenic pulmonary edema. Increased hydrostatic pressure of the pulmonary blood flow resulting from cardiac dysfunction is called *cardiogenic pulmonary edema.*

50. d. With the alveoli kept open during exhalation, positive pressure (CPAP) increases oxygen delivery to the alveoli. Diuretics decrease interstitial fluid by removing them from the system, whereas nitrates exert their effect by dilating the vascular tree.

51. d. Any mechanical obstruction of the pulmonary artery results in a pulmonary embolus. Blood clots originating in the lower leg are the most common. Fat emboli are associated with humeral and femoral fractures, in which fat in the bone marrow is introduced into the circulation.

52. a. Although each of the listed conditions can result in a pulmonary embolus, a clot breaking free from a DVT is the most common. DVTs most often occur in the lower extremities.

53. c. The larger the clot, the larger the portion of the affected lung, resulting in greater impairment of lung perfusion and greater hypoxia. However, chest pain, which is often pleuritic, is the most common presenting complaint. In the event of a large saddle embolus lodging in the pulmonary artery, completely blocking all blood flow from the heart, sudden cardiogenic shock results.

54. c. Because a pulmonary embolus does not block the airway, the lungs are clear.

55. b. Oxygen delivery to the blood is impaired with a pulmonary embolus. The patient should be given 100% oxygen and may require positive pressure ventilation to increase the movement of oxygen into the pulmonary capillaries. Definitive treatment consists of either surgically removing the clot or administering thrombolytics to dissolve it. Neither of these can be performed in the field, and both can be performed only when the patient is delivered to a facility capable of diagnosing and treating the condition.

56. a. Cigarette smoking is the single greatest cause of lung cancer. Never starting is far preferable to merely stopping. Although toxic chemical exposures do result in lung cancer, they represent a much smaller percentage of the overall cases.

57. c. Different types of lung cancers have various degrees of aggressiveness in how quickly they grow and how invasively they spread in the lung and throughout the body. Those that invade the bronchial tree present with hemoptysis, whereas those that invade the lung tissue present with hypoxia. There are no hallmarks of the respiratory distress caused by lung cancer that set it apart from other causes.

58. b. Most upper respiratory infections are caused by viruses. Strep throat and pneumonia are caused by bacteria. Mononucleosis is caused by a virus and results in sore throat and fever but not cough.

59. b. The spontaneous pneumothorax occurs most commonly in young adults with thin stature. Once the lung collapses, the patient experiences pain on breathing and a sensation of shortness of breath. The pneumothorax might not be large enough to result in loss of breath sounds but is still significant as it can enlarge. Pulmonary emboli usually occur in obese persons and those at risk for deep venous thrombosis. The rib fracture will be associated with trauma, and pericarditis has no predilection for any age.

60. **d.** The spontaneous pneumothorax results when the visceral pleura separates from the parietal pleura of the inner chest wall. Usually, only one portion of the lung, such as the apical or superior segment, collapses. Tension pneumothorax occurs when the pressure in the pleural space compresses the lung and heart resulting in shock and rarely occurs from a spontaneous pneumothorax.

61. **b.** Hyperventilation is a response to many stimuli including pain, hypoxia, anxiety, and toxic exposures. Patients who are hyperventilating should be assessed first for an organic cause before concluding that they are merely excited.

62. **a.** As the patient hyperventilates carbon dioxide is blown off. This results in respiratory alkalosis, which causes a shift of calcium in the tissues leading to irritability of the nerves. Decreased cerebral circulation causes a sense of euphoria.

63. **c.** Because hyperventilation may be a response to a serious physical insult such as hypoxia or toxic exposure, the patient should be treated appropriately with oxygen as with any other medical emergency.

64. **b.** Wheezing during an asthma attack occurs because of narrowing of the airways. Normally during inspiration the airways expand. Therefore hearing wheezes during both inspiration and expiration is an indication of severe bronchospasm and should be treated aggressively.

65. **a.** The use of continuous positive airway pressure is indicated in both SCUBA and near-drowning cases by supporting the alveoli and removing fluid from the lung resulting in improved oxygenation. CPAP requires that the patient be able to breathe spontaneously.

66. **b.** It is vital to release the bronchospasm associated with any obstructive airway disease regardless of whether the patient is intubated. This can be accomplished by putting a breathing treatment in-line of the resuscitation bag and the endotracheal tube.

67. **c.** The typical physical changes associated with COPD include the barrel-shaped chest from the progressive increase in the anterior-posterior diameter of the chest and clubbing of the fingernails from chronic cyanosis. Pedal edema would point toward congestive failure. Cyanosis is not specific to any particular cause. Other physical findings might include thin and easily injured skin from chronic steroid use.

68. **d.** During an acute exacerbation of COPD or asthma the patient begins to use the accessory muscles of the chest and neck to aid the active process of breathing in and out. As the attack worsens they will begin to feel fatigue and develop tachycardia from the increased workload and eventually cyanosis as the ability to exchange oxygen diminishes. Patients with these chronic conditions have learned to control their breathing to maintain positive pressure ventilation and their respiratory rate can be slow.

69. **b.** Of the listed causes, the occurrence of a viral upper respiratory infection, which is more common than pneumonia and rebound from prednisone withdraw, precipitates an acute COPD exacerbation. Continuing, not cessation, of smoking is more likely to worsen his condition.

70. **c.** Prior need for intubation significantly increases the likelihood of requiring it again. The other listed causes may be associated with the need for intubation but only if accompanied by other factors.

71. **a.** The adequacy of ventilation is indicated by the ability to deliver the appropriate tidal volume, which is reflected in the ease with which it enters and leaves the chest. The easy rise and fall of the chest indicates minimal resistance. Pulse oximetry is unreliable in the cardiac arrest situation. The presence of vomit will impair your ability to ventilate but cannot be used as a the gauge of its adequacy.

72. **d.** Hyperextension of the neck can result in occlusion of the airway by the pharyngeal soft tissues and the tongue. An O-P airway keeps the tongue out of the way and the Sellick maneuver minimizes the amount of air entering the stomach. Maintaining a tight mask seal against the face increases the amount of air entering the airway.

73. **b.** Clenching of the jaw significantly limits the ability to visualize the cords. Although each

of the other listed factors may contribute to the difficulty of intubation, they can all be overcome with the proper intervention. The competent medic should be skilled in the use of both straight and curved laryngoscope blades.

74. c. Observing the endotracheal tube pass the vocal cords during intubation is the most reliable indication of proper tube placement. A low end-tidal CO_2 reading may indicate an esophageal intubation or the lack of metabolic activity during a cardiac arrest even if the tube is in the trachea. A high CO_2 reading is a secondary indication of tube placement, as is bilateral breath sounds.

75. b. Decompressing the stomach AFTER intubation improves ventilation and the effectiveness of CPR but does not improve intubation success. Leaving the first tube in the esophagus decreases the probability of performing a second esophageal intubation. Repositioning the head may improve visualization of the cords, and choosing a slightly smaller tube facilitates passage through the cords.

MEDICAL EMERGENCIES II: CARDIAC

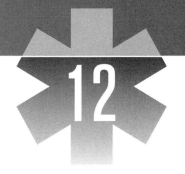

1. Given the following list of components of the conduction system, label Figure 12-1: atrioventricular bundle, atrioventricular node, bundle branches, purkinje fibers, sinoatrial node.

2. The intrinsic firing rate of AV junctional tissue is:
   a. 30 to 40 discharges per minute
   b. 40 to 60 discharges per minute
   c. 60 to 80 discharges per minute
   d. 80 to 100 discharges per minute

3. The most important ions involved in the myocardial action potential include:
   a. iron, potassium, and sodium
   b. potassium, calcium, and magnesium
   c. sodium, calcium, and potassium
   d. chromium, magnesium, and calcium

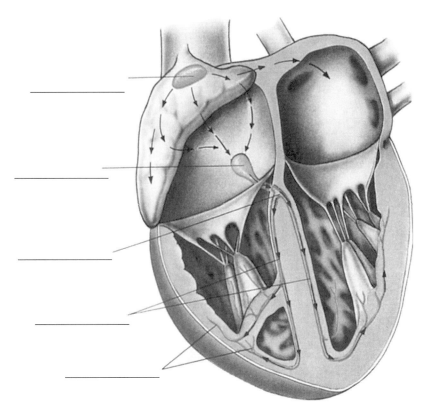

Figure 12-1

4. The clinical significance of Starling's law of the heart is that:
   a. myocardial cells are capable of initiating an electrical impulse
   b. valves close more forcefully when preload is decreased
   c. coronary artery perfusion increases when afterload is decreased
   d. myocardial fibers contract more forcefully when stretched to a point

5. The term *inotropy* pertains to the:
   a. force or energy of muscle contraction, particularly contractions of the heart
   b. ability of heart cells to generate electrical impulses
   c. speed at which the ventricles contract
   d. intrinsic firing rate of various parts of the heart's conduction system

6. Chronotropic medications:
   a. reduce the incidence of ectopy
   b. reduce the irritability of an area of heart muscle
   c. stimulate the heart to contract more forcefully
   d. affect the heart rate

7. Dromotropy pertains to agents that:
   a. increase peripheral vascular resistance
   b. cause vasodilation and venous pooling
   c. affect conduction velocity through the conducting tissues of the heart
   d. increase the sensitivity of the parasympathetic nervous system

8. Two medications that limit the movement of calcium ions into the cell are:
   a. procainamide and lidocaine
   b. digoxin and furosemide
   c. propranolol and atenolol
   d. verapamil and diltiazem

9. The point of maximal impulse (PMI):
   a. is the location at which the apical pulse is most readily seen or palpated
   b. signifies the location of the tricuspid valve when assessing heart sounds
   c. allows for a clearer view of P waves when assessing an ECG
   d. is the area of the heart that is responsible for initiating electrical impulses

10. The first heart sound heard when auscultating the heart relates to:
    a. pumping of blood from the atria to the ventricles
    b. closure of the AV valves during ventricular systole
    c. a turbulent flow of blood into the ventricles
    d. opening of the aortic and pulmonary semilunar valves

11. The heart sound that occurs with closure of the aortic and pulmonic valves is the:
    a. S_1
    b. S_2
    c. S_3
    d. S_4

12. Vagal stimulation results in:
    a. tachyarrhythmias
    b. decreased ventricular ectopy
    c. positive chronotropic effect
    d. a slowing of the heart rate

13. The most common ECG lead used in the prehospital setting is:
    a. lead I
    b. lead II
    c. lead III
    d. aVL

14. On ECG graph paper, the large blocks on the horizontal axis represent a period of:
    a. 0.02 second
    b. 0.04 second
    c. 0.20 second
    d. 0.40 second

15. The heart rate of the ECG shown in Figure 12-2 is approximately:
    a. 60
    b. 70
    c. 80
    d. 90

16. When the "Triplicate Method" is used to determine a heart rate from an ECG tracing, the two number sets used are:
    a. 10-20-30 and 50-75-100
    b. 50-60-70 and 150-160-170
    c. 150-100-50 and 15-10-5
    d. 300-150-100 and 75-60-50

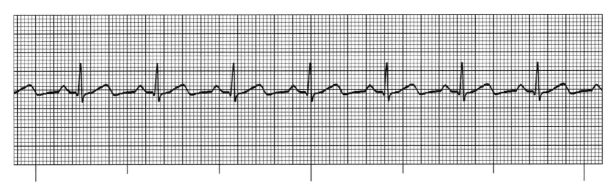

Figure 12-2

17. In an ECG complex, atrial depolarization is represented by the:
    a. P wave
    b. R wave
    c. S wave
    d. T wave

18. When an ECG strip is examined, the QRS complex corresponds to:
    a. atrial depolarization
    b. ventricular depolarization
    c. septal repolarization
    d. ventricular repolarization

19. Mechanical contraction of the heart muscle is related to:
    a. depolarization
    b. repolarization
    c. retrograde conduction
    d. dissociation

20. The normal P-R interval is:
    a. 0.04 to 0.10 second
    b. 0.12 to 0.20 second
    c. 0.20 to 0.25 second
    d. 0.30 to 0.40 second

21. During the absolute refractory period of the heart:
    a. the cardiac muscle is completely insensitive to further stimulation
    b. the cardiac muscle is extremely sensitive to further stimulation
    c. membrane potential gradually drops
    d. depolarization occurs and the ventricles actively force blood into the circulatory system

22. A heart rate greater than 100 beats per minute is referred to as:
    a. bradycardia
    b. tachycardia
    c. bradypnea
    d. tachypnea

23. An acute electrolyte abnormality would most likely be suspected if the ECG shows:
    a. the presence of U waves or peaked T waves
    b. the presence of J waves or ST segment elevation
    c. rounded T waves or a PR interval greater than 0.12 second
    d. ST segment depression or flutter waves

24. Myocardial ischemia would be suspected if an ECG showed:
    a. peaked T waves and widening QRS
    b. a prolonged PR interval and ST segment elevation
    c. ST segment depression and T wave inversion
    d. J waves and U waves

25. Three or more PVCs in a row constitute:
    a. ventricular fibrillation
    b. ventricular bradycardia
    c. ventricular asystole
    d. ventricular tachycardia

26. The width of a normal QRS complex is:
    a. 0.05 to 0.10 second, or 5 to 10 small squares on the graph paper
    b. 0.08 to 0.12 second, or 2 to 3 small squares on the graph paper
    c. 0.12 to 0.20 second, or 3 to 5 large squares on the graph paper
    d. 0.16 to 0.24 second, or 4 to 6 large squares on the graph paper

27. The ECG dysrhythmias that may be defibrillated are:
    a. asystole and ventricular fibrillation
    b. ventricular fibrillation and pulseless ventricular tachycardia
    c. PEA and asystole
    d. pulseless ventricular tachycardia and PEA

28. The absence of electrical activity in the heart is referred to as:
    a. fibrillation
    b. diastole
    c. flutter
    d. asystole

29. The primary pacemaker of the heart, where electrical impulses originate, is the:
    a. AV node
    b. bundle of His
    c. SA node
    d. Purkinje fiber

30. A heart rate less than 60 beats per minute is referred to as:
    a. tachypnea
    b. asystole
    c. bradycardia
    d. AV block

31. A common cause of delayed or blocked electrical impulses that may produce reentry dysrhythmias is:
    a. hyperkalemia
    b. hypercapnia
    c. digitalis toxicity
    d. excess catecholamines

32. Upon examining your patient's ECG, you note wide QRS complexes. The PR interval varies and there is no correlation of P waves to QRS complexes. This best describes a:
    a. first-degree AV block
    b. second-degree AV block Type I (Wenckebach)
    c. second-degree AV block Type II
    d. third-degree AV block

33. Abnormally high leakage of sodium ions into the cell causes ectopy from:
    a. reentry
    b. autonomic conduction
    c. enhanced automaticity
    d. synchronized pacing

34. An ECG that shows dropped QRS complexes but in which the PR interval remains constant for each conducted P wave is:
    a. first-degree AV block
    b. second-degree AV block Type I (Wenckebach)
    c. second-degree AV block Type II
    d. third-degree AV block

35. It is clinically important to recognize a patient with Wolff-Parkinson-White (WPW) syndrome because:
    a. it often leads to ventricular tachycardia
    b. giving calcium-channel blockers may lead to ventricular fibrillation
    c. WPW does not respond to cardioversion
    d. adenosine is contraindicated because it often causes paroxysmal supraventricular tachycardia (PSVT)

36. An ECG characterized by a gradual prolongation of the PR interval and eventually a dropped QRS complex is:
    a. first-degree AV block
    b. second-degree AV block Type I (Wenckebach)
    c. second-degree AV block Type II
    d. third-degree AV block

37. The process by which the myocardium is restimulated by the original impulse is called:
    a. enhanced automaticity
    b. retrograde automaticity
    c. junctional ectopic phenomena
    d. reentry

38. Given the following list of ECG interpretations, label the following ECG strips.
    AC (60-cycle) interference
    accelerated junctional rhythm
    agonal rhythm
    asystole
    atrial fibrillation
    atrial flutter
    first-degree AV block
    junctional escape complexes or rhythm
    pacemaker rhythm
    paroxysmal supraventricular tachycardia (PSVT)
    premature atrial complex (PAC)
    premature junctional complex (PJC)
    premature ventricular complex (PVC)
    second-degree AV block Type I (Wenckebach)
    second-degree AV block Type II
    sinus arrest
    sinus dysrhythmia
    sinus bradycardia
    sinus tachycardia
    third-degree AV block
    ventricular escape complexes or rhythm
    ventricular fibrillation
    ventricular tachycardia
    wandering pacemaker

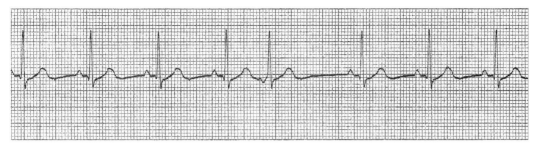

ECG Strip 1 _____

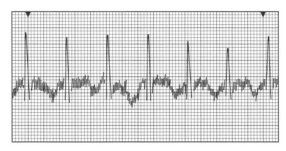

ECG Strip 2 _____

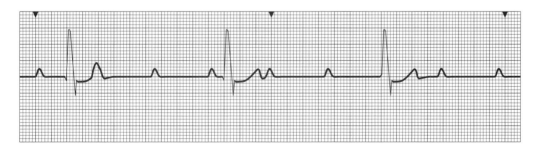

ECG Strip 3 _____

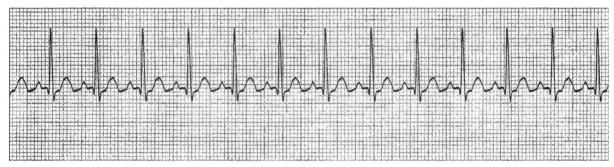

ECG Strip 4 _____

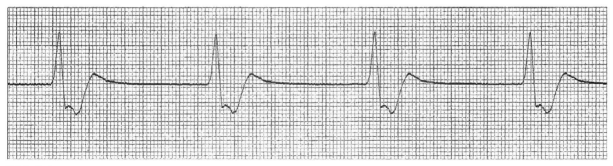

ECG Strip 5 _____

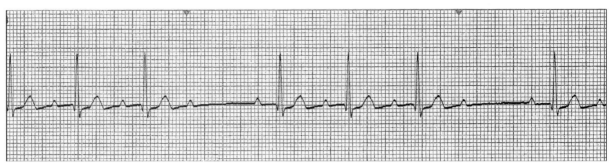

ECG Strip 6 _____

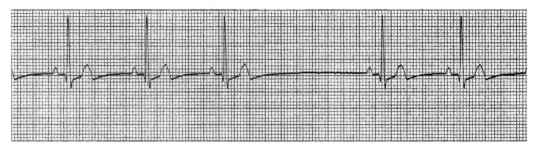

ECG Strip 7 _____

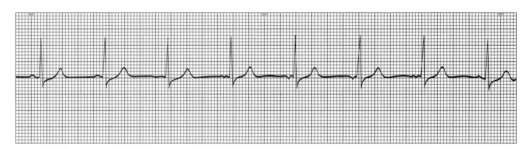

ECG Strip 8 _____

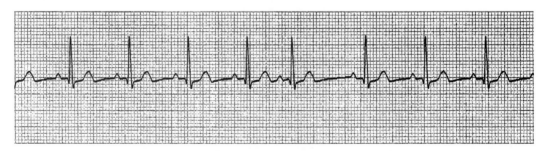

ECG Strip 9 _____

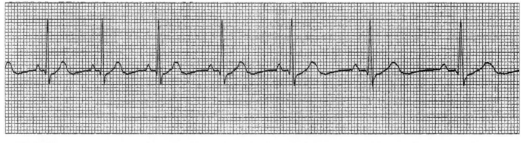

ECG Strip 10 _____

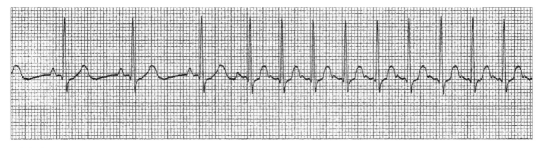

ECG Strip 11 _____

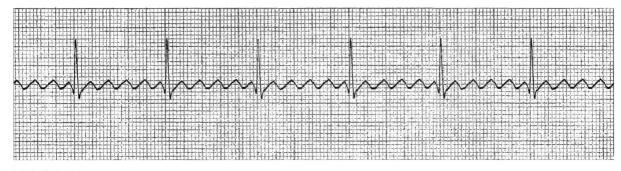

ECG Strip 12 _____

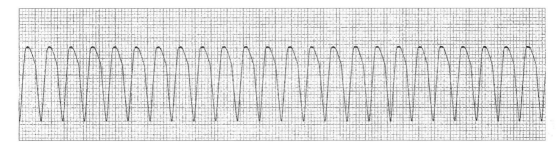

ECG Strip 13 _____

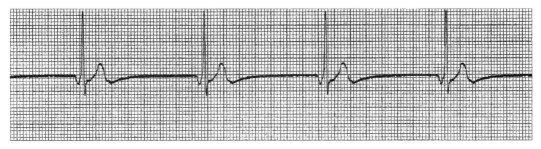

ECG Strip 14 _____

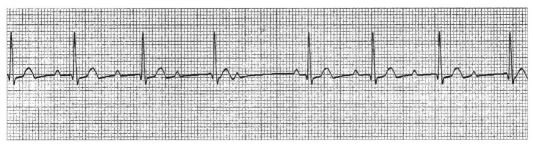

ECG Strip 15 _____

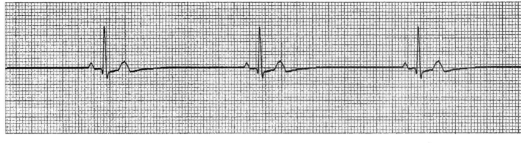

ECG Strip 16 _____

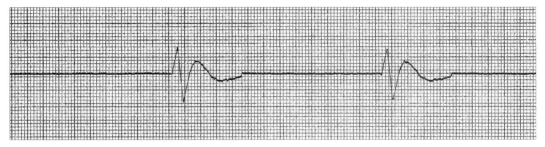

ECG Strip 17 _____

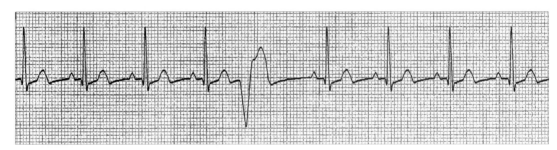

ECG Strip 18 _____

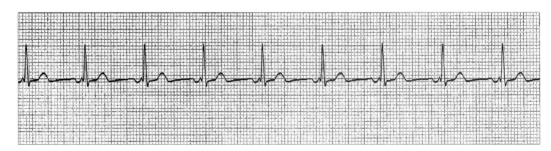

ECG Strip 19 _____

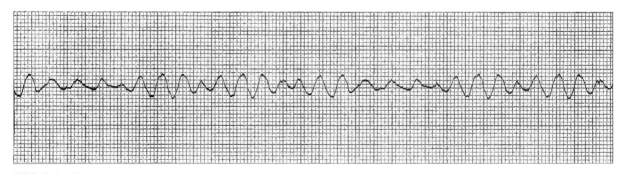

ECG Strip 20 _____

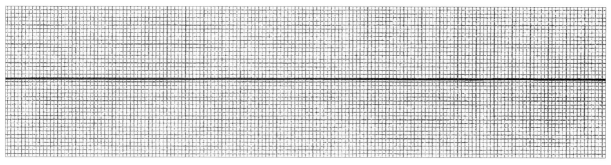

ECG Strip 21 _____

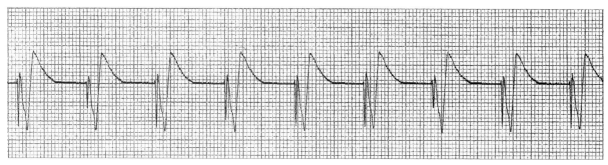

ECG Strip 22 _____

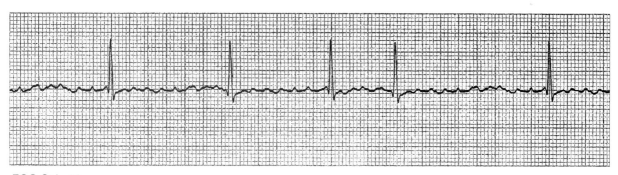

ECG Strip 23 _____

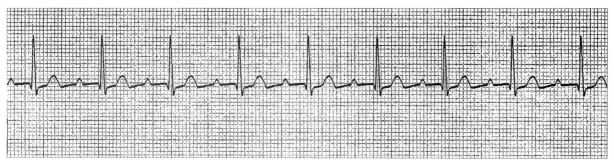

ECG Strip 24 _____

39. A pacemaker that delivers timed electrical stimuli at a selected rate, regardless of the patient's intrinsic cardiac activity, is:
    a. a demand pacemaker
    b. an asynchronous pacemaker
    c. a transvenous pacemaker
    d. a synchronized pacemaker

40. Of the following, the scenario that would benefit most from transcutaneous cardiac pacing involves a patient in:
    a. PEA with normal-looking QRS complexes and a rate of 68
    b. sinus bradycardia with a rate of 56 and a blood pressure of 112/66
    c. ventricular fibrillation who is unresponsive to defibrillation and medications
    d. third-degree block who is unresponsive to atropine and then becomes hemodynamically unstable

41. You have placed a transcutaneous pacemaker on your patient and see pacemaker spikes on the ECG. However, no QRS complexes are seen following the spikes. Your next action would be to:
    a. discontinue pacing because lack of QRS complexes indicates the myocardium is too hypoxic or damaged to respond to external pacing
    b. reposition the pacer electrodes
    c. gradually increase the current until QRS complexes are seen
    d. check the blood pressure to see if the pacer spikes alone are producing adequate cardiac output

42. Of the following patients, the one who would most likely be considered to have stable angina pectoris is:
    a. a 48-year-old male who recently started exercising regularly and after this workout has experienced chest pain for the first time
    b. a 52-year-old male who was working in the yard when his chest pain started, which has been relieved with rest and nitroglycerin
    c. a 60-year-old male who just had an argument with his son and has had pain for the last 20 minutes with no relief from rest
    d. a 63-year-old male who was watching TV when his chest pain started and who had to take three nitroglycerin tablets before the pain subsided

43. A 65-year-old male is complaining of chest pressure and heaviness, which started while he was going for a walk with his grandson. He has a history of angina and has taken two of his nitroglycerin tablets in the last 8 minutes with no relief. Vital signs are within normal limits. Management of this patient should include:
    a. starting an IV and immediately giving morphine because the nitroglycerin was ineffective
    b. having the patient take one more of his own nitroglycerin so that a total of three nitros have been taken
    c. giving the patient additional nitroglycerin carried by the EMS unit
    d. starting an IV and giving prophylactic lidocaine to reduce the likelihood of the patient going into ventricular tachycardia or ventricular fibrillation

44. In the vast majority of myocardial infarctions, the precipitating event is:
    a. acute thrombotic occlusion
    b. reduced myocardial blood flow caused by shock
    c. hypotension that results in reduced coronary artery filling pressures
    d. an increased release of naturally occurring catecholamines, which causes an increase in myocardial oxygen demand

45. Primary differences with the pain/discomfort associated with an acute myocardial infarction as opposed to angina pectoris include:
    a. the pain usually comes on only with exertion
    b. the pain generally does not radiate into other areas of the body
    c. dyspnea is not usually associated with the pain
    d. the pain is generally not alleviated by nitroglycerin

46. ECG changes characteristically seen during the evolution of an acute myocardial infarction include:
    a. a diminished PR interval
    b. ST-segment elevation
    c. the presence of U waves
    d. new onset atrial fibrillation

47. The most common cause of death from myocardial infarction is:
    a. cardiogenic shock
    b. myocardial tissue rupture
    c. congestive heart failure
    d. ventricular dysrhythmias

48. Emergency care for acute myocardial infarction is generally directed at accomplishing all of the following *EXCEPT:*
   a. administering prophylactic lidocaine to reduce the likelihood of the patient going into ventricular tachycardia or ventricular fibrillation
   b. administering supplemental oxygen to increase oxygen supply
   c. decreasing metabolic needs and providing collateral circulation
   d. reestablishing perfusion to the ischemic myocardium as quickly as possible after the onset of symptoms

49. A patient is usually not considered eligible for thrombolytic therapy if he or she:
   a. has high blood pressure that requires daily medication for control
   b. has a history of intracranial bleed or stroke
   c. was successfully defibrillated from witnessed ventricular fibrillation by the second shock
   d. has a history of previous surgery

50. The time frame at which a patient is not considered to be a candidate for thrombolytic therapy is:
   a. more than 3 hours after onset of pain and symptoms
   b. more than 6 hours after onset of pain and symptoms
   c. more than 12 hours after onset of pain and symptoms
   d. more than 15 hours after onset of pain and symptoms

Questions 51 through 56 pertain to the 12-lead ECG.

51. Given the presence of ST segment changes, note the suspected location of the acute myocardial infarction as anterior, inferior, lateral, or septal (*One answer may be used twice*).

   I and aVL _____

   II, III, aVF _____

   V1 and V2 _____

   V3 and V4 _____

   V5 and V6 _____

52. An anterior wall infarct should be suspected if ST segment elevation is noted in leads:
   a. V1 and V2
   b. V3 and V4
   c. V5 and V6
   d. II, III, and aVF

53. The most common area of infarct is the:
   a. anterior wall
   b. inferior wall
   c. lateral wall
   d. septal wall

54. When assessing a 12-lead ECG, remember that:
   a. the 12-lead ECG will always show signs of an active infarct
   b. a myocardial infarction is only present if an abnormal 12-lead ECG is accompanied by chest pain
   c. a myocardial infarction should be suspected only if the same findings are found on two consecutive 12-lead ECGs taken 5 minutes apart
   d. a patient having a myocardial infarction may present with a normal 12-lead

55. When a patient is experiencing an acute myocardial infarction, left coronary artery involvement would most likely be suspected if the location of the infarction is the:
   a. septal wall, anterior wall, or lateral wall
   b. inferior wall, lateral wall, or anterior wall
   c. anterior wall, inferior wall, or septal wall
   d. lateral wall, septal wall, or inferior wall

56. An acute myocardial infarction should be suspected if the patient exhibits:
   a. more than 1 mm of ST segment elevation in two or more anatomically contiguous leads
   b. ST segment depression in the limb leads
   c. a QRS wider than 0.20 second
   d. a P-R interval longer than 0.12 second

57. A patient with right ventricular failure is likely to present with:
   a. pink, frothy sputum
   b. peripheral edema
   c. flat neck veins
   d. severe bradycardia

58. Left ventricular failure would be suspected if a patient presented with:
   a. slow, shallow respirations
   b. pedal edema
   c. pulmonary edema
   d. bradycardia

59. Factors that often precipitate or aggravate heart failure include all of the following *EXCEPT:*
   a. chronic hypertension
   b. valvular disease
   c. myocardial infarction
   d. chronic asthma

60. Acute pulmonary edema is best described as:
a. the accumulation of extravascular fluid in lung tissues and alveoli
b. failure of the lungs to expand normally
c. an excessive excretion and buildup of mucus in the bronchial tree
d. a loss of lung tissue elasticity with associated alveolar breakdown

61. Acute pulmonary edema occurs when:
a. the right ventricle cannot pump enough blood into the lungs
b. the alveolar capillary beds become blocked
c. the left ventricle fails to function effectively as a pump and blood backs up into the pulmonary circulation
d. the right atrium is unable to adequately manage the blood it is receiving from the vena cava

62. In left ventricular failure, an increase in end-diastolic pressure:
a. reduces the pressure in the left atrium, thereby increasing fill volume of the left atrium
b. is the result of blood being delivered to the left ventricle but not being completely ejected from it
c. increases the pressure of blood delivered to the right atrium resulting in increased filling of the right atrium
d. results in an increase of stroke volume and a reduction in organ perfusion

63. An abnormal condition of the respiratory system that is characterized by sudden attacks of shortness of breath that awaken a patient from sleep and that may be accompanied by profuse sweating and tachycardia is:
a. cor pulmonale
b. paroxysmal nocturnal dyspnea
c. pulmonary overpressurization syndrome
d. dyspnea on exertion

64. Edema present in the extremities and sacrum suggests that:
a. the left ventricle is unable to function as an effective forward pump
b. systemic vasodilation has occurred
c. the right heart is unable to pump efficiently, causing back-pressure of blood into the systemic venous circulation
d. the patient is experiencing an incomplete closure of the aortic valve

65. Three pharmacological agents commonly used to manage left ventricular failure include:
a. epinephrine, atropine, and nitroglycerin
b. nitroglycerin, furosemide, and morphine
c. vasopressin, epinephrine, and amiodarone
d. albuterol, furosemide, and diphenhydramine

66. The goal when administering medications to a patient in congestive heart failure is to:
a. decrease contractile function of the myocardium
b. increase blood pressure
c. decrease venous return to the heart
d. increase the workload of the heart

67. Management of hypotension resulting from right ventricular failure may include:
a. placing the patient in the Trendelenburg position to improve cerebral blood flow
b. administering a 250-mL IV bolus of normal saline over 5 to 10 minutes
c. limiting IV fluids to reduce the potential for pulmonary edema to develop
d. immediate initiation of an IV drip of dopamine to raise blood pressure

68. Cardiogenic shock is best defined as:
a. heart failure with systolic blood pressure less than 100 mm Hg
b. shock caused by trauma to the heart
c. low blood pressure associated with an anginal episode
d. the most extreme form of pump failure

69. Generally, the clinical criteria for cardiogenic shock include all of the following *EXCEPT:*
a. pulmonary congestion
b. a systolic blood pressure less than 100 mm Hg
c. altered level of consciousness
d. cool, clammy skin

70. Two commonly used pharmacological agents for cardiogenic shock are:
a. dopamine and lidocaine
b. atropine and epinephrine
c. vasopressin and amiodarone
d. dopamine and dobutamine

71. Cardiac tamponade is best defined as:
a. a weakening of an area of a coronary blood vessel
b. a blockage in a coronary blood vessel
c. catastrophic failure of a heart valve
d. impaired diastolic filling of the heart caused by increased intrapericardial pressure

72. Signs of cardiac tamponade include all of the following *EXCEPT:*
   a. increased systolic pressure
   b. distended neck veins
   c. faint or muffled heart sounds
   d. narrowing pulse pressure difference

73. Field management of cardiac tamponade by EMS personnel may include:
   a. attempting to lower the patient's blood pressure
   b. administering a fluid bolus
   c. inserting a needle into the intrapleural space
   d. administering nitroglycerin to produce vasodilation and reduce the workload of the heart

74. Pulsus paradoxus is characterized by:
   a. the pulse alternating weak and strong
   b. the pulse being weaker or absent in one wrist
   c. an abnormal decrease in systolic blood pressure that occurs during inspiration compared to expiration
   d. pulses that are not felt with each QRS complex seen on the ECG

75. A hypertensive emergency is a condition in which:
   a. the patient has high blood pressure accompanied by other symptoms such as chest pain and/or dyspnea
   b. the systolic blood pressure exceeds 200 mm Hg
   c. the diastolic blood pressure is greater than 70% of the systolic blood pressure
   d. an increase in blood pressure leads to significant, irreversible end-organ damage within hours if not managed

76. A prehospital medication that may be used to manage a hypertensive emergency is:
   a. nitroglycerin
   b. albuterol
   c. atropine
   d. lidocaine

77. Synchronized cardioversion differs from defibrillation in that:
   a. it is timed to deliver a shock on the T-wave
   b. the shock is delivered as soon as the discharge buttons are pressed
   c. it is designed to deliver a shock after the peak of the R-wave
   d. higher energy levels are generally required to terminate the dysrhythmias

78. The energy levels generally used to perform initial defibrillation on an adult patient are:
   a. 100, 200, 300 joules for ventricular fibrillation and 200, 300, 360 joules for pulseless ventricular tachycardia
   b. 200, 300, 360 joules for ventricular fibrillation and 100, 200, 300 joules for pulseless ventricular tachycardia
   c. 200, 300, 360 joules for both ventricular fibrillation and pulseless ventricular tachycardia
   d. 260, 300, 360 joules for both ventricular fibrillation and pulseless ventricular tachycardia

79. The dysrhythmias most likely to respond to cardioversion at lower energy levels are:
   a. atrial flutter and ventricular tachycardia
   b. paroxysmal supraventricular tachycardia and atrial fibrillation
   c. ventricular fibrillation and atrial fibrillation
   d. ventricular tachycardia and paroxysmal supraventricular tachycardia

80. When synchronized cardioversion is performed for ventricular tachycardia, the initial energy level is usually:
   a. 25 joules
   b. 50 joules
   c. 100 joules
   d. 200 joules

81. Referring to Figure 12-3, the correct defibrillator paddle placement is shown in:
    a. part A
    b. part B
    c. part C
    d. part D

82. Your patient is in cardiac arrest. Family members advise you that he has an implantable cardioverter-defibrillator (ICD). When managing this patient:
    a. follow standard ACLS protocols
    b. administer cardiac medications but avoid performing external defibrillation
    c. use standard cardiac medications, but only perform synchronized cardioversion
    d. avoid the use of antidysrhythmic medications

83. You are starting to work a code on a patient who is in asystole. The IV is started and you are ready to push medications. The correct dose for atropine in this situation is:
    a. 0.5 mg every 5 to 10 minutes up to a total of 4 mg
    b. 0.5 to 1.0 mg every 3 to 5 minutes up to a total of 3.0 mg/kg
    c. 1.0 mg every 3 to 5 minutes up to a total of 0.04 mg/kg
    d. 1.0 to 1.5 mg every 5 minutes up to a total of 3 mg

84. You would most likely expect to administer amiodarone to a patient in:
    a. third-degree heart block with wide, bizarre QRS complexes
    b. ventricular fibrillation or pulseless ventricular tachycardia
    c. sinus bradycardia with ventricular escape beats
    d. PEA with a rate between 60 and 80

85. The usual dose for adenosine is:
    a. a 6-mg bolus every 5 minutes up to a total of 3 doses
    b. an initial bolus of 6 mg followed by a second dose of 12 mg if the first dose does not work
    c. a 12-mg bolus given once
    d. a 12-mg loading dose followed by a 0.01 mg/kg/min drip

86. Your patient has been in cardiac arrest for some time and your protocol calls for sodium bicarbonate. In the absence of lab values to guide dosing, the usual dose for sodium bicarbonate is:
    a. 0.5 to 1.0 mg/kg repeated every 10 minutes
    b. 1 mEq/kg repeated at half the initial dose every 10 minutes thereafter
    c. an initial bolus of 50 mEq followed by a 25-mEq bolus every 5 minutes
    d. a single 100-mEg bolus

87. The usual dose for dopamine in the prehospital setting is:
    a. 0.5 to 30.0 µg/min titrated to effect
    b. 2 to 20 µg/kg/min IV drip
    c. 0.5 to 1.0 mg every 3 to 5 minutes
    d. 1 mg/kg IV bolus followed by a 2 to 4 mg/min drip

88. Your patient is in cardiac arrest and your protocol calls for amiodarone. The correct dose is:
    a. 150 mg repeated every 5 minutes
    b. a single dose of 1 mg/kg
    c. an initial dose of 300 mg IV push, with a second dose of 150 mg in 3 to 5 minutes
    d. an initial bolus of 1.5 mg/kg immediately followed by an IV drip of 2.0 to 4.0 mg/min

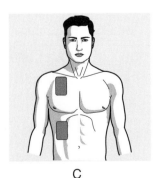
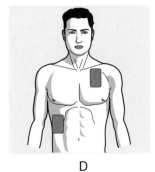

A   B

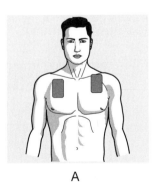
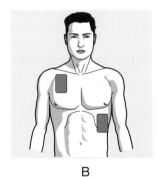

C   D

Figure 12-3

89. Your patient is in sinus bradycardia at a rate of 48 and complains of feeling weak and light headed. Blood pressure is 86/52. The most likely dose for atropine in this case is:
    a. 0.5 mg every 5 to 10 minutes up to a total of 4.0 mg
    b. 0.5 to 1.0 mg every 3 to 5 minutes up to a total of 0.04 mg/kg
    c. 1 mg every 3 to 5 minutes up to a total of 3 mg/kg
    d. 1.0 to 1.5 mg every 5 minutes up to a total of 3.0 mg

90. An adult patient is experiencing pulmonary edema related to left ventricular failure. Your protocol calls for furosemide. The usual dose is:
    a. 0.5 to 1.0 mg/kg
    b. 5 to 10 mg/kg
    c. 10 to 20 mg/kg
    d. 20 to 40 mg/kg

91. Your patient is having chest pain radiating into the left arm suggestive of ischemic pain. He also has dyspnea and is diaphoretic. The dose of aspirin for this patient is:
    a. 160 mg to 325 mg
    b. 325 mg to 500 mg
    c. 500 mg to 650 mg
    d. 650 mg to 1000 mg

92. Of the following, the stroke patient who is most likely to receive fibrinolytic therapy is one who:
    a. woke up with strokelike symptoms
    b. had similar signs and symptoms 1 month ago and was definitively diagnosed at that time as having had a stroke
    c. had an onset of symptoms less than 1 hour ago but has a blood pressure of 170/100
    d. had a seizure 20 minutes ago at the time of stroke onset

93. The proper way to administer adenosine is to:
    a. give it slow IV push to avoid nausea and hypotension
    b. dilute it in 250 mL of normal saline and infuse it over 15 to 20 minutes
    c. push it at a normal speed and follow it with a maintenance drip
    d. give it rapid IV push and follow the drug with a fluid bolus

94. A common side effect noted with the administration of adenosine is:
    a. supraventricular tachycardia
    b. a hot, flushed feeling
    c. hypertension
    d. wheezing

95. The correct IV dose of epinephrine for an adult in cardiac arrest is:
    a. 0.1 mg/kg of 1:1000 solution
    b. 0.5 mg/kg of 1:100 solution
    c. 1 mg of 1:10,000 solution regardless of the patient's weight
    d. 2 mg of 1:1000 solution regardless of the patient's weight

96. While managing a patient in asystole, the two medications most commonly used are:
    a. dopamine and diphenhydramine
    b. epinephrine and atropine
    c. atropine and albuterol
    d. lidocaine and epinephrine

97. A patient is in cardiac arrest and the monitor shows ventricular fibrillation. If lidocaine is used, an acceptable dose in this case is:
    a. an initial dose of 1.0 to 1.5 mg/kg IV with subsequent doses at 0.5 to 0.75 mg/kg IV repeated in 5 to 10 minutes, up to a maximum total dose of 3.0 mg/kg
    b. an initial dose of 1 mg/kg IV followed by a 2 to 4 mg/min maintenance infusion
    c. 1.5 mg/kg given every 3 to 5 minutes for the duration of the arrest
    d. 150 mg given as an IV infusion over 5 to 10 minutes

98. When including vasopressin in the treatment regimen for ventricular fibrillation, administer:
    a. 20 units every 5 minutes
    b. a one-time dose of 40 units
    c. a single dose of 40 units followed 5 minutes later by 1 mg of epinephrine
    d. alternate doses of vasopressin and epinephrine every 5 minutes

99. The highest priority when managing a cardiac arrest patient in pulseless electrical activity (PEA) is:
    a. early defibrillation
    b. rapid IV access to allow administration of medications
    c. searching for a correctable cause
    d. early initiation of transcutaneous pacing

100. Generally, circumstances and situations where resuscitation efforts would not be initiated would include all of the following *EXCEPT*:
   a. family members state the patient signed a Do-Not-Resuscitate order but do not know where it is
   b. rigor mortis is present
   c. injuries are incompatible with life (i.e., decapitation)
   d. the patient shows signs of fixed lividity

101. A situation that would meet the generally accepted inclusion and exclusion criteria for termination of resuscitation efforts would be a:
   a. 12-year-old boy who drowned in the backyard pool and remains in asystole despite appropriate resuscitation measures
   b. 36-year-old overdose patient who took an unknown quantity of tricyclic antidepressants and who is not responding despite 20 minutes of appropriate ALS interventions
   c. 68-year-old emphysema patient in cardiac arrest whom the family wants transported to a hospital despite EMS personnel kindly explaining that further resuscitation efforts will likely be futile
   d. 74-year-old patient with a history of heart problems who is currently in asystole and not responding despite 25 minutes of appropriate ALS interventions

102. The ballooning of an arterial wall, resulting from a defect or weakness in the wall, is:
   a. a claudication
   b. vasculitis
   c. an acute arterial occlusion
   d. an aneurysm

103. The term used to refer to severe pain in the calf muscle resulting from inadequate blood supply is:
   a. claudication
   b. phlebitis
   c. vasculitis
   d. paresthesia

104. You are about to perform synchronized cardioversion on your patient and are instructed to administer 5 mg of diazepam prior to the procedure. The primary reason for administering diazepam is that it:
   a. is an analgesic
   b. enhances electrical conversion
   c. improves blood flow to the heart
   d. is an amnestic

105. The patient you are about to cardiovert suddenly goes limp. You glance over at the cardiac monitor and notice ventricular fibrillation. Your next action is to:
   a. leave the synchronizer on but increase the output to 360
   b. start CPR and attempt to gain IV access if an IV is not already present
   c. turn off the synchronizer and defibrillate at 200
   d. immediately secure the airway, preferably by performing endotracheal intubation

106. Your patient is a 42-year-old female who called 9-1-1 because she had a "funny feeling" in her chest. Upon placing her on a cardiac monitor, you note that she has a heart rate of 180 and narrow QRS complexes. Her blood pressure is 98/72, which she states is a little low for her, and she does say she is feeling a bit weak. The medication of choice for this patient is:
   a. adenosine
   b. albuterol
   c. lidocaine
   d. Valium

107. The appropriate initial dose of medication for this patient is:
   a. 0.5 mg/kg
   b. 2.5 to 5.0 mg
   c. 5 mg/kg
   d. 6 mg

108. If the patient's blood pressure remains stable but the rate does not respond to the first dose of medication, your next action would likely be to:
   a. prepare for immediate synchronized cardioversion
   b. prepare to defibrillate
   c. repeat the medication at 12 mg
   d. administer atropine 0.5 mg

109. You and your partner respond to assess a 68-year-old male who presents with sudden onset of severe dyspnea but denies having any chest pain. His only medical history is recent knee surgery, and he states he has been somewhat immobile during his recuperation. The patient is mildly tachycardic and normotensive and has a respiratory rate of 28 and oxygen saturation of 91%. Breath sounds are present and clear bilaterally. You suspect his dyspnea to be related to:
   a. myocardial infarction with an atypical presentation
   b. pulmonary embolism
   c. tension pneumothorax
   d. chronic obstructive pulmonary disease

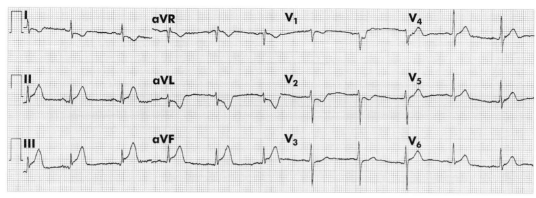

Figure 12-4

110. Your patient has a history of congestive heart failure and is presenting with severe dyspnea. Jugular vein distention is present, and auscultation of breath sounds reveals bilateral crackles and rhonchi. Among the medications you would consider administering are:
   a. albuterol, epinephrine, lidocaine
   b. adenosine, albuterol, atropine
   c. lidocaine, atropine, naloxone
   d. nitroglycerin, furosemide, morphine

111. A 52-year-old male with no history of heart problems presents with crushing substernal chest pain, which is radiating down his left arm, and shortness of breath. He is diaphoretic and, according to his family, appears paler than normal. Treatment of this patient is likely to include:
   a. adenosine, albuterol, atropine (AAA)
   b. adenosine, Benadryl, cordarone (ABC)
   c. lidocaine, atropine, Narcan, epinephrine (LANE)
   d. morphine, oxygen, nitroglycerin, aspirin (MONA)

112. An important consideration when deciding whether to administer furosemide to a patient is that:
   a. the diuretic actions take place quickly and the patient will likely need to urinate before reaching the hospital
   b. very little field benefit is derived from administering the medication because the diuretic actions take time to occur
   c. although the diuretic actions take time to occur, venous pooling may improve the patient's condition
   d. the patient may experience a sharp increase in blood pressure following administration

113. A 68-year-old male patient is complaining of severe pain in his back of sudden onset. He describes the pain as a "ripping" or "tearing" sensation. When checking vital signs, you notice that the blood pressure differs in the two arms. The patient also looks "shocky." You suspect:
   a. a dissecting aortic aneurysm
   b. an acute myocardial infarction
   c. atherosclerotic heart disease
   d. a spontaneous pneumothorax

114. Your patient is experiencing substernal chest pain radiating to the left arm. He is also complaining of moderate dyspnea and fatigue and is pale and diaphoretic. He has a history of angina but this episode of chest pain seems to be worse, and he has taken two nitroglycerin tablets already with no relief. Vital signs are pulse 106, blood pressure of 132/88, respiratory rate of 20, and a pulse oximeter reading of 96% on room air. You obtain a 12-lead ECG, and it reveals what is shown in Figure 12-4. Based on this ECG, you suspect the patient is experiencing:
   a. a lateral wall infarct
   b. an anterior wall infarct
   c. a septal wall infarct
   d. an inferior wall infarct

115. Management of this patient is likely to include:
   a. oxygen, aspirin, prophylactic lidocaine
   b. oxygen, albuterol, furosemide, and morphine
   c. oxygen, additional nitroglycerin, aspirin, and morphine
   d. oxygen, additional nitroglycerin, adenosine, and morphine

ANSWERS TO CHAPTER 12: MEDICAL EMERGENCIES II: CARDIAC

1.

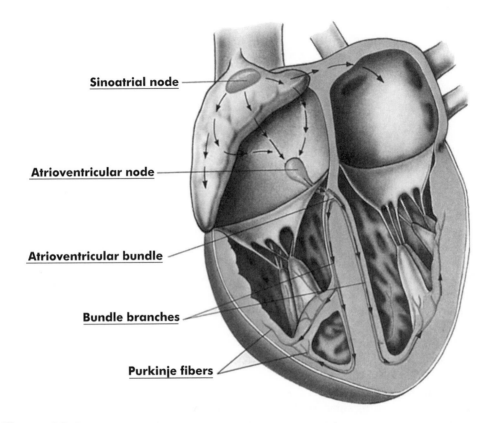

Sinoatrial node

Atrioventricular node

Atrioventricular bundle

Bundle branches

Purkinje fibers

Figure 12-1

2. **b.** The AV junctional tissue has an intrinsic firing rate of 40 to 60 discharges per minute, with the inherent firing rate of the AV node itself being 60. The firing rate of the SA node is 60 to 100 discharges per minute. The ventricles, including the bundle branches and Purkinje fibers, have an intrinsic firing rate of 20 to 40 discharges per minute.

3. **c.** Sodium, calcium, and potassium are the most important ions involved in myocardial action potential.

4. **d.** The clinical significance of Starling's law of the heart is that myocardial fibers contract more forcefully when stretched to a point. Therefore when ventricles receive an increased preload (are filled with larger-than-normal volumes of blood), they contract with greater-than-normal force.

5. **a.** The term *inotropy* pertains to the force or energy of muscle contraction, particularly contractions of the heart. Inotropic drugs that strengthen or increase the force of contraction are referred to as having a positive inotropic effect and include digoxin (Lanoxin), dobutamine (Dobutrex), isoproterenol (Isuprel), and epinephrine. Medications that weaken or decrease the force of contraction are referred to as having a negative inotropic effect and include propranolol (Inderal).

6. **d.** Chronotropic agents affect the heart's rate. Positive chronotropes such as isoproterenol (Isuprel) speed up the heart. Negative chronotropes, such as verapamil (Isoptin), slow it down.

7. **c.** Dromotropy pertains to agents that affect conduction velocity through the conducting tissues of the heart. Medications that speed conduction, such as isoproterenol (Isuprel), are said to have positive dromotropic effects. Medications that delay conduction, such as adenosine (Adenocard) and verapamil (Isoptin), are said to have negative dromotropic effects.

8. d. Verapamil and diltiazem are calcium-channel blockers. Use of such medications allows heart rate and contractility to be manipulated pharmacologically. An understanding of the effects common medications, such as calcium-channel blockers or beta blockers (such as propranolol and atenolol), have on the heart allows EMS personnel to gain some additional insight into the cardiac history of a patient.

9. a. The point of maximal impulse (PMI) is the location at which the apical pulse is most readily seen or palpated, often the fifth intercostal space just medial to the left midclavicular line. It can be used to assess for pulse deficit and also identifies the location of the mitral valve for assessing heart sounds.

10. b. The first heart sound, or S_1, occurs with closure of AV valves during ventricular asystole.

11. b. The second heart sound, or S_2, occurs with closure of aortic and pulmonic valves and signifies the beginning of ventricular diastole. A third and fourth heart sound, S_3 and S_4, related to a turbulent flow of blood into the ventricles, may sometimes be heard and is often a sign of congestive heart failure in adults.

12. d. When the vagus nerve is stimulated, it signals the SA node to decrease the rate of firing. It does not decrease ventricular ectopy, and because it does not have a positive chronotropic effect it does not result in tachyarrhythmias.

13. b. Lead II is the most common ECG lead used in the prehospital setting because it allows P-waves to be more easily visualized. The MCL_1 lead may also prove useful for prehospital cardiac monitoring activity.

14. c. The large blocks on ECG paper represent a time period of 0.20 second. The small blocks represent a time period of 0.04 second. Five small blocks make up one large block.

15. b. The heart rate shown in Figure 12-2 is 70. The space between the first and third long mark at the bottom of the strip represents 6 seconds. There are 7 QRS complexes in this space. Because there are 10 6-second intervals in a minute, the 7 beats are multiplied by 10. This equals 70, which is the heart rate.

16. d. The "Triplicate Method" is used to gain a rapid, approximate determination of heart rate when analyzing a regular ECG rhythm. The two number sets to remember are 300-150-100 and 75-60-50. To use the triplicate method, select an R wave that lines up with a dark vertical line on the ECG graph paper and identify where the next R wave falls with reference to the next six dark vertical lines. These six vertical lines represent heart rates of 300, 150, 100, 75, 60, and 50, respectively.

17. a. The P wave represents atrial depolarization. The T wave represents repolarization of the ventricular myocardial cells and occurs during the last part of ventricular systole.

18. b. The QRS complex corresponds to ventricular depolarization. The R and S waves represent the sum of electrical forces resulting from depolarization of the right and left ventricles.

19. a. The atria and ventricles contract when their cells are depolarized and refill during electrical repolarization.

20. b. The normal P-R interval is 0.12 to 0.20 second.

21. a. The absolute refractory period of the heart allows complete relaxation of the heart muscle to occur before another contraction can be initiated. This provides enough time for the heart to refill. During the absolute refractory period, the cardiac muscle is completely insensitive to further stimulation.

22. b. *Tachycardia* is the term used to refer to a heart rate greater than 100 beats per minute. *Tachypnea* is a rapid breathing rate, and *bradypnea* is a slow breathing rate.

23. a. A peaked T wave may indicate hyperkalemia (excessive potassium levels). Prominent U waves appear when a patient has deficient potassium levels, or hypokalemia. The J wave, or Osborn wave, may be apparent in cases of hypothermia. ST segment elevation indicates myocardial injury.

24. c. Myocardial ischemia would be suspected if an ECG showed ST segment depression and T wave inversion. Recognizing myocardial ischemia is important because if blood supply to ischemic tissue can be restored promptly, permanent myocardial injury can often be avoided. ST segment elevation indicates myocardial injury.

25. **d.** Three or more PVCs in a row constitute ventricular tachycardia.

26. **b.** The width of a normal QRS complex is 0.08 to 0.12 second, which equals 2 to 3 small squares on the graph paper.

27. **b.** Ventricular fibrillation and pulseless ventricular tachycardia are defibrillated.

28. **d.** Asystole is the absence of electrical activity in the heart and is recognized on an ECG as a flat line. Although attempts may be made to resuscitate the patient in asystole, the prognosis for success is poor.

29. **c.** The primary pacemeker of the heart is the SA (sinoatrial) node.

30. **c.** Bradycardia refers to a heart rate that is less than 60 beats per minute.

31. **a.** Hyperkalemia, myocardial ischemia, and certain drugs are common causes of delayed or blocked electrical impulses that may produce reentry dysrhythmias. Excess catecholamines, hypercapnia, and digitalis toxicity may cause non-reentry dysrhythmias that result from enhanced automaticity.

32. **d.** With third-degree AV block, the PR interval varies and there is no correlation of P-waves to QRS complexes because the atria and ventricles are electrically functioning independent of each other. Although wide QRS complexes are often present, in some cases the QRS may be of normal width.

33. **c.** Enhanced automaticity is a mechanism by which ectopic electrical impulses are generated. It is caused by an acceleration in depolarization that commonly results from an abnormally high leakage of sodium ions into the cells. This causes the cells to reach threshold prematurely. The result is that the rate of electrical impulse formation in potential pacemakers increases beyond their inherent rate.

34. **c.** In second-degree AV block Type II, some P waves will not be followed by QRS complexes. However, the PR interval will remain constant for each conducted P wave.

35. **b.** Patients with Wolff-Parkinson-White syndrome have an accessory electrical pathway that provides a ready-made reentry circuit. These patients are highly susceptible to bouts of paroxysmal supraventricular tachycardia (PSVT). Calcium channel blockers (such as verapamil) are contraindicated because they may precipitate very rapid atrial-to-ventricular conduction down the accessory pathway and may lead to ventricular fibrillation and death. Prehospital management may include administration of adenosine and cardioversion.

36. **b.** Second-degree AV block Type I, or Wenckebach, is characterized by a gradual prolongation of the PR interval and then a dropped QRS. The pattern will repeat itself.

37. **d.** Reentry is the reactivation of myocardial tissue for the second or subsequent time by the same impulse. Reentry is the most common mechanism in producing ectopic beats. These include PVCs, ventricular tachycardia, ventricular fibrillation, atrial fibrillation, atrial flutter, and paroxysmal supraventricular tachycardia (PSVT).

38.   The answers to the ECG strip recognition is in order as follows:
    1. premature junctional complex (PJC)
    2. AC (60-cycle) interference
    3. sinus tachycardia
    4. third-degree AV block
    5. ventricular escape complexes or rhythm
    6. second-degree AV block Type II
    7. sinus arrest
    8. wandering pacemaker
    9. premature atrial complex (PAC)
    10. sinus dysrhythmia
    11. paroxysmal supraventricular tachycardia (PSVT)
    12. atrial flutter
    13. ventricular tachycardia
    14. junctional escape complexes or rhythms
    15. second-degree AV block Type I (Wenckebach)
    16. sinus bradycardia
    17. agonal rhythm
    18. premature ventricular complex (PVC)
    19. accelerated junctional rhythm
    20. ventricular fibrillation
    21. asystole
    22. pacemaker rhythm
    23. atrial fibrillation
    24. first-degree AV block

39. b. An asynchronous, or nondemand, pacemaker delivers timed electrical stimuli at a selected rate, regardless of the patient's intrinsic cardiac activity. Demand pacemakers sense the patient's inherent QRS complex and deliver electrical stimuli only when needed. Most external pacemakers used by EMS personnel have the capability to work in either a nondemand or demand mode. The nondemand mode is generally used for asystole and overdrive pacing. Transvenous has to do with the way the pacemaker leads are inserted, not whether it is a nondemand or demand pacer.

40. d. The primary indications for transcutaneous cardiac pacing in the prehospital setting are heart block associated with reduced cardiac output that is unresponsive to atropine, symptomatic bradycardia, asystole, and pacemaker failure. In some EMS systems, third-degree block is immediately managed with pacing because atropine is often ineffective. Always follow local protocols for pacing indications and procedures.

41. c. Your next action would be to gradually increase the current until QRS complexes are seen. There is no need to reposition the electrodes. The current must be sufficient to result in "electrical capture," which is indicated by the QRS following the spike. Pacer spikes alone do not constitute electrical capture and will not produce cardiac output. For that matter, electrical capture may be seen, but even then the heart muscle may be too weak to produce mechanical output.

42. b. Stable angina pectoris usually is precipitated by physical exertion or emotional stress. The pain typically lasts 1 to 5 minutes but may last as long as 15 minutes. The pain associated with stable angina is relieved by rest, nitroglycerin, or oxygen. The attacks usually are similar in nature and are always relieved by the same mode of therapy. Unstable angina denotes an anginal pattern that has changed in its ease of onset, intensity, duration, frequency, quality, or pattern of relief. The pain usually lasts 10 minutes or more and is less promptly relieved by rest or nitroglycerin. Any new onset of angina in a patient who has never experienced chest pain is considered unstable and should be promptly evaluated.

43. c. It is difficult for EMS personnel to know how effective a patient's personal nitroglycerin is. When in doubt as to the stability and strength of the patient's medication, or if the patient has not taken the maximum dose of nitroglycerin allowed by protocol, additional nitroglycerin from the EMS unit's supply should be administered. Nitroglycerin is not an analgesic. It acts as an antiischemic because it is a vasodilator. Therefore for the patient's benefit, further nitroglycerin therapy should be tried before simply going to morphine. Prophylactic lidocaine is no longer indicated when a patient is having chest pain.

44. a. Acute thrombotic occlusion of the coronary arteries is the precipitating event in the vast majority of myocardial infarctions. Other factors that may lead to acute myocardial infarction include coronary spasm, coronary embolism, and severe hypoxia.

45. d. A primary difference with the pain/discomfort associated with an acute myocardial infarction (AMI) as opposed to angina pectoris is that the pain often is constant and is not altered or alleviated by nitroglycerin or other cardiac medications. Also, rest and changes in body position do not usually alleviate the pain. Pain associated with AMI often occurs during rest, whereas with angina pectoris the pain frequently occurs during periods of activity. Patients with AMI often complain of associated dyspnea. Both AMI and angina patients may experience radiation of pain into the arms, neck, jaw, or back.

46. b. ST segment elevation signifies acute injury to the heart muscle. ST segment elevation greater than 0.1 mV (one small square on ECG graph paper) in at least two anatomically contiguous ECG leads indicates acute myocardial infarction. Care must be taken, however, not to rely too much on ECG findings because the initial ECG may not demonstrate ST segment elevation in the patient who is suffering an infarction.

47. d. The most common cause of death from myocardial infarction is ventricular dysrhythmias. Pump failure such as cardiogenic shock or congestive heart failure, and myocardial tissue rupture are other causes of death that result from myocardial infarction but are far less common.

48. a. Emergency care for acute myocardial infarction is generally directed at administering supplemental oxygen to increase oxygen supply, decreasing metabolic needs and providing collateral circulation, and reestablishing perfusion to the ischemic myocardium as quickly as possible after the onset of symptoms. Some of these goals cannot be accomplished in the field, but rapid transportation to a hospital capable of advanced cardiac care allows all the goals to be met quickly. Generally, prophylactic administration of lidocaine or other antiarrhythmics is not indicated.

49. b. There are a number of criteria that would exclude a patient from receiving thrombolytic therapy. Among them are a history of intracranial bleed or stroke, uncontrolled hypertension, or prolonged CPR. Previous surgery is not in and of itself a contraindication. It depends on when the surgery took place and the type of surgery. EMS personnel should be familiar with the general and local inclusion and exclusion criteria for thrombolytic therapy.

50. c. Early treatment with thrombolytics where appropriate can limit infarct size, preserve left ventricular function, and reduce mortality. Ideally thrombolytic agents should be administered within 6 hours after the onset of symptoms, but a reduction of mortality may still be observed 12 hours from onset. A patient is generally not considered to be a candidate for thrombolytic therapy if the onset of symptoms is greater than 12 hours.

51. Given the presence of ST segment changes, note the suspected location of the acute myocardial infarction as anterior, inferior, lateral, or septal (*One answer may be used twice*).
I and aVL—lateral
II, III, aVF—inferior
V1 and V2— septal
V3 and V4—anterior
V5 and V6—lateral

52. b. An anterior wall infarct should be suspected if ST segment elevation is noted in leads V3 and V4. This is important for EMS personnel to remember because this is considered to be the most lethal location of infarct.

53. b. The most common location of infarct is the inferior wall. Inferior wall infarct is characterized by ST segment elevation in leads II, III, and aVF.

54. d. When assessing a 12-lead ECG, remember that a patient having a myocardial infarction may present with a normal 12-lead and may not exhibit ECG changes for an hour or more. Serial monitoring of the ECG is required.

55. a. Left coronary artery involvement would most likely be suspected if the location of the infarction is the septal wall, anterior wall, or lateral wall. Right coronary artery involvement would most likely be suspected if the location of the infarction is the inferior wall or right ventricle.

56. a. An acute MI should be suspected if the patient exhibits more than 1 mm of ST segment elevation in two anatomically contiguous leads. An acute MI should also be suspected if a patient presents with a new or presumably new left bundle branch block (LBBB).

57. b. Signs of right ventricular failure include peripheral edema as the blood entering the right ventricle is slowed, causing a systemic backup. The peripheral edema is often seen in the lower extremities, jugular vein distention, and tachycardia.

58. c. When left ventricular failure occurs, the left ventricle fails to function as an effective forward pump. This causes a back pressure of blood into the pulmonary circulation and results in pulmonary edema and severe respiratory distress. Respirations are often rapid and labored because the patient is hypoxic. The pulse rate is usually rapid to compensate for low stroke volume.

59. d. Factors that often precipitate or aggravate heart failure include chronic hypertension, valvular disease, and myocardial infarction. Right-sided heart failure can also result from chronic obstructive pulmonary disease.

60. a. Acute pulmonary edema refers to the accumulation of extravascular fluid in lung tissues and alveoli, or fluid in the lungs. As pulmonary capillary hydrostatic pressure increases, the plasma portion of blood is forced into the alveoli and mixes with air, resulting in the characteristic finding of pulmonary edema.

61. c. Acute pulmonary edema occurs when the left ventricle fails to function effectively as a pump and blood backs up into the pulmonary circulation. It is associated with left ventricular failure.

62. b. In left ventricular failure, blood is delivered to the left ventricle but not completely ejected from it. This causes an increase in end-diastolic blood volume, which in turn causes an increase in end-diastolic pressure. This increase is transmitted to the left atrium and subsequently to the pulmonary veins and capillaries. The end result is pulmonary edema. Additionally, left ventricular failure results in a reduction of stroke volume.

63. b. Paroxysmal nocturnal dyspnea (PND) refers to a sudden episode of dyspnea that occurs after lying down and that awakens a patient from sleep. It may be accompanied by profuse sweating, tachycardia, and wheezing. It is often associated with left ventricular failure and pulmonary edema.

64. c. When the right heart is unable to pump efficiently, it cannot deal with the blood it is receiving from systemic venous circulation. This causes a back pressure of blood and presents itself as edema in the extremities and sacrum. Sacral edema is more likely to be found in bedridden patients.

65. b. Nitroglycerin, furosemide, and morphine commonly are administered to a patient experiencing left ventricular failure. The medications are useful because they decrease preload, decrease myocardial oxygen demand, decrease pain and anxiety, and have vasodilatory effects.

66. c. When medications are administered to a patient in congestive heart failure, the goal is to decrease venous return to the heart, enhance contractile function of the myocardium, and reduce dyspnea. If the patient is experiencing pain associated with the cardiac event, the pharmacological agents used may also decrease the pain.

67. b. Management of hypotension resulting from right ventricular failure may include administering a 250 mL IV bolus of normal saline over 5 to 10 minutes. This can help normalize left ventricular filling, thereby increasing myocardial strength and improving contractility. The patient should be placed in a sitting or semisitting position.

68. d. Cardiogenic shock is the most extreme form of pump failure. Stroke volume, cardiac output, and blood pressure are markedly decreased. Left ventricular function is so compromised that the heart cannot meet the metabolic needs of the body.

69. b. Generally, patients in cardiogenic shock show clinical evidence of hypoperfusion to vital organs and significant systemic hypotension. Other signs include systolic blood pressure usually less than 80 mm Hg, pulmonary congestion, altered level of consciousness, cool, clammy skin, tachypnea, and sinus tachycardia or other dysrhythmias.

70. d. Pharmacological therapy for cardiogenic shock may include inotropic agents to improve cardiac output. These include dopamine and dobutamine. Dobutamine may be considered for pump problems with systolic blood pressure of 70 to 100 mm Hg and no signs of shock. Dopamine may be considered for pump problems with systolic blood pressure of 70 to 100 mm Hg with signs and symptoms of shock.

71. d. Cardiac tamponade occurs when fluid builds up in the pericardial sac. Diastolic filling of the heart is impaired because of increased intrapericardial pressure.

72. a. Distended neck veins, a narrowing pulse pressure difference, and faint or muffled heart sounds are all signs of cardiac tamponade. Systolic pressure will decrease.

73. b. A fluid bolus may be administered to help support the circulatory system temporarily if the patient becomes hypotensive. However, definitive management often requires inserting a needle into the pericardial sac to drain the fluid. This is referred to as *pericardiocentesis* and is usually done by a physician.

74. c. Pulsus paradoxus is an abnormal decrease in systolic blood pressure that drops more than 10 to 15 mm Hg during inspiration compared to expiration. In pulsus alternans, the pulse alternates between weak and strong.

75. d. A hypertensive emergency is a condition in which an increase in blood pressure leads to significant, irreversible end-organ damage within hours if not managed. As a rule, the diagnosis of hypertensive emergency is based on altered end-organ function and the rate of the rise in blood pressure, not the level of blood pressure itself. Hypertensive emergencies may be accompanied by various symptoms such as nausea and vomiting, restlessness, confusion, visual difficulties, and severe headaches.

76. a. In most cases of hypertensive emergencies, pharmacological therapy is not instituted in the prehospital setting. However, in severe cases of hypertensive encephalopathy or if transport is delayed, nitroglycerin may be ordered by medical command to try to reduce blood pressure because it is a vasodilator.

77. c. Synchronized cardioversion differs from defibrillation in that it is designed to deliver the shock after the peak of the R-wave of the cardiac cycle, thus avoiding the vulnerable relative refractory period.

78. c. The energy levels generally used to perform initial defibrillation for an adult in ventricular fibrillation or pulseless ventricular tachycardia are 200, 300, and 360 joules.

79. b. Paroxysmal supraventricular tachycardia and atrial fibrillation generally respond to lower energy levels. When cardioverting these rhythms, start with 50 joules.

80. c. When synchronized cardioversion is performed, the initial energy level is usually 100 joules. When paroxysmal supraventricular tachycardia and atrial fibrillation are cardioverted, an initial energy level of 50 joules may be used.

81. b. Part B of Figure 12-3 shows the correct location to place the defibrillator paddles.

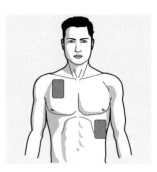

Figure 12-3

82. a. It is important to manage a patient with an implantable cardioverter-defibrillator (ICD) as if he or she did not have a device. Generally, standard ACLS protocols should be followed if the patient is in cardiac arrest or medically unstable in another way.

83. c. When a patient is in asystole, the dose for atropine is 1.0 mg every 3 to 5 minutes up to a total of 0.04 mg/kg.

84. b. Amiodarone is indicated for treatment of ventricular fibrillation and pulseless ventricular tachycardia. It is also useful in managing various tachycardias.

85. b. The initial dose for adenosine is 6 mg. If the first dose does not convert the patient, a second dose of 12 mg may be given 1 to 2 minutes later. In some cases, a third dose and final dose of 12 mg may also be given 1 to 2 minutes after the second.

86. b. When lab values are not available to use as a dosing guide, the usual dose for sodium bicarbonate is 1.0 mEq/kg repeated at half the initial dose every 10 minutes thereafter. Always follow local protocols.

87. b. Dopamine is administered IV drip with the dose based on the patient weight. The dosage range is 2 to 20 μg/kg/min. At low doses of 2 to 5 μg/kg/min, the dopaminergic effect is seen resulting in the dilation of renal and mesenteric vessels. This low of a dose may not increase the heart rate or blood pressure. Moderate doses of 5 to 10 μg/kg/min produce predominantly beta-adrenergic effects, including an increase in the force of contraction, a minimal increase in heart rate, and an increase in cardiac output. At high doses of 10 to 20 µg/kg/min, the alpha-adrenergic response dominates and a vasopressor effect is seen.

88. c. In a cardiac arrest situation, an initial dose of 300 mg of amiodarone is given IV push, with a second dose of 150 mg given in 3 to 5 minutes.

89. b. For hemodynamically unstable bradycardia, the dose for atropine is 0.5 to 1.0 mg every 3 to 5 minutes up to a total of 0.04 mg/kg. Use a shorter dosing interval (e.g., 3 minutes) and a higher dose (e.g., 1.0 mg) in severe clinical conditions.

90. a. The usual adult dose for furosemide is 0.5 to 1.0 mg/kg (usually 20 to 40 mg) given slow IV over 1 to 2 minutes.

91. a. A single dose of 160 to 325 mg of aspirin should be administered as soon as possible to all patients with acute coronary syndromes (ACS), particularly reperfusion candidates. Because it is preferable to have the patient chew rather than swallow the aspirin, children's aspirin is easier for most patients to take. Because children's aspirin normally is an 81-mg tablet, 2 to 4 tablets (162 to 324 mg) are commonly administered. Higher doses of aspirin (1000 mg) interfere with prostacyclin production and may limit the positive benefits.

92. c. For a patient to qualify for fibrinolytic therapy, the time of stroke symptom onset must be well established. Therapy must begin within 3 hours of time of onset. Ideally, systolic blood pressure should be less than 185 mm Hg and diastolic blood pressure should be less than 110 mm Hg. Patients who wake up with stroke symptoms do not qualify because the time of onset of symptoms cannot be accurately identified. Also, patients who had a previous stroke within 3 months or who had a seizure at stroke onset normally do not qualify.

93. d. Adenosine has a short half life and therefore must be pushed as quickly as possible. After pushing the medication, administer a rapid fluid flush of at least 20 mL of normal saline and elevate the extremity.

94. b. There are numerous common side effects noted with the administration of adenosine. Among them are a hot, flushed feeling, hypotension, and transient periods of sinus bradycardia, sinus pause, or bradyasystole. The patient also may complain of chest pain or discomfort and a feeling of impending doom.

95. c. Adult patients receive 1.0 mg of epinephrine IV every 3 to 5 minutes regardless of weight. Normally, a 1:10,000 concentration is used.

96. b. Epinephrine and atropine are the two primary pharmacological agents used to treat asystole.

97. a. If lidocaine is used during a cardiac arrest situation, an acceptable dosing regimen is an initial dose of 1.0 to 1.5 mg/kg IV with subsequent doses at 0.5 to 0.75 mg/kg IV repeated in 5 to 10 minutes, up to a maximum total dose of 3.0 mg/kg. IV maintenance infusions are not indicated in the arrest setting.

98. b. Vasopressin is a potent peripheral vasoconstrictor. For cardiac arrest situations, it is only given to ventricular fibrillation patients and is given as a one-time dose of 40 units. Because it has a relatively long half life, it is recommended that epinephrine not be given until at least 10 to 20 minutes after vasopressin is administered.

99. c. When managing a cardiac arrest patient in pulseless electrical activity (PEA), give high priority to searching for and identifying correctable causes of the arrest. The cause must be reversed for the patient to survive.

100. a. Generally, resuscitation efforts would not be initiated if rigor mortis is present, if there are injuries incompatible with life (i.e., decapitation), or if the patient shows signs of fixed lividity. Resuscitation efforts also would not be started if a valid Do-Not-Resuscitate (DNR) order was present, not simply if the family said the patient had DNR orders.

101. d. Generally, resuscitation efforts may be terminated when the patient remains in asystole despite appropriate resuscitation measures for at least 10 minutes or more. Appropriate efforts include suitable CPR, successful intubation with adequate oxygen delivery, successful IV access, appropriate pharmacological therapy, and other modalities called for by local protocols. When the patient is young, when the family wants the patient transported, or when unusual situations such as drug overdoses or hypothermia are present, field termination of resuscitation efforts is usually not appropriate. Always follow local protocols regarding termination of resuscitation efforts in the field.

102. d. An aneurysm is the ballooning of an arterial wall, resulting from a defect or weakness in the wall.

103. a. Claudication is severe, cramplike pain in the calf muscle due to inadequate blood supply. It typically occurs with exertion and subsides with rest. Phlebitis is inflammation of a vein, often accompanied by formation of a clot. Vasculitis is inflammation of blood vessels. Paresthesia is a sensation of numbness, tingling, or burning.

104. d. Diazepam is not an analgesic. It is given prior to cardioversion because it causes sedation and is an amnestic, which causes the patient not to remember the procedure. The patient may still feel the pain of cardioversion but may not remember it.

105. c. Early defibrillation is the best treatment for ventricular fibrillation. In this case, as soon as ventricular fibrillation is recognized, the synchronizer should be turned off and the initial defibrillation energy level of 200 J should be delivered. Although airway control, CPR, and IV access are important, early defibrillation is the first priority.

106. a. Adenosine is indicated for the pharmacological conversion of symptomatic narrow-complex tachycardias. The medication is normally administered after trying vagal maneuvers.

107. d. The initial dose of adenosine is 6 mg.

108. c. If the patient does not respond to the initial dose of adenosine, a repeat dose of 12 mg may be administered 1 to 2 minutes after the first dose of 6 mg. A third dose of 12 mg may be given 1 to 2 minutes after the second dose if needed.

109. b. The patient's presentation and history suggest he may have a pulmonary thromboembolism. Clues are the sudden onset of severe and unexplained dyspnea and recent surgery with immobility.

110. d. Nitroglycerin, furosemide, and morphine are commonly used to manage pulmonary edema associated with congestive heart failure.

111. d. When a patient with a suspected myocardial infarction is treated, the acronym MONA can be used to remember the medications commonly used. These medications are morphine, oxygen, nitroglycerin, and aspirin. Although the acronym MONA is used, the medications are not usually given in that order. Oxygen, nitroglycerin, and aspirin are administered first and can be given almost simultaneously. Morphine is normally given later, primarily if there is little to no relief of pain.

112. c. Furosemide works as a diuretic and also dilates the venous system. Although the diuretic effects may not be seen for 15 to 20 minutes and may only provide minimal benefits during transport, venous dilation occurs within 5 minutes and the venous pooling may improve the patient's condition en route to the hospital.

113. a. This patient is presenting with signs and symptoms of a dissecting aortic aneurysm. Signs and symptoms may include sudden onset of abdominal or back pain often described as tearing or ripping, hypotension, absent or reduced pulses, different blood pressures in the two arms, and syncope. If the aneurysm involves the abdominal aorta, a pulsatile, tender mass may be palpated in the abdomen.

114. d. Based on the location of ST-segment elevation (leads II, III, and aVF) shown in Figure 12-4, this patient is likely experiencing an inferior wall myocardial infarction.

115. c. Management of this patient is likely to include oxygen, additional nitroglycerin, aspirin, and morphine.

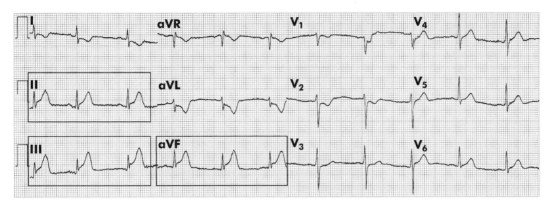

Figure 12-4

MEDICAL EMERGENCIES III: ENDOCRINE

1. The primary means by which hormones are distributed throughout the body is:
   a. the lymphatic system
   b. the nervous system
   c. the bloodstream
   d. the gastrointestinal system

2. The most important factor affecting the specificity of a hormone's action is:
   a. the receptor number and affinity for that hormone on target organs and tissue
   b. the concentration of the hormone in the body
   c. the speed of secretion
   d. the rate of metabolism

3. The primary purpose of the endocrine system is to:
   a. control the blood sugar level
   b. maintain homeostasis and respond to environmental stress
   c. control the blood pressure
   d. control body temperature

4. Hormones can only exert their effect on cells by interacting with receptors on the cell surface.
   a. true
   b. false

5. As levels of a hormone rise in the bloodstream, the organ that secreted the hormone decreases production. This is an example of a(n) _____ feedback mechanism.
   a. negative
   b. positive
   c. inhibitor
   d. stimulatory

6. All of the following are examples of endocrine glands *EXCEPT*:
   a. ovaries
   b. pituitary
   c. gallbladder
   d. thyroid

7. Diabetes mellitus results from pancreatic dysfunction affecting more than 15 million Americans and is:
   a. potentially lethal
   b. associated with juvenile arthritis
   c. only a disorder of glucose metabolism with little effect on other organs
   d. easily diagnosed based on history alone

8. Match the hormone with its associated gland.
   a. insulin   1. thyroid
   b. growth hormone   2. parathyroid
   c. norepinephrine   3. pancreas
   d. thyroxin   4. adrenal gland
   e. calcitonin   5. pituitary

9. The endocrine cells of the pancreas are contained within the islets of Langerhans. Which of the following is true?
   a. Insulin is secreted by the delta cells.
   b. Beta cells secrete somatostatin.
   c. The islets are connected to the pancreatic duct.
   d. The alpha cells secrete glucagon.

10. Insulin does all of the following *EXCEPT*:
    a. decreases liver glycogen levels
    b. increases glucose transport into cells
    c. increases glucose metabolism by cells
    d. decreases blood glucose levels

11. When serum glucose levels fall:
    a. glucagon stimulates increased absorption of glucose from the GI tract
    b. glucagon stimulates release of glucose stores from the liver
    c. insulin production increases
    d. gluconeogenesis occurs to move glucose into the adipose tissue

12. An increased level of glucose is the only means by which insulin production is stimulated.
   a. true
   b. false

13. Growth hormone is a polypeptide hormone that is:
   a. secreted by the posterior pituitary
   b. stimulated by the release of somatostatin
   c. required for the proper function of glucagon
   d. stimulated by hypoglycemia and acts as an insulin antagonist

14. There are only two types of diabetes: Type 1, which is due to impaired insulin production, and Type 2, which is a combination of decreased insulin production and diminished tissue sensitivity to insulin.
   a. true
   b. false

15. Differences in Type 1 and Type 2 diabetes include all of the following *EXCEPT*:
   a. Type 1 requires lifelong use of insulin injections
   b. Type 2 is more common in obese, older patients, whereas Type 1 occurs at an early age
   c. Type 2 never requires the use of insulin
   d. Type 2 is usually managed with diet, exercise, and drugs to improve cellular sensitivity to insulin

16. In Type 1 diabetes the patient is born without sufficient numbers of insulin-producing cells.
   a. true
   b. false

17. Decreased levels of glucose result in an altered level of consciousness because:
   a. the brain uses up its supply of glycogen, leading to cerebral hypoglycemia
   b. elevated insulin levels in the brain lead to ketone formation
   c. decreased levels of glucose lead to cerebral gluconeogenesis, which results in acid formation that decreases cerebral function
   d. the brain has no glycogen stores and therefore relies solely on the body to regulate blood glucose levels within a narrow range

18. Which of the following mechanisms is NOT involved in achieving adequate blood glucose regulation?
   a. the liver removes excess glucose from the blood and stores it as glycogen
   b. insulin and glucagon are produced in a feedback mechanism depending on the level of glucose
   c. the sympathetic nervous system stimulates glucagon production to increase blood glucose levels
   d. growth hormone and cortisol respond to prolonged hypoglycemia

19. A 13-year-old male presents with weight loss and fatigue. His mother states that he has been urinating frequently and drinks water constantly. These symptoms are caused by:
   a. elevated glucose levels in the blood, which lead to cerebral impairment and cause this abnormal behavior
   b. loss of glucose in the urine, resulting in an osmotic diuresis and thirst
   c. polydipsia as a reflex to dilute the blood glucose level
   d. not eating properly (fatigue only)

20. The 3 *P*s of diabetes include the following *EXCEPT*:
   a. polyuria
   b. polydipsia
   c. polyphasia
   d. polyphagia

Questions 21 through 25 refer to the following scenario:

A 37-year-old insulin-dependent diabetic presents with an altered level of consciousness. He complains of abdominal pain and is vomiting. His respiratory rate is 26, and his breath has a fruity odor.

21. Important questions to ask include:
   a. When was the last time he ate?
   b. When and how much insulin did he last take?
   c. Has he been ill lately?
   d. All of the above

22. Which of the following is true as it relates to his altered mental status?
    a. Diabetic ketoacidosis can result in coma as profound as hypoglycemia.
    b. His increased respiratory rate is a reflex to hypoxia from increased metabolic demand.
    c. Ketone formation from glycogenolysis results in metabolic acidosis, which affects the brain.
    d. All of the above

23. The fruity odor of his breath is the result of:
    a. elevated glucose in his system, which is spilled in his respiratory tract making his breath smell sweet
    b. acetone, which is excreted in his breath
    c. chewing spearmint gum prior to your arrival
    d. respiratory alkalosis from hyperventilation

24. All of the following accurately reflect the role of gastrointestinal upset in diabetic ketoacidosis *EXCEPT*:
    a. vomiting and diarrhea lead to dehydration, which worsens the condition
    b. the diabetic may inappropriately decrease his insulin intake because the vomiting has kept him from eating
    c. the vomiting can be a result of the acidosis alone
    d. the diarrhea is a result of the inability of the body to absorb dietary glucose

25. Kussmaul's respirations are:
    a. an attempt to remove carbon dioxide in response to the metabolic acidosis
    b. an attempt to blow off excess acids secreted into the lung
    c. exemplified by fast and shallow respirations
    d. a response to decreased cerebral glucose metabolism

26. The most appropriate prehospital therapy for diabetic ketoacidosis after ensuring the ABCs is:
    a. have the patient breathe into a paper bag to resolve hyperventilation
    b. establish two large-bore IVs and run wide open
    c. assist the patient in administering his own insulin to decrease hyperglycemia
    d. administer sodium bicarbonate to reverse the metabolic acidosis

27. The most common electrolyte abnormality found in diabetic ketoacidosis is:
    a. hypernatremia
    b. hyperkalemia
    c. hyperglycemia
    d. hypercalcemia

28. Which of the following best differentiates hyperosmolar hyperglycemic nonketotic (HHNK) coma from diabetic ketoacidosis (DKA)?
    a. HHNK results in greater mental status changes than DKA.
    b. HHNK occurs more often in Type 2 diabetes.
    c. Dehydration and electrolyte imbalance occur more often in DKA.
    d. None of the above are correct.

29. Diabetes is a systemic disease with many long-term complications. Which of the following best describes some of these complications?
    a. Cardiovascular disease and stroke are increased because of repeated injury to small vessels.
    b. Wound infections occur because increased blood sugar promotes bacteria growth.
    c. Up to 10% of all diabetics develop some form of kidney disease including renal failure.
    d. Blindness occurs from increased cataract formation.

Questions 30 through 35 refer to the following scenario:

An obese 55-year-old woman with Type 2 diabetes mellitus states that she has been feeling "weak all over for a few days." She has generalized edema, including edema of the hands, legs, and eyelids. You check her blood glucose and get a reading of 492. Her blood pressure is 190/110, heart rate 110, respiratory rate 12. She admits to not seeing her doctor regularly or taking her medication. Her ECG is depicted in Figure 13-1.

30. Hyperkalemia is demonstrated on her ECG by:
    a. flattening of the ST segments
    b. tall peaked P waves
    c. narrowing of the QRS
    d. tall peaked T waves

31. What complication of diabetes would account for her edema and hypertension?
    a. congestive heart failure
    b. renal failure
    c. DKA
    d. HHNK

32. All of the following medications are used in the treatment of Type 2 diabetes *EXCEPT:*
    a. Diabinese
    b. Actos
    c. insulin
    d. Pancrease

33. With weight loss, exercise, and the proper diet it is possible for Type 2 diabetes to be controlled to the point of no longer requiring medication.
    a. true
    b. false

34. The appropriate prehospital treatment for this woman's condition would be:
    a. treat her hypertension with nitroglycerin
    b. supportive only and transport
    c. treat her volume overload with furosemide
    d. treat her hypertension with labetalol

35. The treatment of her hyperglycemia would consist of:
    a. intravenous fluid bolus of normal saline
    b. assist her in the administration of her medication
    c. insulin administration
    d. none of the above

Questions 36 through 40 refer to the following scenario:

A 26-year-old man with Type 1 diabetes took his insulin but forgot to eat breakfast. As he arrives at work he begins to feel shaky and faint. On arrival you find him incoherent with a blood pressure of 80/20, heart rate 140, respiratory rate 12. His skin is cold and clammy.

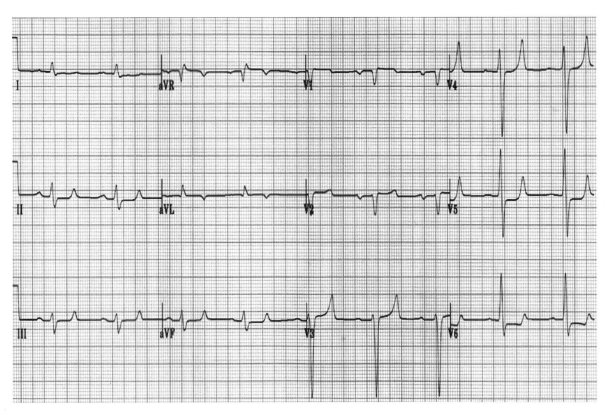

Figure 13-1

36. His cold, clammy skin and shakiness are due to:
    a. hypotension
    b. hypoglycemia
    c. epinephrine
    d. hyperinsulinemia

37. In the absence of a blood glucose level the administration of dextrose should be withheld because it could worsen his condition if he is hyperglycemic.
    a. true
    b. false

38. His blood glucose is checked and found to be 40. Which of the following best describes the decision process of how dextrose should be administered to the patient?
    a. An IV should be started and D_{50} given even if he is awake and talking.
    b. Glucagon always works and should be relied on if an IV cannot be established.
    c. D_{50} should be administered VERY slowly and stopped as soon as LOC improves.
    d. None of the above are correct.

39. Which of the following is a complication of D_{50} administration?
    a. Extravasation can result in tissue necrosis.
    b. It can cause seizures.
    c. It can result in hyperglycemia precipitating DKA.
    d. It can precipitate Wernicke's encephalopathy in opiate addicts.

40. You administer 25 g of dextrose and the patient fails to improve. Your next step would be to:
    a. administer naloxone 2 mg IV
    b. administer an additional 25 g of dextrose
    c. await arrival to the hospital to check blood sugar
    d. administer IV glucagon

41. A condition that results in hyperfunction of the thyroid presenting with significant physiological manifestations is called:
    a. hyperthyroidism
    b. thyrotoxicosis
    c. goiter
    d. hyperparathyroidism

42. The thyroid gland functions normally by:
    a. secreting thyroxine (T4) and triiodothyroxine (T3) after stimulation from the adrenal gland
    b. regulatory feedback from the pancreas
    c. regulatory feedback from the parathyroid gland
    d. secreting iodine-containing hormones following stimulation from the pituitary gland

43. The thyroid gland is located:
    a. at the angle of the jaw in the upper neck
    b. in the lower neck, just below the larynx
    c. at the base of the tongue
    d. at the base of the neck behind the sternum

44. Hyperthyroidism results from all the following conditions *EXCEPT*:
    a. infection of the thyroid
    b. autoimmune disorders
    c. surgical removal of the pituitary
    d. pituitary gland tumors

45. The primary purpose of thyroxine is to:
    a. control body metabolism
    b. control serum calcium levels
    c. control body temperature
    d. none of the above

46. Thyroid storm, a name given to an acute hyperfunction of the thyroid, will demonstrate itself with all of the following signs and symptoms *EXCEPT*:
    a. tachycardia
    b. agitation
    c. abdominal pain
    d. weight gain

47. A 46-year-old woman presents with agitation, tachycardia, and delirium. On exam you notice that you can see the whites of her eyes completely around her iris, and it appears as if her eyeballs are protruding from the sockets. All of the following are true *EXCEPT*:
    a. this is consistent with Graves' disease, an autoimmune disorder
    b. generalized enlargement of the thyroid gland is called a "gizzard"
    c. the condition of protruding eyes is called exophthalmos
    d. you would expect to find swelling of her lower neck

48. Proper prehospital management of thyroid storm consists of:
a. administration of beta-blockers to blunt the physiological effects of thyroxine
b. administration of antithyroid medications to reduce hormone secretion
c. searching for other possible causes of adrenergic hyperactivity such as cocaine or amphetamine use, hypoglycemia, and alcohol withdrawal
d. administration of Tylenol for fever control

49. A rare condition that occurs from a deficiency of thyroid hormone is:
a. called myxedema coma
b. more common in young men
c. treated with iodine
d. not life threatening

50. Typical signs and symptoms of hypothyroidism consist of each of the following *EXCEPT*:
a. weight gain
b. depression
c. constipation
d. hair loss

51. Excess corticosteroid secretion is a condition of hyperfunction of the adrenal gland and is:
a. called Cushing's syndrome
b. common following the use of corticosteroids for an allergic reaction
c. only caused by a tumor in the adrenal gland
d. not associated with any particular physical findings

52. Your patient states she has Cushing's syndrome. What physical signs and symptoms would you expect to find?
a. hump on the back of the neck called a "hunch-back"
b. obese, round, red face called "moon-face"
c. loss of body hair
d. yellow jaundiced skin

53. Addison's disease, a rare, potentially life-threatening disorder, is caused by:
a. adrenal hypersecretion similar to Cushing's syndrome
b. a response of the adrenal gland to cortisone levels
c. any process that destroys the adrenal cortex
d. any process that destroys the adrenal medulla

54. Common symptoms associated with Addison's disease include all of the following *EXCEPT*:
a. progressive weakness, weight loss, and anorexia
b. GI disturbances such as nausea, vomiting, and diarrhea
c. hypotension
d. skin hypopigmentation

55. Your 65-year-old patient's family states he has Addison's disease. You find him unconscious with a blood sugar of 30, blood pressure of 60/P, with thin wasted skin, and he appears to be markedly dehydrated. This condition is a result of:
a. Addisonian crisis
b. diabetes mellitus
c. drug overdose
d. none of the above

ANSWERS TO CHAPTER 13: MEDICAL EMERGENCIES III: ENDOCRINE

1. c. Hormones are secreted from the endocrine glands directly into the bloodstream, which then carries them throughout the body to exert their effect on various organ systems.

2. a. Although each of the listed factors affects the speed and efficiency of a hormone's action, it can only act on organs that have receptors for it. The greater the number of receptors, the greater the ability of the hormone to exert its effects.

3. b. Homeostasis is the ability of the body to reach a point of balance between the internal needs of the body and the external stresses of the environment. Although the endocrine system is involved in blood sugar, blood pressure, and body temperature control, these are only a few of the many actions involved in homeostasis.

4. b. False. Hormone receptors exist both inside and outside of the cell.

5. a. The regulation of hormone activity can be through either a negative or positive feedback mechanism. Negative feedback is most common and occurs when higher hormone levels inhibit further secretion. In the positive feedback mechanism the lower hormone level stimulates hormone secretion.

6. c. Endocrine glands secrete their products directly into the bloodstream, whereas exocrine glands secrete their products into ducts. The gallbladder secretes bile into the bile duct then into the GI tract. The pancreas is both an endocrine and exocrine gland sending insulin into the bloodstream and amylase into the GI tract.

7. a. Diabetes is potentially lethal if left untreated and can be very difficult to diagnose without a full history and physical along with diagnostic tests. Although glucose metabolism is the root of the defect its effects are bodywide, and it is the effects on organ systems that lead to the associated complications. Arthritis is not one of these associated complications.

8. a. pancreas; b. pituitary; c. adrenal gland; d. thyroid; e. parathyroid.

9. d. The islets of Langerhans are composed of three cell types. Alpha cells secrete glucagon, beta cells secrete insulin, and delta cells secrete somatostatin, which inhibits the secretion of growth hormone from the pituitary. The pancreatic duct carries the exocrine gland production of amylase and lipase for digestion.

10. a. The primary functions of insulin are to increase glucose transport into cells, increase glucose metabolism by cells, increase liver glycogen levels, and decrease blood glucose levels.

11. b. As serum glucose levels fall the body responds with the process of gluconeogenesis, which moves glucose out of the adipose tissue and the liver to raise the blood glucose levels. Glucagon has no effect on the GI tract. Insulin production is decreased.

12. b. False. The secretion of insulin is stimulated not only by increased glucose levels but also by proteins released from the GI tract and neural impulses from the parasympathetic nervous system in response to dietary intake.

13. d. During prolonged hypoglycemia as in fasting or starvation, growth hormone is released from the anterior pituitary to increase glucose levels by inhibiting insulin production. Somatostatin inhibits the secretion of growth hormone.

14. a. Although Type 1 and Type 2 diabetes make up the majority of cases of diabetes, there are other conditions that result in diabetes that are essentially impairments in glucose metabolism. Gestational diabetes occurs during pregnancy from an impaired production of insulin and usually resolves after delivery but can recur years later.

15. c. Type 1 diabetes presents in teenagers and young adults, whereas Type 2 occurs later in life as a result of decreased sensitivity of the tissues to the patient's insulin. Type 2 patients tend to be obese and, if diet, exercise, and medications are ineffective, will require the administration of insulin to control blood sugar levels.

16. b. False. Type 1 diabetes has a heritable component and is a result of an autoimmune response in which the body attacks and destroys its own insulin-producing cells, leading to impaired insulin production.

17. d. Insulin has no effect on the brain tissue to increase glucose uptake. The brain uses glucose only for energy and does not store reserves as glycogen. Because there are no glycogen stores in the brain, gluconeogenesis does not occur there. However, gluconeogenesis in the body results in ketone body production, which results in acidosis that impairs cerebral function.

18. c. The sympathetic nervous system is stimulated to produce epinephrine and norepinephrine as a response to hypoglycemia. Both chemicals act directly on the liver to promote glycogenolysis similar to glucagon.

19. b. As serum glucose levels increase the excess is spilled in the urine. These large molecules cause water to shift with them resulting in polyuria. Polydipsia is in response to this diuresis and an attempt to maintain hydration. Fatigue results from the body's inability to metabolize the glucose leading to starvation of the tissues, which require glucose to function.

20. c. Polyuria is increased urination from glucosuria. Polydipsia is a response to thirst from polyuria. Polyphagia is increased dietary intake to compensate for poor utilization of glucose. Polyphasia is from talking too much in class.

21. d. The patient may be suffering from diabetic ketoacidosis, which may result from insufficient insulin intake, poor dietary intake, or infection.

22. c. The patient with DKA seldom becomes comatose as with severe hypoglycemia but often has an altered LOC as a result of the severe metabolic acidosis from ketone body formation.

23. b. Acetone is one of the ketone bodies produced by glycogenolysis and has a fruity smell. It can also occur from severe dehydration without hyperglycemia.

24. d. The diabetic often regulates insulin administration based on dietary intake and blood glucose levels and may inappropriately lower the dose thinking that there is insufficient carbohydrate intake because of GI distress. Dehydration results not only from the diarrhea but from the diuresis as well, and vomiting and abdominal pain can be the result of metabolic acidosis.

25. a. Metabolic acidosis results in a compensatory hyperventilation to create a respiratory alkalosis. Driving carbon dioxide out of the system allows more metabolic acids to be converted to

carbonic acid then to carbon dioxide, which is exhaled. It is not controlled by the brain. Kussmaul's respirations are deep and rapid to increase the efficiency of carbon dioxide removal.

26. b. Proper initial treatment of DKA consists of rapid volume replacement with normal saline to correct dehydration and dilute the metabolic acidosis. Insulin and sodium bicarbonate administration should be reserved until volume replacement has been accomplished and should be guided by laboratory data.

27. b. During metabolic acidosis hydrogen ions move into the cells pushing potassium out and into the bloodstream. This results in hyperkalemia, which can result in cardiac dysrhythmias.

28. b. The primary difference between HHNK and DKA is the lack of ketone formation in HHNK, which does not result in the level of acidosis seen in DKA. Both conditions can result in severe changes in mental status because of dehydration and hyperglycemia.

29. a. Diabetes is considered a small-vessel disease because the long-term elevation in glucose levels leads to destruction and obstruction of capillary beds. Therefore tissues that rely on rich capillary perfusion are those most prone to damage from diabetes. Blindness occurs as a result of impaired retinal perfusion, wound infection from peripheral neuropathies leading to unrecognized injuries, and poor perfusion leading to diminished immune response. The patient with diabetes is two to four times more likely to develop heart disease and two to six times more likely to have a stroke. Because the kidney requires a rich perfusion of the glomeruli, renal injury is common.

30. d. In the setting of hyperkalemia, the T waves may start to become increasingly tall and peaked at a serum potassium level of 5.5 mmol/L. The QRS complex may begin to widen at a serum potassium level of 6.5 mmol/L. The P wave may begin to flatten at a serum potassium level of 7 mmol/L. Note the PR prolongation. PR prolongation caused by hyperkalemia is primarily due to an increase in the P wave duration. This patient has a first-degree atrioventricular (AV) block. At a serum potassium level of 8 mmol/L, the P wave may become invisible. This patient had a serum potassium level of 7.1 mmol/L.

31. b. Renal failure results in the inability to properly excrete water and electrolytes. The decrease in renal perfusion stimulates the production of angiotensin, which results in hypertension. This patient's creatinine level was 4.5.

32. d. Pancrease is an enzyme that is ingested to assist in digestion. Diabinese, Actos, and insulin are medications that move glucose into the cells.

33. a. True. Type 2 diabetes, unlike Type 1, can be controlled without medication if the patient adheres to a strict diet with weight loss and exercise. The patient's own insulin production becomes sufficient for glucose control.

34. b. Supportive care is all that is required in the absence of congestive heart failure or a hypertensive crisis. Diuretics would be poorly effective in the presence of renal failure.

35. c. Insulin would be used to reduce the blood glucose levels. This would be performed in the emergency department based on diagnostic tests. Intravenous fluids would further worsen her volume overload.

36. c. Although his underlying condition is hypoglycemia, most of his symptoms are secondary to release of epinephrine from the adrenal gland. Epinephrine is released in response to the hypoglycemia and acts similar to glucagon in generating gluconeogenesis. It also acts as an alpha agonist resulting in tachycardia, tremors, and diaphoresis.

37. b. False. If a blood glucose level cannot be obtained and altered mental status is thought to be from diabetes, the empiric administration of dextrose is indicated. If the patient is hypoglycemic, he will improve. If he is hyperglycemic, the additional 25 g of glucose will not add significantly to his total blood glucose level.

38. d. If the patient is able to maintain his airway he should be given glucose containing agents by mouth. It is appropriate to start an IV in the event that he worsens. If D_{50} is given there is no need to titrate its effects. Glucagon will not be effective in alcoholics or those with liver disease as they have poor glycogen stores.

39. a. Intravenous dextrose is a highly concentrated osmotic agent, which if extravasated into the tissue can result in necrosis. DKA occurs slowly over time and is not a direct result of the hypoglycemia but of the acidosis from glycogenolysis. Administration of dextrose in alcoholics without pretreatment with thiamin can precipitate Wernicke's encephalopathy.

40. b. If you are confident that you are treating an insulin reaction, it would be appropriate to administer an additional 25 g of dextrose. Naloxone would be indicated if you suspected opiate ingestion, but this is not the case. Waiting to arrive at the hospital could delay appropriate treatment if the patient is still hypoglycemic. Although glucagon may be given intravenously, IV dextrose is much more effective and reliable in reversing hypoglycemia.

41. b. Thyrotoxicosis is the general term used to describe all the conditions that result in a toxic condition from thyroid hyperfunction. Hyperthyroidism is a less severe condition of hyperfunction but does not cause significant, acute, life-threatening conditions. A goiter is a thyroid growth that may precipitate thyrotoxicosis. The parathyroid gland is involved in calcium and phosphate control and is embedded in the thyroid gland.

42. d. The thyroid gland is normally controlled by a negative feedback mechanism from the pituitary that secretes thyroid-stimulating hormone (TSH) in response to decreased levels of thyroxin (T4) and triiodothyroxine (T3), which are the iodine-containing hormones produced by the thyroid gland. There is no hormonal interaction between the parathyroid and thyroid glands.

43. b. The thyroid gland is composed of two lobes joined by a small portion called the isthmus and is located in the lower anterior neck just below the larynx.

44. c. Hyperthyroidism can result from any condition that increases secretion of thyroid hormones. Infection, thyroiditis, autoimmune disorders, pituitary gland tumors that secrete TSH, and other conditions such as genetic disorders and congenital defects can cause hyperthyroidism.

45. a. The thyroid hormones play an important role in controlling body metabolism and are required for normal physical and mental development in children. Calcitonin, which is secreted from the parathyroid gland, is involved in serum calcium levels. Body temperature is controlled by the hypothalamus in the brain.

46. d. Thyroid storm refers to the constellation of signs and symptoms associated with thyrotoxicosis. Elevated thyroxine levels present with signs and symptoms similar to adrenergic hyperactivity such as tachycardia, tremulousness, agitation, abdominal pain, hyperthermia, delirium, and even coma. Weight loss rather than gain is secondary to the elevated metabolic rate.

47. b. This woman has Graves' disease, an autoimmune disorder of the thyroid gland, that results in thyroid hyperfunction. Exophthalmos results from increased intraocular pressure and can be associated with vision loss. Thyroid enlargement is called a "goiter," which would be noticed as swelling of the lower neck.

48. c. The treatment for thyrotoxicosis is undertaken in the hospital setting and consists of the use of beta-blockers and antithyroid medications. Tylenol will be ineffective in reducing fever. It is important not to miss other causes of adrenergic hyperactivity when caring for such a patient.

49. a. Myxedema coma is a rare condition from severe thyroid hormone deficiency and can be life threatening if left untreated. It is more common in older women and is treated with thyroxine.

50. b. Although hypothyroidism may cause loss of initiative and somnolence, it does not result in clinical depression. Because of depressed metabolic activity, the patient gains weight, retains water, is cold intolerant, and has dry coarse skin and hair loss.

51. a. Cushing's syndrome is a condition of excessive corticosteroid secretion by the adrenal gland. It can occur from an adrenal tumor, prolonged steroid use, and corticotropin-secreting pituitary tumors.

52. b. Cushing's syndrome has several characteristic physical signs and symptoms such as a fat pad on the back of the neck called a "buffalo hump"; round, red, obese "moon-faced"; increased body hair; bronze skin; weight gain; and thin, easily injured skin.

53. c. Addison's disease occurs from loss of the adrenal cortex production of cortisol and aldosterone such as hemorrhage or infarction, infection (TB, fungal, viral), and autoimmune disorders. Most cases are idiopathic from hormone secretion inadequate to meet the metabolic requirements of the body. The adrenal medulla produces epinephrine and norepinephrine.

54. d. Skin hyperpigmentation occurs as a result of adrenal stimulation of the pituitary gland to secrete melanin. Each of the other listed symptoms occurs slowly and progressively with the disorder.

55. a. Addisonian crisis occurs in patients with Addison's disease who are physically stressed and unable to produce sufficient adrenal cortisol and aldosterone. This leads to an inability to retain sodium, which causes dehydration. Blood sugar drops and cardiovascular instability occurs, which must treated aggressively or death may occur. Treatment consists of dextrose, volume replacement, and cortisone administration.

MEDICAL EMERGENCIES IV: NEUROLOGY

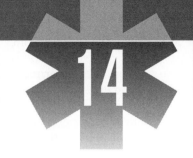

14

1. The initial step in the neurological exam begins with:
   a. ensuring a patent airway
   b. ensuring the patient is breathing
   c. ensuring the patient has a pulse
   d. determining level of consciousness

2. When taking the history from a patient with a neurological complaint, which of the following is true?
   a. The events that preceded it such as headache, seizure, and body position should be determined, particularly if a loss of consciousness occurred.
   b. A history of seizures makes the condition straightforward.
   c. The patient's family rarely has useful information.
   d. None of the above are correct.

3. The reason for obtaining several sets of vital signs from a patient with altered LOC is that:
   a. it is standard practice in all patients
   b. they can change rapidly indicating early changes in intracranial pressure
   c. they can indicate what type of seizure occurred
   d. they will indicate the presence or absence of illicit drugs

4. Which of the following is true regarding the effect of rising ICP on vital signs?
   a. In the early stages of increased ICP, the systolic blood pressure lowers.
   b. Hypotension is an early sign of increased ICP.
   c. Cushing's triad consists of a widened pulse pressure, elevated BP and slow pulse.
   d. Body temperature drops as ICP increases.

5. Significant neurological emergencies may be associated with abnormal posturing of the limbs. Which of the following is true?
   a. Decorticate rigidity is worse than decerebrate rigidity.
   b. Decorticate rigidity involves an abnormal extension of the arms and flexion of the legs.
   c. Decerebrate rigidity involves an abnormal flexion of the arms and flexion of the legs.
   d. None of the above are correct.

6. You examine a 12-year-old boy who has fallen off his bike and landed on his head. He is awake and alert. On exam you find that his left pupil is fixed and dilated. Which of the following is true regarding your findings?
   a. This represents a dire emergency and indicates rising intracranial pressure.
   b. It is not possible for only one pupil to be affected.
   c. Control of pupillary size involves the brain stem.
   d. Pupils are controlled by the second cranial nerve.

7. Extraocular eye movements should be assessed in the patient with an altered LOC because:
   a. they will indicate the potential for orbital fractures
   b. strokes will always cause the eyes to look toward the side of injury
   c. a disconjugate gaze may be the result of a structural lesion to one of the peripheral nerves of the eye
   d. conjugate gaze to one side or the other indicates a brain stem lesion

8. Which of the following is true regarding stroke?
a. It has a 10% to 15% mortality.
b. It is the third leading cause of death in the United States.
c. It is a sudden interruption of blood flow to the brain resulting in neurological deficit.
d. All of the above are correct.

9. The blood supply to the brain is delivered by two carotid arteries and two vertebral arteries. Which of the following is true regarding this blood supply?
a. The two vertebral arteries supply 80% of the blood flow.
b. The two vertebral arteries join to form the basilar artery.
c. The anterior circulation from the carotid arteries is joined to the posterior circulation of the vertebral arteries by the circle of Willis.
d. There is excellent collateral blood flow between the lobes of the brain and deep in the brain structure.

10. Which of the following is most characteristic of ischemic strokes?
a. They are less common than hemorrhagic strokes.
b. They develop more suddenly than hemorrhagic strokes.
c. They are associated with valvular heart disease and atrial fibrillation.
d. They usually occur with stress or exertion.

11. A transient ischemic attack is:
a. less serious than a regular stroke and can be ignored
b. defined as a focal cerebral dysfunction that resolves within 24 hours
c. not associated with an increased risk of complete stroke
d. treated with thrombolytic therapy

Questions 12 through 15 refer to the following scenario:

A 75-year-old man develops acute loss of speech and right-sided weakness while getting dressed. On arrival he is alert and able to answer questions by nodding and shaking his head. His blood pressure is 180/110, heart rate 136 and irregular, respiratory rate 12 and unlabored.

12. Important questions to ask him include:
a. Exactly when did the symptoms appear?
b. Does he have a headache?
c. Is he on anticoagulants?
d. All of the above are correct.

13. While performing the neurological exam, you note that the right side of his face droops when he smiles, his right arm drifts downward when both arms are held out, and he closes his eyes, and when asked to say, "You can't teach an old dog new tricks," his words are slurred. You have just completed what is known as the:
a. DOT-approved stroke neurological exam
b. Cincinnati Prehospital Stroke Scale
c. Pronator drift
d. Rhomberg exam

14. Appropriate prehospital management of a stroke patient is most likely to consist of all of the following *EXCEPT*:
a. administering supplemental oxygen if hypoxic
b. establishing IV access
c. checking blood glucose level
d. administering nitroglycerin or labetalol per protocol to treat his hypertension

15. After connecting him to the ECG you would not be surprised to find him in what cardiac rhythm?
a. sinus tachycardia
b. ventricular tachycardia
c. atrial fibrillation
d. Mobitz type II heart block

16. Which of the following is true regarding seizures?
a. They are always caused by epilepsy.
b. They result from increased neuronal membrane permeability leading to depolarization.
c. Febrile seizures and epilepsy are the same.
d. None of the above are correct.

17. Which of the following are causes of seizures?
a. stroke, head injury, brain tumors, and abscesses
b. drug and alcohol withdrawal, infection, shock
c. hypoglycemia, hypoxia, and other metabolic abnormalities
d. all of the above

18. The generalized seizure is characterized by:
a. sudden loss of consciousness followed by a tonic-clonic phase
b. absence of an aura warning of the imminent seizure
c. clonic activity of only one part of the body
d. none of the above

19. Differences between the tonic and clonic phase of a generalized seizure include:
   a. the clonic phase begins first
   b. bowel and bladder incontinence occur during the tonic phase
   c. the clonic phase is characterized by somnolence
   d. none of the above

20. Petit mal, or absence seizures, are a type of partial seizure.
   a. true
   b. false

21. The partial seizure differs from the generalized seizure in that:
   a. the partial seizure is always preceded by an aura
   b. the partial seizure never leads to a generalized seizure
   c. the mental status is relatively normal in the partial seizure
   d. the partial seizure lasts longer than the generalized

22. Partial seizures are characterized by:
   a. arising from an identifiable focal cortical lesion
   b. motor activity of one specific part of the body
   c. sensory activity such as tingling, numbness, and visual and auditory symptoms
   d. all of the above

23. The complex partial seizure is characterized by:
   a. sudden loss of consciousness
   b. temporal lobe, psychomotor, activity with behavioral changes
   c. prolonged postictal phase
   d. lack of an aura

24. Partial seizure activity, which spreads in an orderly fashion to surrounding areas and across the body, is known as a Jacksonian seizure.
   a. true
   b. false

25. When assessing the patient who has suffered a seizure, which of the following mnemonics is helpful to use?
   a. TIPS
   b. SEIZURE
   c. FACTS
   d. AEIOU

26. Important things to look for on the physical exam of a seizure victim include:
   a. presence of urine or feces
   b. level of consciousness
   c. presence of cardiac dysrhythmias
   d. all of the above

Questions 27 through 30 refer to the following scenario:

A 26-year-old woman with a history of epilepsy suffers a generalized seizure while riding on the bus. Upon your arrival she is postictal and has vomited and suffered urinary incontinence. Her blood pressure is 110/86, heart rate 110, respiratory rate 16, and she is diaphoretic. There is no sign of head trauma.

27. Appropriate initial treatment would include all of the following *EXCEPT*:
   a. establish intravenous access
   b. obtain blood glucose level
   c. administer high flow oxygen
   d. administer 1.0 mg of lorazepam or 5.0 mg of diazepam intravenously

28. The patient states she is taking anticonvulsants for her condition. Likely agents she may be prescribed include all of the following *EXCEPT*:
   a. Tegretol—carbamazepine
   b. Depakote—valproic acid
   c. Dilantin—phenytoin
   d. Xanax—alprazolam

29. You check her blood glucose level and get a reading of 70. Of the following causes for seizures, which is the most likely in this case?
   a. she has not been compliant in taking her medications
   b. hypoglycemia
   c. substance abuse
   d. breakthrough seizure

30. While assessing the patient she suffers another seizure lasting 3 minutes followed by a short postictal phase then seizes again. This is called:
   a. epilepticus continuous
   b. status epilepticus
   c. grand mal seizure
   d. petit mal seizure

31. All of the following are true statements regarding status epilepticus *EXCEPT:*
   a. it is a true emergency that, without treatment, can result in permanent brain damage
   b. long bone fractures may occur
   c. the convulsions are more violent than other forms of epilepsy
   d. aspiration may occur

32. When initiating medication administration to control seizure activity, which of the following should be considered?
   a. Lorazepam is associated with less respiratory suppression than diazepam.
   b. Respiratory status must be constantly assessed regardless of agent used.
   c. Seizure activity may continue despite the amount of any agent used.
   d. All of the above are correct.

33. Which of the following is true regarding the difference between a syncopal episode and a seizure?
   a. Syncope can occur with any position.
   b. Tachycardia is more common with seizures.
   c. The seizure is associated with a feeling of lightheadedness.
   d. It is almost impossible to tell the difference.

34. When assessing the unconscious patient the mnemonic AEIOUTIPS is useful. What do each of the letters refer to?

A _____
E _____
I _____
O _____
U _____
T _____
I _____
P _____
S _____

35. Headaches are extremely common; 40% of all Americans will have a serious headache sometime in their lives. Which of the following types is the most common?
   a. tension
   b. migraine
   c. cluster
   d. sinus

36. Migraines can be differentiated from other causes of headaches by:
   a. migraine symptoms are secondary to histamine release
   b. vascular spasm occurs as a result of serotonin or hormone fluctuations
   c. migraines tend to present with bilateral head pain
   d. none of the above

37. When caring for a patient complaining of a headache, important factors to consider include all of the following *EXCEPT:*
   a. prior history of headaches or migraines
   b. presence or absence of altered mental status
   c. how often a patient has been to the emergency department to get "a shot"
   d. suddenness of headache onset

38. The most common symptom(s) of brain tumors and abscesses is(are):
   a. nausea and vomiting
   b. altered mental status
   c. numbness and weakness
   d. headache

39. All of the following are true regarding muscular dystrophy *EXCEPT:*
   a. it is a progressive disease of the central nervous system
   b. it is inherited and only affects males
   c. it is usually diagnosed in childhood
   d. death usually results from pulmonary complications

40. All of the following are true regarding multiple sclerosis *EXCEPT:*
   a. it is the most common acquired disease of the nervous system in young adults
   b. it is an autoimmune disease of the myelin in the central nervous system
   c. symptoms include uncontrollable shaking of the head and hands
   d. it is characterized by relapses and long symptom-free periods

41. A 76-year-old man has fallen at church. His wife says he is very unsteady on his feet and often loses his balance. On exam his head bobs up and down rhythmically, and you notice a tremor in his hands that appears as if he is rolling a pill repeatedly between his index finger and thumb. These symptoms are most characteristic of:
    a. Bell's palsy
    b. Parkinson's disease
    c. Lou Gehrig's disease
    d. dystonia

42. A 23-year-old woman presents with left facial weakness that she noticed when she awoke. You can differentiate Bell's palsy from a stroke by which of the following?
    a. She is too young to have a stroke.
    b. Strokes will never affect only the face.
    c. In Bell's palsy the eyebrow on the affected side will not rise on command.
    d. All of the above are correct.

43. Amyotrophic lateral sclerosis is:
    a. also known as Lou Gehrig's disease
    b. a rare disorder of the motor nerves within the brain and spinal cord
    c. often fatal within 2 to 4 years of diagnosis
    d. all of the above

44. Peripheral neuropathy refers to any disease or disorder that leads to damage of the peripheral nerves resulting in loss of perception to pain, pressure, heat, and cold and is associated with the perception of phantom pain. It can occur from which of the following conditions?
    a. diabetes
    b. alcoholism
    c. uremia
    d. all of the above

45. The condition in which a child is born with a congenital defect of the vertebra that results in an unprotected opening over the spinal cord is called spina bifida. Which of the following is true regarding this condition?
    a. Mental retardation is common.
    b. The most common location of the defect is in the cervical spine.
    c. There are four types of which two are associated with severe handicaps.
    d. None of the above are correct.

46. Polio is an inherited disease that has been eradicated by the education and counseling of affected persons who carry the gene.
    a. true
    b. false

ANSWERS TO CHAPTER 14: MEDICAL EMERGENCIES IV: NEUROLOGY

1. d. After the ABCs have been secured, the paramedic may move on to the specific assessments for a given organ system. For the neurological exam that first step is to determine the level of consciousness. The unconscious and unresponsive patient must be presumed to have an unprotected airway until proven otherwise.

2. a. A complete history should be taken after any life threat has been identified. The chief complaint and a detailed listing of pertinent medical history should be obtained, including drug and alcohol use. The events leading up to the altered LOC can give significant clues to its etiology.

3. b. Vital signs in a patient with an altered LOC must be repeated often because they may be the only and earliest indicators of changes in the patient's intracranial pressure. However, they are not specific to any particular etiology or precipitating event.

4. c. In the early stages of increased ICP the systolic blood pressure increases, pulse pressure widens, and pulse slows. This is Cushing's triad. In the terminal stages, as ICP continues to rise, body temperature rises, pulse rate continues to slow, then blood pressure drops as herniation occurs.

5. d. Abnormal posturing is thought to result from structural impairment of certain cortical regions of the brain. Abnormal flexion of the arms and extension of the legs is called decorticate posturing. Abnormal extension of the arms and legs is called decerebrate posturing. Decerebrate posturing is worse than decorticate because it involves impairment deeper in the brain.

6. c. Exam of the pupils is most helpful in patients with an altered level of consciousness but should be part of the routine exam in all trauma patients. In the awake and alert patient, the presence of a unilaterally dilated pupil indicates a traumatic injury to the third, oculomotor, cranial nerve instead of a central nervous system abnormality. The pupils are controlled by parasympathetic fibers, which originate in the brain stem and travel with the oculomotor nerve.

7. d. The extraocular eye movements are controlled by three cranial nerves: the oculomotor, the abducens, and the trochlear. The gaze is coordinated by the brain stem to ensure that both eyes track together. Strokes in the cerebral hemispheres will not affect the gaze unless they extend into the brain stem. Disconjugate and conjugate gazes refer to the position of the eyes at rest, not when exercised to their full range of movement. Any abnormality, whether conjugate, where both eyes look together, or disconjugate, where each eye looks in a different direction, indicates the possibility of a brain stem injury.

8. d. Stroke affects 500,000 Americans each year, and the ability to recognize it and provide appropriate therapy is critical. It occurs from blockage of a cerebral artery resulting in ischemia and death of brain cells.

9. b. The two carotid arteries provide 80% of the cerebral blood flow and the two vertebral arteries, which join to form the basilar artery, the remaining 20%. The circle of Willis is the major connection between the anterior and posterior circulation, but beyond this there is no collateral circulation between the lobes or deep in the brain tissue itself.

10. c. Several characteristics differentiate the ischemic from hemorrhagic stroke. They are more common, develop slowly, are associated with diffuse atherosclerosis of the cerebral vessels, and occur from debris released from abnormal heart valves and atrial fibrillation. Hemorrhagic strokes generally occur with stress and exertion and are associated with hypertension and aneurysms.

11. b. A transient ischemic attack (TIA) is often referred to as a "mini stroke" and presents in the same manner as a complete stroke, but the symptoms resolve within a matter of minutes or hours but always within 24 hours. They forecast the potential for the development of a complete stroke. A total of 5% of TIAs will develop into a complete stroke within 1 month and 30% within 1 year. Because their symptoms slowly improve, TIAs are not routinely treated with thrombolytics but do require aggressive evaluation for their cause.

12. d. When assessing the stroke patient, several important elements of their history are vital.

The benefits of thrombolytic therapy are greatest within 3 to 6 hours of symptom onset. The presence of a headache and the use of anticoagulants are more often associated with a hemorrhagic stroke, which is potentially life threatening. Other important questions to ask include the existence of previous strokes or TIA, history of diabetes and hypertension, and any precipitating events.

13. b. The Cincinnati Prehospital Stroke Scale evaluates the three most common physical findings during a stroke: facial droop, arm drift indicating hemiparesis (pronator drift), and speech deficits. An abnormality in any of the three components indicates the possibility of a cerebrovascular accident. The Rhomberg test evaluates balance.

14. d. The initial treatment for stroke includes oxygen, IV access, and blood glucose determination. Treatment of hypertension is not recommended unless cardiovascular compromise occurs. Rapid transport to an appropriate facility with the capability to perform a CAT scan and administer thrombolytics is critical to improved outcome.

15. c. The presence of atrial fibrillation and atrial flutter are common precipitators of stroke because they both promote the development of a mural thrombus within the atria, which is then released as small debris to lodge in the cerebral vessels.

16. b. About 6% of the population will suffer a seizure at some time in their lives. Although the exact cause is not known, it is thought to be related to increased permeability of the neural membranes to the movement of sodium and potassium, which results in depolarization of the axon. Epilepsy refers to a condition in which seizures from any cause occur repeatedly over a period of time. Febrile seizures are related to changes in core body temperature and are not related to epilepsy.

17. d. In the prehospital setting, determining the origin of the seizure activity is less important than managing its complications and recognizing whether it can be stopped with therapy.

18. a. Generalized seizures are characterized by a sudden loss of consciousness followed by a tonic phase sequence of extensor muscle tone activity, which then leads to a clonic phase of rigidity alternating with relaxation. An aura, whether olfactory or auditory, may precede the seizure. Clonic activity of only one part of the body is typical of the partial or focal seizure.

19. b. During a generalized seizure the tonic phase begins first and is followed by several minutes of clonic rigidity and relaxation of the body. Incontinence occurs during the tonic phase. The clonic phase is associated with a massive autonomic discharge resulting in hyperventilation, salivation, and tachycardia. The period of somnolence after the seizure is called the postictal phase.

20. b. Petit mal seizures occur most often in children and are characterized by a brief lapse of consciousness without loss of posture along with some isolated clonic activity such as eye blinking or lip smacking. They are grouped with generalized seizures because they have no discernable focus in the brain.

21. c. The primary difference between generalized and partial seizures is that little change in mental status occurs with partial seizures, whereas the generalized seizure always has a markedly altered level of consciousness. A partial seizure can spread throughout the body to become a generalized seizure. The partial seizure usually lasts less than a minute.

22. d. The partial seizure is focal in that it arises from an identifiable lesion in either the motor or sensory cortex of the brain. It will be demonstrated by activity of the area controlled by the affected area of the brain including motor, sensory, or both.

23. b. The complex partial seizure arises from a focal seizure involving the temporal lobe and manifests with behavioral changes such as repetitive motor activity such as lip smacking, chewing, or swallowing, during which the patient is amnestic to the events. It is usually preceded by an aura and lasts less than a minute.

24. a. True. The progression of the seizure activity across the body is known as the Jacksonian march.

25. c. The mnemonic FACTS is useful when assessing the patient who has suffered a seizure. F—focus, what body part was affected? A—activity, what movements took place? C—color, did the patient become cyanotic? T—time, how long did the seizure last? S—secondary information, did the patient bite his or her tongue, lose consciousness, have incontinence, or experience an aura?

26. d. The presence of urine or feces suggests incontinence. Cardiac dysrhythmia suggests a syncopal episode from hypotension. The level of consciousness, including the presence of amnesia, assists in determining the likely cause of the seizure.

27. d. An IV should be established in the event that the seizure recurs necessitating the administration of medication. Oxygen should be administered to reverse any hypoxia that may have occurred during the seizure. Blood glucose should be measured to determine whether hypoglycemia contributed to the cause of the seizure or resulted from the seizure activity. The administration of an anticonvulsant is usually not indicated once the seizure has stopped.

28. d. Alprazolam is a benzodiazepine sedative and not considered a primary anticonvulsant. Each of the others, as well as gabapentin (Neurontin) and phenobarbital, is a common anticonvulsant.

29. a. The most common cause of a seizure in the patient taking anticonvulsants is noncompliance to therapy with missed or improper dosing resulting in subtherapeutic blood levels of the agent. Despite proper therapy, some patients will have the occasional or "breakthrough" seizure. Although hypoglycemia and substance abuse may be involved, there is nothing in the history to suggest this.

30. b. Status epilepticus is defined as seizure activity lasting longer than 30 minutes or recurrent seizures without an intervening period of alertness.

31. c. Status epilepticus is life threatening. The convulsions are no more violent than in other types of epilepsy but may be sufficiently intense to result in long bone fracture and spinal injury. The prolonged muscular activity can result in hyperthermia, hypoxia from apnea, and hypoglycemia. Rhabdomyolysis from muscular contraction can lead to renal failure, and the unguarded airway is prone to aspiration.

32. d. The two primary prehospital agents used to control seizure activity are lorazepam (Ativan) and diazepam (Valium). Midazolam (Versed) has also been found to be effective. Both lorazepam and midazolam have less respiratory suppression than diazepam; however, any agent can result in respiratory insufficiency and therefore the airway and ventilatory status must be constantly assessed. Despite the administration of an anticonvulsant, the patient may continue to seize and will require aggressive life support at the hospital.

33. b. The primary means to differentiate syncope from seizure relates to the symptoms immediately before and after the seizure activity. The short, choppy movements seen with syncope are called myoclonic jerks and not full tonic-clonic contractions. Syncope usually occurs while in the standing position. Because of the autonomic discharge, tachycardia is more common in seizure, whereas bradycardia from increased vagal tone is more common in syncope.

34. When assessing the unconscious patient the mnemonic AEIOUTIPS is useful. What does each of the letters refer to?

A acidosis, alcohol
E epilepsy
I infection
O overdose
U uremia
T trauma
I insulin (hypoglycemia)
P psychosis
S stroke

35. a. Muscle tension headache is caused by muscle contractions of the face, neck, and scalp and usually treated with analgesics such as ibuprofen and aspirin. Vascular migraines are related to dilation and spasm of cerebral vessels. Cluster headaches occur around the eyes in the middle of the night and are associated with nasal congestion and tearing. Sinus headaches are related to inflammation of the sinuses, usually the maxillary sinuses.

36. b. Vascular migraines are severe, incapacitating headaches that are associated with visual and GI disturbances. They are usually unilateral and the patient complains of retroorbital pain, which is pain behind the eye. Cluster headaches occur in the early morning and are associated with histamine release.

37. c. The patient complaining of a headache may be considered to be drug seeking. This can cause the EMT to miss important features that may indicate a serious underlying medical condition. A sudden onset of headache, particularly with an altered mental status, is consistent with an intracerebral hemorrhage.

38. d. Brain neoplasms and abscesses occur with greater frequency past the seventh decade and are associated with signs and symptoms of increased intracranial pressure. Headache is the earliest sign common to both etiologies.

39. a. Muscular dystrophy is a degenerative disease of the muscle fibers that leads to the inability to walk. Only males are affected, although women can carry the gene.

40. c. Multiple sclerosis (MS) is a progressive disease of the central nervous system affecting 1 in 1000 persons. Symptoms range from numbness and tingling to paralysis. Damage to the white matter in the brain leads to fatigue, vertigo, unsteady gait, slurred speech, double vision, and pain.

41. b. Parkinson's disease is related to degeneration of the basal ganglia in the brain, leading to loss of dopamine production, which controls muscle contraction. The Parkinson's patient often has a shuffling gait, which leads to loss of balance and falls. This patient demonstrates the classic "pill rolling" tremor of his hands.

42. c. The facial nerve has two CNS branches, the facial and the ocular. A stroke will usually affect the facial portion sparing the ocular. Bell's palsy results in complete paralysis of the seventh (facial) cranial nerve. Therefore the patient with Bell's palsy will be unable to raise the eyebrow.

43. d. Amyotrophic lateral sclerosis (ALS) came to be recognized when diagnosed in the great baseball player Lou Gehrig. It is a rapidly progressive disorder of the motor neurons presenting with involuntary quivering of the hands and arms. The process spreads to all four extremities and death occurs once the muscles of respiration are involved.

44. d. Peripheral neuropathy can occur from a host of diseases. Diabetes, renal failure, and alcoholism lead the list. Rheumatoid arthritis, lupus, and other autoimmune disorders are also involved. Peripheral neuropathies result in unrecognized injuries and subsequent infections, as well as falls from poor perception.

45. c. Spina bifida is divided into four types: occulta, which is the most common and least serious; meningocele, in which the covering of the spinal cord protrudes through the defect but has no nerve defect; myelomeningocele, in which the spinal cord is deformed and damaged resulting in severe physical handicaps, particularly to the legs; and encephalocele, the rarest and most lethal form, where the defect occurs in the skull. The most common site of spina bifida is in the lumbar spine.

46. b. False. Polio is a disease caused by poliovirus hominis. Its incidence has declined in the United States since the introduction of the Salk vaccine in the 1950s; however, it remains a major public health threat in the Middle East, Africa, and Asia, as well as in the United States in immigrants and indigent children who have not been immunized.

MEDICAL EMERGENCIES V: ENVIRONMENTAL AND ALLERGIES

15

1. The thermoregulatory center of the body is located in the:
   a. thalamus
   b. hypothalamus
   c. pituitary
   d. cerebellum

2. Nerve centers that are stimulated by changes at the skin surface are called:
   a. skin arterioles
   b. efferent nerves
   c. adrenal medulla
   d. peripheral thermoreceptors

3. There are more warm receptors than cold receptors in the body.
   a. true
   b. false

4. The skin receptors and some mucous membranes send input to the thermoregulatory center. What other area sends input to this center?
   a. the areas in or near the anterior hypothalamus
   b. the midbrain
   c. the limbic system
   d. the sixth cranial nerve

5. Information from receptors in the skin are sent to the posterior hypothalamus by:
   a. efferent nerve pathways
   b. afferent nerve pathways
   c. the cerebellum
   d. the vagus nerve

6. _____ react directly to alterations in the temperature of the blood.
   a. Peripheral thermoreceptors
   b. Cold receptors
   c. Warm receptors
   d. Central thermoreceptors

7. Skeletal muscle is innervated by descending pathways and:
   a. somatic motor nerves
   b. release of hormones from the thyroid
   c. the sympathetic nervous system
   d. central thermoreceptors

8. Central thermoreceptors affect vasomotor tone, sweating, and:
   a. hormone release
   b. wake-sleep cycle
   c. metabolic rate
   d. thermal gradient

9. The primary purpose of the thermoregulatory center is to maintain:
   a. constant core body temperature
   b. thermogenesis
   c. thermolysis
   d. transfer of heat to environment

10. Body temperature can be increased through production of heat, which is called:
    a. thermolysis
    b. thermogenesis
    c. convection
    d. thermal gradient

11. The body can generate heat in response to cold through mechanical, metabolic, and chemical activities. Another system the body uses to generate heat is the:
    a. endocrine system
    b. respiratory system
    c. renal system
    d. gastrointestinal system

12. Heat production is controlled chemically by:
    a. calcium
    b. reticular activating system
    c. sodium
    d. cellular metabolism

13. The body's defenses against cold include all
    EXCEPT:
    a. shivering
    b. hydration
    c. dry skin
    d. rapid, shallow respirations

14. The temperature difference between the body and
    the environment is known as the:
    a. ambient temperature
    b. equivalent temperature
    c. thermal gradient
    d. thermal conduction

15. Heat from the body is lost to the environment pri-
    marily through:
    a. breathing
    b. skin
    c. urination
    d. perspiration

16. A patient's age is a factor in the body's ability to
    generate heat.
    a. true
    b. false

17. Ambient temperatures and _____ affect
    evaporative heat loss from moisture on skin or lin-
    ings of the respiratory tract.
    a. wind chill
    b. cellular metabolism
    c. cold receptor stimulation
    d. relative humidity

18. Which of the following occur(s) in response to
    hyperthermia?
    a. decreased hormone secretions
    b. decreased appetite
    c. decreased heat production
    d. all of the above

19. Muscle pain associated with heat cramps is a result of:
    a. lack of potassium
    b. loss of water and sodium
    c. poor muscle conditioning
    d. eating large meals prior to exercise

20. Patients experiencing heat cramps usually present:
    a. alert, with hot sweaty skin, tachycardia, and
       normal core body temperature
    b. confused, with hot dry skin, tachycardia, and
       hypertension
    c. alert, with cool moist skin, normal heart rate,
       and hypotension
    d. confused, with warm moist skin, tachycardia,
       and elevated core body temperature

21. A severe heat injury characterized by nausea,
    headache, irritability and known as heat exhaustion:
    a. is another name for heat cramps
    b. is difficult to reverse
    c. always results in orthostatic pressure changes
    d. can progress to heat stroke if left untreated

22. Increased body temperature in heat stroke can be
    treated with medications used to treat fever.
    a. true
    b. false

23. Which of the following is true regarding cardiac
    output associated with heat stroke?
    a. It is rarely more than twice the normal
       amount.
    b. Heat stroke does not affect cardiac output.
    c. It can be four to five times the normal
       amount.
    d. It usually is only slightly greater than normal.

24. Treatment for heat stroke may include:
    a. airway management, tepid water immersion,
       IV fluids, and diazepam
    b. airway management, ice water immersion,
       vigorous fluid administration
    c. fanning of patient, IV fluids, diazepam, and ice
       water immersion
    d. rapid transport of patient without attempting
       to cool, airway management

25. Shivering ceases in hypothermia when the core
    body temperature drops below:
    a. 95° F
    b. 90° F
    c. 86° F
    d. shivering does not cease in hypothermia

26. Hypothermia will initially cause:
    a. the heart rate, respiratory rate, and blood
       pressure to decrease
    b. the heart rate to decrease and the respiratory
       rate and blood pressure to increase
    c. the heart rate, blood pressure, and respiratory
       rate to increase
    d. the heart rate and blood pressure to remain
       unchanged while the respiratory rate decreases

27. Thermoregulatory mechanisms can be impaired by:
    a. alcohol
    b. excessive aspirin use
    c. trauma
    d. all of the above

28. Patients with diabetic ketoacidosis are usually not at risk for hypothermia because their metabolism is keeping the skin warm.
a. true
b. false

29. The most important thing to remember when dealing with hypothermia is:
a. give the patient warm fluids to drink
b. put the patient in a hot environment
c. maintain a high index of suspicion for its presence
d. give the patient oxygen by nasal cannula at 3 LPM

30. Hypovolemia can develop in hypothermia.
a. true
b. false

31. Patients with moderate to severe hypothermia require prehospital providers to:
a. give appropriate ventilatory assistance, perform passive rewarming, and minimize patient movement
b. use an oral or nasal airway, hyperventilate, and perform rapid and aggressive rewarming of the patient
c. perform endotracheal intubation with hyperventilation and rapid rewarming
d. use airway adjuncts, high-flow oxygen, and IVs of lactated Ringer's running wide open to treat hypovolemia

32. Patients with severe hypothermia should be transported:
a. in the semi-Fowler position
b. sitting up to increase their metabolism
c. in reverse Trendelenburg
d. horizontal and supine

33. Severely hypothermic patients can be presumed dead when:
a. they have no vital signs such as pulse, blood pressure, and respiratory effort
b. the pupils are fixed and dilated
c. the core body temperature is at least 95° F, there is no perfusing rhythm, and all resuscitative measures have failed
d. the patient's muscles are stiff and rigid

34. Afterdrop phenomenon occurs in hypothermia when:
a. the patient's heart rate decreases
b. there is a sudden return of acidotic blood and waste products to the body's core
c. the peritoneal lavage is attempted with solutions that are not the right temperature
d. the body is passively rewarmed

35. During a hypothermic cardiac arrest lidocaine, epinephrine, and procainamide are often:
a. given in larger than normal doses because of the slow metabolic rate
b. given more frequently so that levels can build up in the body
c. withheld when the patients core temperature is less than 86° F
d. always used to treat cardiac arrhythmias in hypothermic patients

36. Most of the damage to tissue from frostbite occurs when:
a. ice crystals, which are sharp and damage cells, form in the skin
b. the skin is rewarmed too quickly
c. water is drawn out of the cells and electrolyte levels become toxic
d. the frostbitten tissue is submerged in tepid water

37. In addition to extreme temperature, wind, and humidity, predisposing factors to frostbite include all of the following *EXCEPT*:
a. loose-fitting, layered garments
b. preexisting psychiatric illness
c. alcohol consumption
d. atherosclerosis

38. Most patients with superficial frostbite usually can expect all of the following *EXCEPT*:
a. edema after rewarming
b. vesicle formation within 3 to 24 hours
c. skin that turns black and hard within a week
d. probable amputation of affected limb

39. Although frozen tissue should not be massaged, palpating the tissue to distinguish between superficial or deep injury is acceptable.
a. true
b. false

40. Trench foot is similar to frostbite and should be treated as follows:
    a. trench foot occurs at temperatures above freezing so no treatment is necessary
    b. cover the affected area with sterile dressings and keep it dry and warm
    c. submerge the area in sterile warm water
    d. have the patient massage area to promote the return of circulation

41. In deeply frostbitten tissue the disrupted capillary flow is never restored.
    a. true
    b. false

42. Treatment for deep frostbite once patients arrive in a stable environment includes all of the following *EXCEPT*:
    a. elevating and protecting the affected extremity
    b. removing restrictive and wet clothing
    c. rapid rewarming of the frozen part by immersion in hot water
    d. slow rewarming with blankets or other warm objects

43. The difference between fresh and salt water must be considered in the initial management of submersion incidents.
    a. true
    b. false

44. Aspiration and laryngospasm in submersion events lead to:
    a. cardiac dysrhythmias
    b. hypoxemia
    c. hypercapnia
    d. all of the above

45. In submersion events, the laryngospasm is never severe enough to stop aspiration.
    a. true
    b. false

46. Submersion injuries can affect which of the following body systems?
    a. cardiovascular
    b. renal
    c. pulmonary
    d. all of the above

47. Initial management of patients with submersion incidents should begin with:
    a. subdiaphragmatic thrusts to remove water from the airways
    b. high-flow oxygen
    c. spinal precautions while victim is still in the water
    d. establishing IV access

48. All of the following statements regarding barotrauma associated with diving are true *EXCEPT*:
    a. barotrauma is the most common affliction of scuba divers
    b. barotrauma results from compression or expansion of gas spaces
    c. the mechanism of barotrauma during ascent is the same as during descent
    d. air trapped in chambers is compressed, leading to a vacuum-type effect and hemorrhage of exposed tissue

49. The most common cause of barotrauma is:
    a. failure to clear the Eustachian tubes during descent
    b. emphysema
    c. breath-holding
    d. air embolism

50. If a diver suddenly loses consciousness after surfacing, the rescuer should suspect:
    a. air embolism
    b. the bends
    c. nitrogen narcosis
    d. subcutaneous emphysema

51. If definitive airway management is required in dive-related conditions and the patient is being transported to a hyperbaric chamber, the rescuer should:
    a. use only a nasal or oropharyngeal airway with bag-valve-mask ventilation because the patient's distal airway usually constricts
    b. use a blind insertion airway to save time because aspiration from stomach contents is rare in divers
    c. use an endotracheal tube filling the balloon with more air than normal to prevent dislodgement when moving the patient from the environment
    d. use an endotracheal tube, filling the balloon with normal saline to avoid extubation during recompression

52. The patient with a suspected air embolism should be transported:
    a. supine with head and lower extremities elevated to at least 45 degrees
    b. in the Trendelenburg position
    c. prone to allow secretions to drain from lungs
    d. in the left lateral recumbent position with the head lower than the heart.

53. A patient suffers decompression sickness while diving in a remote area with only a small community hospital available. The action that would most benefit this patient is:
    a. ground transport to a major trauma center
    b. transport by rotary winged aircraft at low altitude to a trauma center
    c. rapid transport in a fixed wing aircraft without controlled cabin pressure
    d. maintain patient at community hospital until symptoms resolve

54. Hyperbaric medicine has been proven effective in which of the following conditions?
    a. decompression sickness
    b. carbon monoxide poisoning
    c. crush injuries
    d. all of the above

55. The areas of the body most commonly affected by decompression sickness are the:
    a. heart and brain
    b. spinal cord and joints
    c. lungs
    d. hollow organs

56. Oxygen toxicity and nitrogen narcosis are both reversed with ascent to the surface.
    a. true
    b. false

57. Prevention of high-altitude illness includes all of the following *EXCEPT:*
    a. eating a high-protein diet
    b. taking steroids
    c. using a gradual ascent (days)
    d. sleeping at lower altitudes each night

58. The signs and symptoms of acute mountain sickness (AMS) and high-altitude cerebral edema (HACE) are very different making their distinction obvious.
    a. true
    b. false

59. Ataxia is the most common early sign of:
    a. HACE
    b. HAPE
    c. AMS
    d. ALS

60. Which of the following binds to antigens to facilitate neutralization and removal from the body?
    a. allergen
    b. leukotrienes
    c. antibodies
    d. thromboxanes

61. Previous exposure to a specific antigen that causes an increased physiological response is known as:
    a. localized allergic reaction
    b. sensitization
    c. urticaria
    d. erythema

62. Anaphylactoid reactions present like anaphylaxis; therefore they should be treated with the same medications.
    a. true
    b. false

63. Hypersensitivity reactions are divided into four distinct types. Which of the following is the most dramatic and may lead to anaphylaxis?
    a. Type I
    b. Type II
    c. Type III
    d. Type IV

64. Histamines that are released during a systemic reaction can cause:
    a. an increase in gastric, nasal, and lacrimal secrections
    b. contraction of nonvascular smooth muscle
    c. increased vascular permeability
    d. all of the above

65. The loss of intravascular volume in anaphylaxis is caused by plasma leaking into the interstitial space.
    a. true
    b. false

66. Which of the following causes the most potent bronchoconstriction?
    a. neutrophil chemotactic factor
    b. kinins
    c. leukotrienes
    d. heparin

67. Signs and symptoms of a severe allergic reaction or anaphylaxis are so specific it is not necessary to take time considering a differential diagnosis.
    a. true
    b. false

68. Dysrhythmias associated with anaphylaxis are common and generally associated with:
    a. hypoxia from bronchospasm
    b. hypoglycemia
    c. vasodilation
    d. rhinorrhea

69. The pharmacological treatment of choice for the initial management of anaphylaxis in an adult is:
    a. epinephrine 0.1 to 0.5 mg (1:10000) IV
    b. epinephrine 0.3 to 0.5 mg (1:1000) SC
    c. diphenhydramine 25 to 50 mg IM
    d. decadron 0.25 to 0.5 mg/kg dose IV

ANSWERS TO CHAPTER 15: MEDICAL EMERGENCIES V: ENVIRONMENTAL AND ALLERGIES

1. b. The hypothalamus, part of the diencephalon, regulates body temperature, water balance, sleep-cycle, appetite, and sexual arousal. The thalamus acts as a sensory relay station from the body to the cerebral cortex. The pituitary is the gland that regulates release of hormones that regulate many body functions. The cerebellum is the second largest part of the human brain responsible for gross motor coordination.

2. d. Peripheral thermoreceptors are nerve endings that are stimulated by either higher or lower skin surface temperatures. Efferent nerves are pathways back to the periphery in response to stimulus to the posterior hypothalamus. The adrenal medulla is the gland that releases epinephrine and norepinepherine to prolong and intensify the sympathetic nervous response during stress.

3. b. There are up to 10 times as many cold receptors as warm ones.

4. a. The central thermoreceptors are located in, or near, the anterior hypothalamus and send input to the thermoregulatory center.

5. b. Afferent nerve pathways carry impulses from the periphery to the brain. Efferent carry impulses from the brain to the periphery.

6. d. Central thermoreceptors are temperature sensitive neurons that react directly to changes in the temperature of the blood. Cold and warm receptors are peripheral thermoreceptors that are stimulated by skin surface temperatures.

7. a. Muscle is innervated through the nervous system. Thyroid hormones control metabolism. The sympathetic nervous system is involved in preparing the body for activity.

8. c. Metabolic rate is affected through sympathetic nerve output.

9. c. To maintain an optimum environment for normal cell metabolism, it is necessary to keep the core body temperature fairly constant.

10. b. Thermogenesis (*thermo* meaning temperature, and *genesis* meaning creation) allows the body to increase temperature through several mechanisms. Thermolysis, meaning destruction of heat, allows the body to dissipate heat by radiation, evaporation, conduction, or convection.

11. a. The endocrine system, utilizing the thyroid and adrenal medulla, releases hormones. Epinephrine and norepinephrine and the activity of the sympathetic nerves that connect to adipose tissue, increase the metabolic rate and augment heat production. The respiratory system can be a source of heat loss, with external cold air inhaled. The loss of body substances through the gastrointestinal system is another form of heat loss. The renal system by producing urine is another source of heat loss through excretion.

12. d. Oxidation of energy sources contributes to heat production. The body needs calcium to conduct nerve impulses and enable cardiac and other body systems to function. Sodium is the principal extracellular osmotic cation of the body. The reticular activating system is essential for consciousness.

13. d. Shivering can increase heat production by as much as 400%. Dry skin can prevent heat from evaporating, and hydration will maintain body systems for a longer period of time. Rapid, shallow respirations or panting increases heat loss.

14. c. Ambient temperature describes the temperature of the environment surrounding the patient. Equivalent temperature is used to determine cooling power of wind on exposed flesh. Thermal conduction is the exchange of heat by the transfer of energy.

15. b. The surface of the body constantly emits heat in the form of infrared rays. Some heat is lost through breathing and through elimination of waste products and perspiration.

16. a. Elderly patients do not have the reserve adipose tissue to metabolize into energy, and their skin is more fragile allowing greater heat loss. The very young have a greater body surface to weight ratio and therefore relatively greater area to lose heat.

17. d. Relative humidity is the ratio of the actual amount of moisture in the air to the greatest amount that the air can hold at a specified temperature. Diaphoresis can markedly increase evaporative heat loss, provided that the relative humidity is low enough that the sweat can evaporate.

18. d. A decrease in hormone secretions and appetite will lower metabolism by lowering activity in the gastrointestinal tract. The body compensates by limiting all activities of the body to decrease heat production.

19. b. Heat cramps are caused primarily by a rapid change in extracellular fluid osmolarity, which results from sodium and water loss. Additional electrolyte loss can cause other complications of heat-related injuries. Poor muscle conditioning can result in cramping of muscles during exertion without the complication of hyperthermic conditions.

20. a. Persons with heat cramps sweat profusely and replenish water without replenishing the salt lost through perspiration. They typically are tachycardic but have a normal core body temperatures.

21. d. Rapid recovery from heat exhaustion is possible with removal from the hot environment and fluid replacement. If left untreated, hyperthermia will rapidly progress to heat stroke. The body has limited compensatory mechanisms to sustain homeostasis. Orthostatic pressure changes are seen in severe cases of heat exhaustion.

22. b. In fever, which is caused by toxins produced by the bacteria and viruses causing the infection, the use of antipyretics to lower the body temperature is appropriate. However, working alone in customary doses, these medications will not lower the core body temperature from heat stroke.

23. c. Peripheral vasodilation results from increased temperature. If it is untreated, decreased vascular resistance and shunting occur. High output cardiac failure is common.

24. a. As always, airway management is the initial treatment. Tepid water will help to cool the skin temperature by convection and conduction. IV fluids should begin with an initial fluid challenge of 500 mL over 15 minutes. Vigorous fluid administration can precipitate pulmonary

edema, especially in older adults. Diazepam (Valium) can be given for sedation and seizure control. Heat stroke almost invariably ends in death if left untreated. Ice water submersion can cause shivering or seizures, which would ultimately increase body temperature.

25. c. Shivering continues until the core body temperature reaches about 86° F, glucose or glycogen is depleted, or insulin is no longer available.

26. c. Initially there is immediate vasoconstriction in the peripheral vessels and an increase in sympathetic nervous discharge, catecholamine release, and basal metabolism.

27. d. Trauma can damage areas around the thermoregulatory center. Alcohol and other depressants can affect the response to cold. Aspirin can lower body temperature abnormally and interfere with the mechanisms needed to generate heat.

28. b. Acid-base imbalances that occur during ketoacidosis can affect thermostability by decreasing heat production and increasing heat loss.

29. c. Failure to recognize and properly manage hypothermia can increase the rate of morbidity and mortality. By maintaining a high index of suspicion, you should consider hypothermia in the differential diagnosis or as a complication of other illness. Management of patients with moderate to severe hypothermia begins with airway management and circulatory support. Maintain body temperature by moving the patient to a warm environment. Fluids by mouth are acceptable if the patient's level of consciousness allows. Otherwise, warm IV fluids, and rapid and gentle transport to a definitive care facility is appropriate.

30. a. Hypovolemia can develop when there is a shift of fluid out of the vascular space with increased loss of fluid through urination (cold diuresis).

31. a. The use of oral or nasal airway adjuncts, including intubation, can produce ventricular dysrhythmias. Overzealous ventilatory assistance can induce hypocapnia and ventricular irritability. Minor physical activity can bring on dysrhythmias.

32. d. Horizontal positioning of the patient can avoid aggravating hypotension.

33. c. Prolonged resuscitation can be beneficial in severely hypothermic patients, and CPR is indicated even if signs of death are present. After rewarming to at least 95° F, the rescuer should confirm a nonperfusing rhythm (VF, pulseless VT, or asystole) by ECG monitoring for a minimum of 30 to 45 seconds; then CPR can be initiated if there are no vital signs. Continued rewarming should continue to the hospital where peritoneal and pleural lavage have also been used to successfully manage patients with hypothermia and cardiac arrest.

34. b. When the body is warmed too rapidly, the cold by-products of anaerobic metabolism enter the body's core and can cause the body temperature to continue to drop.

35. c. Medications can accumulate to toxic levels in the peripheral circulation if they are administered repeatedly in the severely hypothermic patient. For this reason medications are often withheld in patients with core temperatures that are less than 86° F. If temperature is greater then 86° F these medications may be given but at increased intervals between doses. Medical Control should be contacted for guidance in administration.

36. c. When ice crystals form in tissue, microvascular abnormalities occur, which result in cell injury. Along with this injury, ice crystals can cause direct mechanical destruction of tissue. Further destruction of blood vessels produces ischemia.

37. a. Loose-fitting layered garments trap warmed air, forming an insulation of the body. The consumption of alcohol and some psychiatric medications can predispose patients to frostbite because of the inability to maintain normal body temperature. Atherosclerosis causes poor circulation, which fails to normally circulate warm blood to periphery.

38. d. Amputation is a very rare outcome in superficial frostbite. Usually some underlying disease process must be present to result in such severe outcome. In most patients with superficial frostbite, the initial symptoms are coldness and numbness in the affected area, followed by pain during rewarming. Edema usually appears within 3 hours, followed by formation of vesicles within 3 to 24 hours. Once the blisters begin to resolve (within a week or so), the skin blackens into a hard eschar and eventually peels away.

39. a. Regardless of the depth of injury, the area may appear to be frozen. Palpation may distinguish between superficial and deep injury. In superficial injury the underlying tissue springs back on compression, whereas in deep injury the underlying tissue is hard and not compressible.

40. b. The signs and symptoms of trench foot (immersion foot) are similar to frostbite but occur at temperatures above freezing. The affected area should never be massaged because this can cause deep tissue damage. The area should be kept warm and dry and covered with sterile dressings because infection can rapidly develop.

41. a. In deep frostbite the affected area remains cold, mottled, and discolored after rewarming. After the first 9 to 15 days, dark hard eschar is formed. Unlike superficial frostbite, edema is slow to develop. Eventually, nonviable skin and deep structures mummify and slough off.

42. d. Slow rewarming can actually be injurious. Removing tight or wet clothing is important for rewarming and improving circulation. Rapid rewarming of the frozen part by immersion in hot water (104° F maximum) is the most effective therapeutic measure for preserving viable tissue.

43. b. Although there are theoretical differences between the effects of different submersion fluids, they are not clinically significant in the initial management of submersion victims. Aspiration and hypoxia with resulting hypoxemia and acidosis need the same resuscitative measures regardless of submersion liquid.

44. d. Hypoxemia and acidosis lead to cardiac dysrhythmias and CNS anoxia. Carbon dioxide builds up in the body, resulting in hypercapnia.

45. b. In 15% of drowning victims, the laryngospasm is severe enough that very little fluid is aspirated in what is known as "dry drowning."

46. d. Cardiovascular injuries can occur secondary to hypoxia and acidosis, resulting in dysrhythmias and decreased cardiac output. Renal dysfunction is unusual but can progress to acute renal failure as a result of hypoxic injury. The pulmonary system suffers complications such as fluid in the alveoli and interstitial spaces, loss of surfactant, contaminants in the alveoli and tracheobronchial tree, and damage to the alveolar-capillary membrane and vascular endothelium.

47. c. After gaining access to the victim, the paramedic should take spinal precautions while the patient is still in the water and begin rescue breathing if necessary. High-flow oxygen administration is indicated for treatment of hypoxia, and IV access can be valuable if further resuscitative measures are indicated. Subdiaphragmatic thrusts are controversial and generally not recommended unless a foreign body airway obstruction is suspected.

48. c. Barotrauma during descent, also known as "the squeeze," results from compression of gas in enclosed spaces as the ambient pressure increases. Barotrauma during ascent occurs through reverse squeeze, assuming that air-filled cavities of the body have equalized during descent. The volume of air trapped in this pressurized space expands as ambient pressure decreases. If air is not allowed to escape, the expanding gases distend the tissues surrounding them.

49. c. Breath-holding due to running out of air during a long dive or due to panic can cause barotrauma. It is the most common cause and in rare situations can cause pulmonary overpressurization syndrome (POPS). This can lead to alveolar rupture and extravasation of air into extraalveolar locations.

50. a. Air embolism is the most serious complication of pulmonary barotrauma and the major cause of death and disability in sport divers. Divers are at risk for this when they ascend too rapidly or hold their breath during ascent. Expanding air enters the systemic arterial supply. The most common presentation of air embolism is similar to stroke.

51. d. BLS and ALS measures should be used for treatment of these patients. If definitive airway management is necessary, the rescuer should fill the balloon with normal saline because filling it with air will result in the balloon shrinking during recompression in the chamber.

52. d. This position minimizes the potential for the air embolus to move further into the pulmonary circulation.

53. b. Management of the patient with a decompression sickness requires treatment in a facility that has the capability for hyperbaric medicine. The most rapid mode of transport for this patient would be indicated as long as the aircraft is pressurized to sea level or by rotary-winged aircraft that can fly at low altitude so that the existing intraarterial bubbles do not expand further.

54. d. Hyperbaric medicine has expanded to treatment of injuries and disease processes other than dive injury. Hyperbaric chambers allow for the administration of oxygen at a greater-than-normal atmospheric pressure. This can be used to overcome the natural limit of oxygen solubility in blood, thereby reducing intravascular bubble volume and restoring tissue perfusion. Rescuers should be familiar with the location of the nearest hyperbaric treatment facility.

55. b. Nitrogen bubbles can form in any tissue. Lymphedema, cellular distention, and cellular rupture can also occur. The net effect of these processes is poor tissue perfusion and ischemia. The joints and spinal cord are the anatomic areas most often affected because it takes longer for the nitrogen to wash out during decompression.

56. a. Nitrogen narcosis affects all divers but is better tolerated by experienced divers. The narcotic effects of nitrogen are reversed with ascent. The syndrome is a common factor in diving accidents and may be responsible for memory loss. Oxygen toxicity occurs from prolonged exposure to oxygen or exposure to excessive concentrations of oxygen. Seizures and altered level of consciousness can occur.

57. a. A diet high in carbohydrates is effective along with other measures in preventing high-altitude illness. All medications are controversial; however, steroids can help prevent inflammation at altitude. Gradual ascent and sleeping at lower level than climbed during the day help to acclimate climber over time.

58. b. High-altitude cerebral edema (HACE) is characterized by the progression of global cerebral signs in the presence of acute mountain sickness (AMS) that are probably related to increased intracranial pressure from cerebral edema and swelling. The distinctions between AMS and HACE are inherently blurred. The progression from mild AMS to unconsciousness associated with HACE can be as fast as 12 hours. However, it usually requires 1 to 3 days of exposure to high altitudes.

59. a. Ataxia is associated with high-altitude cerebral edema. Because of swelling, the cerebellum can be affected, causing gait disturbances.

60. c. Antigens are substances that induce the formation of antibodies. Antigens can enter the body by injection, ingestion, inhalation, or absorption. The antibodies bind to the antigen that produced them and facilitate antigen neutralization and removal from the body.

61. b. An allergic reaction is indicated by an increased response to an antigen after a previous exposure (sensitization) to the same antigen. Urticaria is a skin reaction characterized by wheals and itching. Erythema is a reddening of the skin or mucous membranes as a result of dilation of capillaries near the skin surface.

62. a. Anaphylactoid reactions are allergic reactions that are not mediated by an antigen-antibody reaction. However, the distinction between this and anaphylaxis are unimportant in relation to the treatment of an acute attack.

63. a. Type I, IgE-mediated allergic reaction, also known as *immediate hypersensitivity reaction*, is the most dramatic with its rapid onset. Type II is a tissue-specific reaction, Type III is an immune complex–mediated reaction, and cell-mediated reactions are Type IV. The allergic reaction is initiated when a circulating antibody (IgG or IgM) combines with a specific foreign antigen, resulting in hypersensitivity reactions or with antibodies bound to mast cells, or basophils (IgE).

64. d. Histamines promote vascular permeability and cause dilation of capillaries and venules and contraction of nonvascular smooth muscle especially in the gastrointestinal tract and bronchial tree.

65. a. The increased capillary permeability allows plasma to leak into the interstitial space, decreasing the intravascular volume available for the heart to pump.

66. c. Leukotrienes have a much longer duration of action than histamines. They are the most potent bronchoconstrictors, causing wheezing. These chemical mediators also cause coronary vasoconstriction and increased vascular permeability. It is believed that eosinophils contain an enzyme that can deactivate leukotrienes.

67. b. Conditions that can mimic anaphylaxis include foreign body airway obstruction, aspiration, epiglottitis, angioedema, ACE inhibitor use, panic disorders, asthma, COPD, bronchitis, seizures, hypoglycemia, cardiac dysrhythmias, and shock from any cause or infection.

68. a. Hypoxia and intervascular hypovolemia in anaphylaxis are the main causes of cardiovascular difficulties. Hypoxia is caused by bronchospasm and hypersecretion of mucus. Respiratory symptoms can develop rapidly.

69. b. Epinephrine 0.3 to 0.5 mg of a 1:1000 solution should be given SC initially and repeated after 5 to 10 minutes if there is improvement. IV epinephrine should be given only when there are profound, immediately life-threatening presentations and when there are no delays in obtaining IV access. Diphenhydramine (Benydryl) is used as an adjunctive therapy with epinephrine. Decadron (dexamethasone) is a synthetic steroid that suppresses acute and chronic inflammation. Although it is appropriate as another adjunct to epinephrine, the dose listed is the pediatric dose.

MEDICAL EMERGENCIES VI: TOXICOLOGY, RENAL, AND INFECTIOUS DISEASE

16

Toxicology

1. All of the following are routes of poisoning *EXCEPT*:
   a. absorption
   b. inhalation
   c. ingestion
   d. diffusion

2. A heroin addict whose habit requires daily use to avoid withdrawal is demonstrating _____ to the drug.
   a. dependence
   b. tolerance
   c. potentiation
   d. synergism

3. The most common drug of abuse and addiction is:
   a. cocaine
   b. heroin
   c. alcohol
   d. LSD

4. A combination of signs and symptoms associated with similar poisons is referred to as a:
   a. toxidrome
   b. syndrome
   c. classic presentation
   d. constellation

5. After accidentally inhaling an unknown powder, your patient complains of a headache and dizziness. His heart rate is 40, he is drooling and tearing, and he is incontinent of both urine and feces. This is consistent with what toxidrome?
   a. amphetamines
   b. cholinergic
   c. hallucinogens
   d. opiates

6. The combination of salivation, lacrimation, urination, defecation, gastrointestinal upset, and emesis (SLUDGE) is characteristic of _____ poisoning.
   a. crack cocaine
   b. methamphetamine
   c. organophosphate
   d. cyanide

7. The pharmacological treatment of a sarin gas exposure would include all of the following *EXCEPT*:
   a. oxygen
   b. cyanide kit
   c. atropine
   d. diazepam

8. The most important factor that must be considered when treating a victim of a hazardous material is:
   a. removing contaminated material from the patient
   b. preventing rescuer contamination
   c. giving the correct antidote
   d. removing the victim from the contaminated area

9. The most appropriate means to decontaminate a victim exposed to an organophosphate pesticide powder is to:
   a. administer atropine 1 mg every 2 minutes until symptoms improve
   b. flush the patient with copious quantities of water to remove all residue
   c. have the patient, if able, remove clothing and place it in an appropriate container and use a brush to gently sweep away any residual material from the skin
   d. use a high-pressure hose to blow away all particulate matter from the patient's clothing and skin

10. A 16-year-old male ingested 100 tablets of 25-mg diphenhydramine. He is delirious and tachycardic. His skin is hot and dry. This is due to what pharmacological effect?
   a. anticholinergic
   b. acidosis
   c. uncoupling of oxidative phosphorylation
   d. hypoxia

11. All of the following are true regarding narcotic overdose *EXCEPT*:
   a. most opiates last longer than naloxone
   b. can occur from all routes of entry
   c. always requires naloxone treatment
   d. reversal may precipitate seizures

12. Which of the following signs and symptoms is most consistent with an acute opiate overdose?
   a. agitation and restlessness
   b. hypoxia leading to cardiac arrest
   c. sluggish and constricted pupils with decreased mental status and depressed respiratory activity
   d. delirium and hallucinations

13. Match the agent with its common street name.
   a. cocaine   1. downers
   b. marijuana   2. crosses
   c. heroin   3. weed
   d. amphetamines   4. snow
   e. barbiturates   5. smack

14. Cocaine overdose is associated with all of the following *EXCEPT*:
   a. seizures
   b. myocardial infarction
   c. nosebleeds
   d. poisoning of the hemoglobin molecule

15. All of the following are physiological complications of intravenous drug use *EXCEPT*:
   a. HIV and hepatitis B and C
   b. life of crime to acquire money for drugs
   c. endocarditis
   d. pulmonary embolus

16. Match the substance with its antidote.
   a. carbon monoxide   1. Narcan
   b. cyanide   2. flumazenil
   c. heroin   3. atropine
   d. valium   4. amyl nitrite and sodium thiosulfate
   e. organophosphates   5. hyperbaric oxygen

17. Cyanide poisoning can occur from each of the following *EXCEPT*:
   a. laetrile overdose
   b. brake pad dust
   c. nitroprusside infusion
   d. circuit board electroplating

18. A 4-year-old spending the weekend with his elderly aunt is found unresponsive, hypotensive, and bradycardic. Empty prescription bottles are present. The most likely agent responsible is:
   a. cardiac medication
   b. psychiatric medication
   c. anticoagulants
   d. antibiotics

19. Regarding the first aid for caustic ingestions, one of the most important treatment priorities is:
   a. avoidance of vomiting
   b. administration of milk
   c. administration of the proper antidote
   d. early intubation

20. A 22-year-old schizophrenic drinks a glass of drain cleaner containing hydrochloric acid. Which of the following is true?
   a. Administration of baking soda will neutralize the acid.
   b. Administration of activated charcoal will limit absorption.
   c. Severe lung injury may occur if the patient vomits.
   d. Acid ingestions generally result in more damage than alkali ingestions.

21. An unresponsive woman is removed from the basement of a burning building. She appears unharmed but is not breathing. Which of the following is most correct?
   a. Carbon monoxide poisoning is the most likely cause.
   b. Cyanide poisoning is commonly involved in smoke inhalation victims.
   c. Hypoxia is a result of carbon monoxide inhalation, which prevents oxygen from passing through the alveoli.
   d. Her unresponsiveness is caused by extreme heat exposure.

22. A 38-year-old woman has overdosed on amitriptyline. She is unresponsive and seizing, and the monitor shows a wide complex tachycardia. Which of the following is most correct?
    a. Administration of sodium bicarbonate inactivates the drug.
    b. Widening of the QRS correlates reliably with the severity of the overdose.
    c. Diazepam is not indicated for the seizures.
    d. There is no need to check blood glucose level if you suspect amitriptyline overdose.

23. A 40-year-old is found unresponsive after ingesting an unknown amount of her Valium prescription. Which of the following is most correct?
    a. It is unlikely that the prescription bottle contained enough pills to harm her.
    b. Administration of flumazenil may cause seizures.
    c. Women are more likely to succeed in their suicide attempts.
    d. Immediate gastric lavage is indicated.

24. A patient complains of severe pain in his left foot after being bitten by a black widow spider and begins to have muscle spasms in his leg. Definitive treatment consists of:
    a. tourniquet application
    b. administration of epinephrine and diphenhydramine
    c. incision over the bite site and application of gentle suction
    d. rapid transport to a facility with antivenin

25. Antivenin is available for all of the following *EXCEPT:*
    a. hornets
    b. diamond back rattlesnakes
    c. black widow spider
    d. pit vipers

26. A 20-year-old college student has overdosed on Lomotil, which is used to treat diarrhea. You read the ingredients and find belladonna listed. On exam, she is delirious. Her skin is hot, dry, and flushed. Her pupils are dilated and she is tachycardic. You would suspect which of the following toxidromes?
    a. cholinergic
    b. anticholinergic
    c. SLUDGE
    d. opiate

27. A chronic alcoholic quit drinking 2 days ago and is now hallucinating, tremulous, tachycardic, and hypertensive. This is known as:
    a. the shakes
    b. Wernicke's encephalopathy
    c. delirium tremens
    d. Korsakoff's psychosis

28. The primary difference between overdoses in children and adults is:
    a. symptom onset is quicker in children
    b. adult overdoses usually consist of only one agent
    c. childhood overdoses are usually accidental
    d. antidotes are based on adult weights

29. Jellyfish, sea anemones, and fire coral are examples of a class of aquatic creatures called coelenterates that have which of the following features in common?
    a. gelatinous outer layers containing venom
    b. nematocysts, which can be inactivated with hot water
    c. presence of long spiny processes containing venom
    d. tentacles, which contain nematocysts filled with venom

30. Echinoderms are aquatic animals that inject venom by the use of long sharp spines. Examples include all of the following *EXCEPT:*
    a. stingrays
    b. sea urchins
    c. starfish
    d. sea cucumbers

31. A young man who spent the weekend camping in the woods presents with restlessness and complains of tingling in his hands and feet. You notice that he has loss of deep tendon reflexes in his legs. This is consistent with what tick-borne condition?
    a. Rocky Mountain spotted fever
    b. tick paralysis
    c. Lyme disease
    d. dengue fever

32. The mechanism of action of amyl nitrite and sodium nitrite in the treatment of cyanide poisoning involves:
a. creation of methemoglobin, which has a higher affinity for cyanide than normal hemoglobin
b. displacement of cyanide from the red blood cells
c. improving the delivery of oxygen to the tissues
d. inactivating the cyanide by stimulating the enzyme cyanidase

33. Which of the following is not one of the initial steps in the treatment of cyanide poisoning?
a. oxygen administration
b. amyl nitrite inhalation
c. sodium bicarbonate for acidosis
d. sodium thiosulfate administration

34. A rare but life-threatening form of food poisoning resulting from improperly canned foods is:
a. pseudomembranous colitis
b. shigellosis
c. botulism
d. campylobacter

35. An alcoholic is found unresponsive with a bottle of antifreeze at his side. The treatment of this ethylene glycol poisoning would consist of all of the following *EXCEPT*:
a. administration of ethanol infusion
b. gastric lavage to limit absorption
c. thiamine to degrade glycolic acid to nontoxic metabolites
d. calcium gluconate to manage hypocalcemia

36. You enter a house to examine a patient complaining of headache and feeling ill for the past several days. You notice amber stains on the kitchen walls, various measuring devices, a Bunsen burner, and a Pyrex-type meatloaf container. You should immediately:
a. open all doors and windows
b. turn on all lights to improve visualization of your patient
c. administer IV diazepam to prevent seizures
d. suspect the presence of a methamphetamine lab, get out, and call the authorities

37. Which of the following concerns cocaine toxicity and its treatment?
a. Freebase cocaine is less potent than standard street cocaine.
b. Benzodiazepines are the mainstay of treatment.
c. Acute myocardial infarction associated with cocaine toxicity is due to hypertensive crisis.
d. Crack cocaine is usually snorted.

38. Phencyclidine (PCP) is:
a. an analgesic originally used as a veterinary tranquilizer
b. a derivative of ketamine
c. only available in a liquid form
d. reversed with naloxone

39. Which of the following is true regarding hallucinogens?
a. Mescaline is derived from mushrooms.
b. Peyote cactus contains the ingredients for LSD.
c. MDMA or "Ecstasy" has become one of the most popular "designer" drugs.
d. Prehospital care consists mainly of keeping the patient awake through various means of stimuli.

40. Chronic alcoholics may develop Wernicke-Korsakoff syndrome, which is due to a thiamine deficiency from malnutrition combined with the inability to utilize thiamine. Which of the following is a true statement?
a. Wernicke's encephalopathy is characterized by apathy, poor memory, dementia, and confabulation.
b. Korsakoff's psychosis is characterized by ataxia, nystagmus, and neuropathy.
c. In treating such patients, the administration of glucose may result in coma if not preceded by thiamine administration.
d. Both are reversible with the proper administration of thiamine.

41. A hiker is bitten on the calf by a small spider. Over the ensuing week the bite becomes necrotic with a deep ulcer. Eventually he requires skin grafting to cover the defect in his leg. Which of the following is true?
a. He should have received antivenin early.
b. Hot compresses to the wound along with lymphatic tourniquets would have decreased absorption of the venom.
c. This is a typical presentation for a black widow spider bite.
d. None of the above are true.

42. Following inhalation of an organophosphate the patient experiences all the classic SLUDGE symptoms. After administration of 2 mg of atropine the patient continues to drool uncontrollably. The next step in treatment would be to:
a. administer additional doses of atropine until the patient is "dry"
b. administer 2 mg Valium
c. administer 1 to 2 g of pralidoxime (2-PAM chloride) over 15 to 30 minutes
d. arrange for hemodialysis

Renal

43. Your 30-year-old patient complains of acute onset of left flank pain that radiates into his groin. He is restless and vomiting. Vital signs are blood pressure 120/70, pulse 120, respiratory rate 16 and afebrile. His presentation is most consistent with:
a. acute appendicitis
b. dissecting aortic aneurysm
c. pyelonephritis
d. kidney stone

44. Acute onset of flank pain that comes in waves and may radiate into the lower abdomen and/or groin associated with a kidney stone is referred to as:
a. biliary colic
b. renal colic
c. parietal pain
d. gastrointestinal colic

45. A 22-year-old woman presents with a fever of 101° F, flank pain, nausea, and vomiting, which followed 1 week of painful and frequent urination. This is most consistent with:
a. pyelonephritis
b. appendicitis
c. cholecystitis
d. gastroenteritis

46. An uncomplicated urinary tract infection (UTI) may be distinguished from pyelonephritis by:
a. painful urination more common with pyelonephritis
b. UTI is complication of pyelonephritis
c. absence of systemic symptoms such as fever, nausea, and vomiting
d. UTI never occurs in males

47. Classifications of the causes of acute renal failure include all of the following *EXCEPT:*
a. prerenal
b. postrenal
c. perirenal
d. renal

48. Common causes of acute renal failure include all of the following *EXCEPT:*
a. diabetes
b. shock
c. infection
d. trauma

49. The common feature shared by both acute and chronic renal failure is:
a. 50% mortality rate
b. both are often reversible
c. diabetes is a common cause
d. buildup of the waste products of metabolism resulting in a condition called uremia

50. The symptoms from acute renal failure:
a. begin once the patient completely ceases urine production (anuria)
b. do not include mental status changes
c. are caused by the inability of the kidney to retain water
d. can occur within hours

51. Common causes of chronic renal failure include all of the following *EXCEPT:*
a. shock
b. diabetes
c. hypertension
d. autoimmune disorders

52. A 65-year-old man with chronic renal failure was unable to make his dialysis appointment on Friday because of weather. Sunday morning you are called to his home with the complaints of shortness of breath and weakness. His physical exam will be similar to that for:
a. COPD
b. pneumonia
c. congestive heart failure
d. pulmonary embolus

53. A renal failure patient suffers a cardiac arrest. The electrolyte disturbance most often associated with this condition is:
a. hyperkalemia
b. hyperglycemia
c. hypercalcemia
d. hypocalcemia

54. Chronic renal failure results in symptoms in which of the following systems?
a. psychiatric and neurological
b. gastrointestinal
c. cardiopulmonary
d. all of the above

55. The use of dialysis for the treatment of both acute and chronic renal failure:
    a. is performed with both hemodialysis and peritoneal dialysis
    b. relies on the circulation of blood across a semi-permeable membrane and the diffusion of waste products out of the blood
    c. is associated with few risks and side effects
    d. is required daily to remove sufficient toxins

56. Common complications of dialysis consist of each of the following *EXCEPT*:
    a. vascular access problems
    b. hypothermia from cold dialysate solutions
    c. hypotension
    d. hemorrhage

57. Severe hyperkalemia in renal failure:
    a. is demonstrated on the ECG by shortened PR intervals, flattened T waves, and bundle branch blocks
    b. is not related to dietary intake of potassium
    c. may result in cardiac arrest and is treated with the administration of calcium and sodium bicarbonate
    d. is caused by the use of the incorrect dialysate solution

58. Your chronic renal failure patient is complaining of chest pain, and you suspect an acute myocardial infarction. Important issues to consider when treating him include:
    a. avoidance of taking blood pressures and starting IVs on the arm with the dialysis shunt
    b. avoidance of volume overloading him with IV fluids
    c. administration of the usual and customary nitrates and oxygen
    d. all of the above

59. A hemodialysis patient has just completed dialysis and is complaining of a headache and appears confused. This condition is most likely due to:
    a. disequilibrium syndrome caused by osmotic shift of water across the blood-brain barrier resulting in cerebral edema
    b. intracerebral hemorrhage from the administration of heparin in the dialysate
    c. hypoglycemia
    d. hypotension

60. Your 16-year-old male patient complains of acute onset of severe left scrotal pain after lifting weights in the gym. He is restless, vomiting, and diaphoretic. Which of the following is most correct?
    a. This is most likely due to a hernia and may be treated conservatively.
    b. This is caused by twisting of a portion of the testicle called the epididymitis.
    c. This is most likely testicular torsion, which requires emergency surgery within 4 to 6 hours.
    d. This can be treated with manual reduction in the field.

61. Prehospital treatment of kidney stones may include the administration of all of the following *EXCEPT*:
    a. furosemide to promote urination
    b. morphine for analgesia
    c. an antiemetic for nausea
    d. ketorolac for renal colic

62. A 60-year-old man presents with severe lower abdominal pain and inability to urinate. Which of the following conditions can result in acute urinary retention?
    a. prostatic hypertrophy
    b. the prescription use of the antidepressant Elavil
    c. foreign body obstruction of the urethra
    d. all of the above

63. A 56-year-old man with renal failure is found in cardiac arrest. The monitor shows v-tach. Appropriate treatment would consist of all of the following *EXCEPT*:
    a. administration of antiarrhythmics such as lidocaine or amiodirone
    b. immediate defibrillation
    c. insulin and sodium bicarbonate
    d. calcium gluconate and sodium bicarbonate

Infectious Disease

64. You are preparing to intubate a patient during CPR. Suction is required to clear the vomit and oral secretions so that the cords can be visualized. All of the following forms of personal protective equipment should be worn during the procedure *EXCEPT*:
    a. disposable gloves
    b. protective eyewear
    c. gown
    d. mask

Questions 65 through 68 refer to the following scenario:

You are caring for a 35-year-old man who is found unresponsive. Your first attempt at establishing an IV is unsuccessful, and while placing the needle into the sharps container you feel a prick in your finger. You discover that someone left the tip of a needle pointing up and out of the container. You remove your glove and discover a puncture wound at the tip of your finger, which is bleeding.

65. Which of the following immunizations is most likely to protect you against infection from a needle stick?
  a. tetanus toxoid
  b. hepatitis B vaccine
  c. hepatitis C vaccine
  d. hepatitis A vaccine

66. Which of the following is the most likely infection to be transmitted by a needle stick to a health care worker?
  a. HIV
  b. hepatitis A
  c. hepatitis B
  d. hepatitis C

67. After delivering your patient to the ER, which of the following steps should you take regarding this incident?
  a. Wash the wound with peroxide and force it to bleed so that the virus will be flushed out.
  b. Look through the logbook to find out who left that needle pointing out.
  c. Follow the instructions in your service's exposure control plan.
  d. Rest and elevate the extremity.

68. All of the following will be considered when determining the proper postexposure prophylaxis to use *EXCEPT:*
  a. whether or not you are sexually active
  b. whether or not you have received the hepatitis B vaccine
  c. whether or not the source of the contaminated blood is known
  d. whether or not the needle stick is considered to represent a significant exposure

69. HIV, the virus that causes AIDS, attacks and injures the body by:
  a. infecting the red blood cells, leading to severe anemia and infection
  b. infecting the liver, heart, and lungs resulting in their failure
  c. infecting the white blood cells known as T-helper cells
  d. all of the above

70. HIV may be transmitted by all of the following *EXCEPT:*
  a. blood transfusion with infected blood
  b. sexual intercourse
  c. sharing of needles by IV drug users
  d. contact with urine and tears

71. The blood of an unknown source is checked and found to be negative for HIV antibodies. This means the blood is absolutely safe for administration.
  a. true
  b. false

72. Which of the following forms of hepatitis does not result in a chronic infection of the liver?
  a. hepatitis A
  b. hepatitis B
  c. hepatitis C
  d. all of the above can result in chronic hepatitis

73. Which of the following is true regarding tuberculosis (TB)?
  a. The widespread use of public health detection and treatment has significantly reduced the incidence of TB.
  b. The patient with HIV is 40 times as likely to have TB because both agents are transmitted by blood.
  c. The highest incidence of TB is found in correctional facilities, homeless shelters, and nursing homes.
  d. Foreigners entering the country are routinely screened for TB.

74. The most effective means to decrease the likelihood of contracting tuberculosis while transporting a patient is to:
   a. wear a surgical mask when transporting any patient with a cough
   b. have a high index of suspicion for the disease when transporting any patient with a cough
   c. have any patient with a cough wear a HEPA mask
   d. have a yearly TB skin test performed

75. Meningitis refers to an inflammation of the membranes surrounding the spinal cord and brain. The most common cause of meningitis is:
   a. meningococcal
   b. *H. influenza*
   c. viral
   d. streptococcal

76. One of the most serious and potentially fatal forms of meningitis is meningococcal caused by the *Neisseria meningitides* bacteria. It is spread by:
   a. contact with contaminated blood
   b. exposure to upper respiratory secretions
   c. infected mosquito bites
   d. consumption of contaminated food

77. Prophylactic postexposure medication is given in an attempt to prevent contraction of the suspected infection. It is available for each of the following infectious agents *EXCEPT:*
   a. HIV
   b. hepatitis A and B
   c. any type of meningitis
   d. tuberculosis

ANSWERS TO CHAPTER 16: MEDICAL EMERGENCIES VI: TOXICOLOGY, RENAL, AND INFECTIOUS DISEASE

Toxicology

1. d. Poisoning may occur from many routes. Poisons may be absorbed directly through the skin as with hydrofluoric acid and organophosphates, inhalation as with chlorine, and ingestion as in prescription medications and alcohol. Diffusion occurs when a substance moves throughout a liquid or gas and is not a form of poisoning.

2. a. Dependence refers to the physical and/or psychological need of a drug to avoid withdrawal symptoms. Tolerance refers to the need to use greater and greater amounts of a drug to acquire the same level of response. Potentiation occurs when the mixing of two or more drugs results in an effect greater than the sum of the two drugs. Synergism is similar to potentiation.

3. c. Although each of the listed agents is a drug of addiction, it is vital to recognize the prevalence of alcohol use and appreciate its role as a drug of addiction. It is estimated that more people are addicted to alcohol than all other agents combined. Persons addicted to nonalcohol agents frequently are alcoholics as well.

4. a. Several agents cause certain physical signs and symptoms that are so specific as to suggest their presence merely by the combination of these signs and symptoms.

5. b. Cholinergic agents stimulate the parasympathetic nervous system resulting in the symptoms of salivation, lacrimation, urination, defecation, GI upset, and emesis.

6. c. The SLUDGE toxidrome is consistent with the cholinergic effect of organophosphate pesticides. Cholinergic symptoms are due to stimulation of the parasympathetic nervous system, which involves the organs of long-term survival such as the gastrointestinal and urinary systems. Parasympathetic stimulation causes salivation or drooling, lacrimation or tearing, the loss of bowel and bladder control. Overactivity of the GI tract results in nausea and vomiting.

7. b. Sarin gas is a nerve agent that results in cholinergic response. The application of oxygen is always appropriate. Atropine is used to dry the mucous membranes and counter the cardiotoxic effects of the gas. Diazepam may be required should seizures occur. Cyanide treatment is not involved in sarin gas exposure.

8. b. As with any EMS encounter scene safety is paramount. When dealing with the exposed patient, the rescuers must ensure that they do not become contaminated or exposed to the hazardous material. Simply removing the material may not be sufficient because the area in which the patient is found may still contain the hazardous material. Therefore first assess the situation and make sure that it is safe to approach the patient.

9. c. The proper method of removing any particulate toxic substance is to first limit the potential for exposure to the rescuer. If the patient is conscious, have the patient disrobe. Use a gentle brush to brush away any material. The use of water will result in dissolving the material, which can then be absorbed through the skin. The use of a high-pressure device will aerosolize the material and increase the risk of inhalation. The administration of atropine is indicated for the treatment of symptoms and does nothing to decontaminate the patient.

10. a. Diphenhydramine is commonly known as Benadryl, an antihistamine. Overdose of this agent results in signs and symptoms consistent with an overdose of atropine, an anticholinergic. Acidosis and hypoxia alone will not result in all the listed symptoms. Uncoupling of oxidative phosphorylation is involved in cyanide poisoning.

11. c. Naloxone is an opiate antagonist and works rapidly to displace opiates from their receptor sites. However, its half-life is shorter than most narcotics leading to the possibility of it wearing off before the narcotics are metabolized. Naloxone is indicated when the level of consciousness threatens airway patency. Its administration may precipitate seizures in the addicted patient by throwing them into withdrawal.

12. c. Agitation is more commonly associated with amphetamines, PCP, and cocaine. Hypoxia may be caused by carbon monoxide poisoning or cyanide. Delirium and hallucinations are typical of mushrooms or agents such as LSD and Ecstasy.

13. a. snow; b. weed; c. smack; d. crosses; e. downers

14. d. The stimulant effect of cocaine can result in seizures and other forms of hyperactivity. Because it is often snorted, long-term use results in thinning of the nasal mucosa and bleeding. Cocaine can induce coronary artery spasm leading to an acute MI as well as tachydysrhythmias. Poisoning of the hemoglobin molecule is characteristic of carbon monoxide exposure.

15. b. The sharing of needles is the major cause of HIV and hepatitis transmission in this population. Endocarditis occurs when bacteria enter the bloodstream and infect the heart, most often the valves. Pulmonary embolus occurs from the particulate matter used to "cut" the drug such as talc, which travels into the pulmonary vasculature lodging in vessels and becoming a nidus for infection. Although crime is clearly linked to IV drug use, other than assaults by those owed money, it is not considered a physiological complication.

16. a. hyperbaric oxygen; b. amyl nitrite and sodium thiosulfate; c. Narcan; d. flumazenil; e. atropine

17. b. Older brake pads were made of asbestos, which resulted in lung cancer. The metabolic breakdown of Laetrile, an illegal medication for the treatment of some cancers, is cyanide. Nitroprusside metabolism can result in cyanide accumulation but is rare. The chemicals used to etch electronic circuit boards often contain cyanide.

18. a. The accidental ingestion by children of adult prescription medications is quite common. Therefore it is vital to obtain a history not only for the patient but of the caretakers as well. Cardiac glycosides such as digoxin and more commonly calcium channel blockers and beta-blocker medication can result in catastrophic cardiovascular collapse. Diabetic medications such as glucophage and others can induce profound hypoglycemia and bradycardia. Psychiatric medications often result in altered mental status such as agitation, delirium, and seizures. Anticoagulants will cause bleeding,

and antibiotics usually result in nausea and vomiting.

19. a. The most serious complication from caustic ingestions occurs if the patient vomits and aspirates. All attempts should be made to decrease this likelihood including the use of antiemetics. Milk may dilute the caustic agent but may also precipitate vomiting. There are no antidotes for caustic ingestions, and early intubation may further increase the risk of vomiting and aspiration.

20. c. The ingestion of acids is generally better tolerated than alkaline material because acid burns tend be more superficial. The concept of neutralizing the acid with a base sounds intuitive, but the reaction is exothermic, meaning that it creates heat, which can worsen the injury. The aspiration of either an acid or alkali can result in severe pulmonary injury.

21. a. Although it is true that the by-products of combustion of many materials in home construction can result in the release of cyanide, this is fairly rare. Carbon monoxide is clearly the most common by-product and, in the absence of other causes of decreased level of consciousness, should always be suspected. The effect of the carbon monoxide is to "poison" the hemoglobin and does not interfere with oxygen transport across the alveoli. Severe heat exposure can result in loss of consciousness but rarely apnea.

22. b. Amitriptyline is highly toxic to the heart and nervous system. It is rapidly absorbed by the fat cells of the body giving it a long half-life. It is has been shown that the widening of the QRS pattern by 50% along with tachycardia is a reliable indicator of its presence. The administration of sodium bicarbonate is intended to drive more of the drug into the fat cells where it can be released more slowly and hopefully with less deleterious side effects. Seizures from any cause are best treated with a benzodiazepine, and the approach to the unconscious victim should always include an assessment of blood glucose.

23. b. Valium prescriptions are often filled in sufficient numbers to result in death, particularly if ingested along with other respiratory depressants such as alcohol. Statistically, women attempt suicide more often by overdosing but are far less successful than men who tend to use more reliably fatal means. Gastric lavage should not be performed until the patient's airway is secure. The administration of flumazenil, while an approved antidote for benzodiazepine overdose, is not indicated because acute reversal of the benzodiazepine may lower the patient's seizure threshold.

24. **d.** The initial care for venomous bites remains controversial and relies on factors such as distance to definitive care and the location of the bite and severity of the envenomation. The primary effect of black widow spider bites is generally local and associated with pain and paresthesias. Tourniquet application will not decrease these effects, and the amount of venom is usually insufficient to justify the classic snake bite remedies. Epinephrine and diphenhydramine may be appropriate in the presence of allergic reaction but will not decrease the effects of the venom. Only the administration of antivenin at an appropriate facility will be useful.

25. **a.** Hornets, wasps, and bees do not have a common chemical basis to their venom and usually the severity of the sting is related to an allergic reaction rather than the effect of a venom. All pit vipers (such as the diamondback rattlesnake) and some spiders such as the black widow have commercially available antivenins.

26. **b.** Belladonna is a natural form of atropine, which is an anticholinergic agent. The anticholinergic toxidrome is characterized by the patient being "mad as a hatter and dry as a bone" with delirium, urinary retention, and hot, dry skin. Treatment includes diazepam and rarely physostigmine in severe cases.

27. **c.** "The shakes" is usually seen the day following binge drinking and is generally not life threatening. It is a result of the loss of the sedative effect of alcohol precipitating anxiousness and tremors. Delirium tremens is a serious and frequently fatal condition and should be treated aggressively with sedatives and hospitalization. It can result in seizures and cardiac arrest. Wernicke's encephalopathy and Korsakoff's syndrome are mental status and cognitive disturbances that result from long-term alcohol use.

28. **c.** Children usually ingest a toxic substance accidentally as a result of easy access to the agents or simple experimentation. The speed of onset of any ingested agent is related to its relative toxicity and the amount or concentration ingested. It is not affected by age. Adult ingestions are usually intentional and combined with multiple agents in an attempt to be more successful in their suicide attempt or to gain a greater "high" from the experience. Antidotes are based on the patient's weight and are not age adjusted.

29. **d.** All coelenterates contain small cysts or nematocysts containing neurotoxin. Long spiny creatures constitute the echinoderms. The nematocysts reside in the soft tentacles of the animal, not in their main body mass. The neurotoxins are heat stable.

30. **a.** Echinoderms inject their venom from long sharp spines as is seen in sea urchins and starfish. The sea cucumber has a sharp spike at the anal end and can inject a very painful sting. The venom from echinoderms is generally less severe than that of the coelenterates and usually produces a local painful reaction. Stingrays have a sharp barb near the end of their tail, which does not contain venom but causes injury from the penetrating trauma and the retention of foreign material in the wound, which leads to infection.

31. **b.** Tick paralysis results from a prolonged bite by a female wood tick. It is due to a neurotoxin secreted by the tick and symptoms present within 6 days of the bite. Removal of the tick results in rapid improvement and resolution of the symptoms but if left untreated can be fatal.

32. **a.** Because cyanide diffuses throughout the body via the circulatory system the first order of treatment is to bind it to something that will aid in its removal. Amyl nitrite changes the hemoglobin molecule into methemoglobin, which has a much higher affinity for cyanide than normal hemoglobin. The second step is to administer sodium thiosulfate, which converts the methemoglobin into a water-soluble compound that can be eliminated from the system via the urinary tract.

33. **c.** Because cyanide interrupts the ability of the tissue to utilize oxygen it is always appropriate to

administer additional oxygen at 100%. Amyl nitrite and sodium thiosulfate are the main ingredients in the cyanide kit. Sodium bicarbonate is not necessary unless other causes of severe metabolic acidosis exist and its administration will not improve the effectiveness of the above listed medications

34. c. Botulism is a toxin produced by the soil bacteria *Clostridium botulinum* and is found in improperly canned foods. Botulism sickness occurs from neurotoxic effects, which result in severe abdominal pain.

35. b. The primary ingredient in antifreeze is ethylene glycol. It is highly neurotoxic and is metabolized by the liver through the same mechanism as alcohol; however, the products of metabolism are more toxic than the substance itself. It is highly water soluble, and by the time of patient presentation little remains in the stomach and gastric lavage is not indicated. By administering intravenous ethanol, the enzymes utilized to metabolize it preferentially attack the ethanol, and the ethylene glycol is excreted in the urine. Thiamine is given to enhance the urinary excretion. Severe hypocalcemia is common and must be treated with supplemental calcium administration.

36. d. Many volatile and hazardous chemicals are utilized in the production of illicit drugs such as methamphetamine. Solvents are the primary means of distilling the active ingredients and the vaporization results in staining of walls and ceilings. Bunsen burners, flasks, and other Pyrex-type containers are frequently used. Noticing this apparatus should alert you to the fact that you are in a very hazardous environment. Operators of such clandestine labs place booby traps such as a match and striker plate on windows and doors and fill light bulbs with gasoline. The rule of thumb when entering such an establishment: "If it's off leave it off, if it's on leave it on." More important, get out and call for law enforcement backup.

37. b. Benzodiazepines reduce the anxiety associated with acute cocaine toxicity and are useful in the event of cocaine-induced seizures. Freebase cocaine is significantly more potent because it is a purified form of street cocaine. Crack cocaine is usually smoked. The sympathetic response to cocaine toxicity results in coronary artery spasm leading to myocardial infarction.

38. a. PCP is a dissociative agent originally used in veterinary medicine. Ketamine is a derivative of PCP and has become a popular drug of abuse. PCP and ketamine are available in various forms including liquid and powder. Naloxone is indicated for opiate ingestion and useless for PCP.

39. c. Ecstasy has become very popular at "rave" parties and can be deadly. Mescaline is derived from the peyote cactus, whereas LSD is manufactured in the laboratory. Prehospital care of all of these ingestions is to keep the patient calm with the use of sedatives and soft lights with minimal disturbance.

40. c. Coma can result from the administration of glucose before thiamine because the thiamine deficiency commonly associated with alcoholism impairs the ability of glucose to enter the central nervous system. The definitions of Wernicke's encephalopathy and Korsakoff's psychosis are reversed. The administration of thiamine does not affect the degree or severity of the syndrome.

41. d. This is a typical presentation for a brown recluse spider bite. There is no antivenin available, and the application of ice rather than heat decreases absorption. Obstruction tourniquets are not helpful in spider bites. The bite of a black widow spider results in severe muscle spasms and rigidity along with systemic signs and symptoms such as perspiration, salivation, and headache. A commercial antivenin is available for black widow spider bites but should only be given in the emergency department.

42. a. The patient with SLUDGE toxidrome is "wet"; therefore treatment is designed to "dry" them out with the administration of the anticholinergic drug atropine. Such patients may require massive doses to counteract the organophosphate. Valium is only indicated if seizures occur, and hemodialysis is ineffective against this agent. Pralidoxime corrects the biochemical process that the organophosphates create but works slowly to reverse the signs and symptoms. Often atropine alone is sufficient.

Renal

43. d. The pain of renal colic associated with the passage of a kidney stone is one of the most intense pains imaginable. The pain causes the patient to be restless in an attempt to find a comfortable position. The pain of appendicitis is due to peritoneal irritation of the abdominal wall, which is worsened with movement. Fever may or may not be present. The dissecting aneurysm is described as a burning, tearing pain in the back and usually associated with hypertension. Pyelonephritis is an infection of the kidney that usually presents with flank pain and fever. It usually presents slowly rather than acutely.

44. b. Renal colic is due to obstruction and the resultant spasm of the ureter. Renal pole and upper ureter obstruction results in pain in the flank. Obstruction of the middle third of the ureter refers pain from the flank to the lower abdominal area. Obstruction in the distal third of the ureter refers pain to the groin.

45. a. Urinary tract infections are divided into lower, affecting the bladder, and upper, affecting the kidney. Simple lower urinary tract infections present with dysuria and no fever. Pyelonephritis is an inflammation of the kidney from infection and can occur as a complication of untreated lower tract infections or from bacteremia.

46. c. Lower urinary tract infections present with signs and symptoms of urinary bladder irritation such as urinary spasm, dysuria, and increased urinary frequency. Systemic symptoms are more consistent with upper tract infections.

47. c. Acute renal failure results when there is a sudden and marked decrease in filtration of the renal glomeruli, leading to the accumulation of salt, water, and nitrogenous wastes in the body. Prerenal failure results from inadequate perfusion of the kidney as seen in hypovolemia or obstruction of the renal arteries. Postrenal failure occurs from obstruction of the ureter or urethra. Renal causes consist of those that result in injury to the renal parenchyma such as hypertension, autoimmune diseases, and pyelonephritis.

48. a. Acute renal failure develops over a matter of days or weeks, whereas chronic renal failure results from prolonged insult from various diseases such as diabetes, hypertension, and autoimmune disorders, which generally affect the small vessels of the parenchyma.

49. d. Both acute and chronic renal failure results in dysfunction of the kidney's ability to eliminate the waste products of metabolism, which are primarily composed of urea. The urea builds up in the system resulting in uremia, which can manifest itself in multiple organ systems. Acute renal failure has a high mortality rate of 50% but is reversible if treated early. Chronic renal failure commonly requires dialysis or renal transplant. Diabetes is associated with chronic renal failure.

50. d. When acute renal failure occurs, the buildup of urea affects many organ systems including the CNS, leading to mental status changes. Renal failure can exist even though urine continues to be excreted (oliguria) and does not require the complete cessation of urine production. The primary dysfunction is retention of water secondary to inability to control excretion of electrolytes and proteins.

51. a. Shock is a prerenal cause of acute renal failure from poor perfusion of the kidney. Diabetes, hypertension, and autoimmune disorders cause small vessel disease, which results in chronic renal failure from prolonged insult.

52. c. The purpose of dialysis is to normalize the blood chemistry and remove excess water from the system. This patient will have signs and symptoms consistent with volume overload similar to congestive heart failure. However, it is important to recognize that the primary problem is one of renal excretion; therefore routine CHF treatment with diuretics will not be as effective.

53. a. Hyperkalemia results from missed dialysis treatments and poor dietary control. It can result in fatal dysrhythmias and therefore should be considered in the renal failure patient in cardiac arrest.

54. d. The volume overload and uremia resulting from renal failure affects almost every organ system. It can cause anxiety, delirium, and altered mental status. It causes anorexia, nausea, and vomiting. The heart is affected by hypertension, pericarditis, and pulmonary edema. It also affects the endocrine system with electrolyte disturbances and anemia.

55. b. Dialysis for renal failure entails passing blood through a dialysate, which extracts the waste products from it. It can result in several complications such as infection, electrolyte disturbance, and volume depletion. The usual course of dialysis occurs every other day or once or twice a week. Peritoneal dialysis is used only for chronic renal failure.

56. b. The vascular access or shunt can become clotted off or infected. If too much fluid is removed the patient may become hypotensive. The anticoagulants used can result in bleeding problems. The dialysis machine maintains proper fluid temperature.

57. c. Elevated potassium levels (hyperkalemia) result from poor dietary control and are demonstrated on the ECG with prolonged PR intervals and tall spiked T waves. The potassium can be "pushed" into the cells, decreasing the blood level, by the administration of calcium and sodium bicarbonate. The dialysate concentration affects the amount of water removed and is more likely to result in hypokalemia if the wrong concentration is used.

58. d. The use of any compression on the arm containing the shunt can result in damage to the shunt including thrombosis. Volume overload can occur with even customary IV fluid administration. The treatment of the ischemia with nitrates and oxygen is indicated just as with any patient with acute coronary syndrome.

59. a. Following dialysis, fluid shifts can occur from the extracellular space into the brain because of an osmotic gradient between them. This influx of fluid into the brain can result in cerebral edema and mental status changes. Intracerebral hemorrhage would only occur if massive amounts of heparin were given. Hypoglycemia is not associated with dialysis and hypotension and would not be associated with these symptoms but should be checked if the patient is diabetic.

60. c. Testicular torsion presents with acute onset of pain and often occurs with strenuous effort. It

is a relenting pain similar to renal colic but located in the scrotum. A hernia gives pain in the inguinal area but is generally of less severity. The epididymis is a gland on the testicle that secretes a large portion of the ejaculate and can become infected but does not get twisted. Testicular torsion represents a real emergency because surgical reduction must be performed quickly to ensure the survival of the testicle.

61. a. The treatment of renal colic is consistent with the routine management of pain including opiates and antiemetics. Ketorolac, a nonsteroidal anti-inflammatory, has been shown to be useful in reducing the spasm of renal colic. Forced diuresis is not indicated and may actually worsen the pain.

62. d. Acute urinary retention occurs when the outlet to the bladder is obstructed. This can occur from mechanical causes such as urethral stricture, enlargement of the prostate, and foreign bodies in the urethra. Dysfunction of the central nervous system and use of medications with anticholinergic side effects such as tricyclic antidepressants can result in urinary retention.

63. c. The initial approach to the renal failure patient in cardiac arrest consists of the routine use of rapid defibrillation and drugs to extinguish the dysrhythmia. All such patients are assumed to be hyperkalemic and should be treated with calcium gluconate and sodium bicarbonate. The combination of these two agents work to move the potassium into the cells and out of the bloodstream.

Infectious Disease

64. c. The use of protective equipment for body substance isolation should be consistent with the potential for exposure. During endotracheal intubation the potential for splashing of secretions is increased, particularly during CPR. A protective gown is generally required only during childbirth and while caring for a bleeding wound, which is spurting blood uncontrollably.

65. b. A series of three hepatitis B vaccine injections will generally result in immunological protection against hepatitis B if taken early enough before exposure. A needle stick is unlikely to result in tetanus exposure, which generally occurs from exposure to soil-contaminated wounds. There is no vaccine against hepatitis A or C.

66. **d.** Hepatitis C results in a chronic hepatitis that remains infectious. Because there is no vaccine for it, this form of hepatitis has become increasingly prevalent. Most health care workers are immunized against hepatitis B. Hepatitis A is transmitted by consumption of contaminated food and/or fecal-oral transmission. HIV exposure from a needle stick is extremely rare.

67. **c.** Every EMS service and health care facility must have an Exposure Control Plan outlining what steps should be followed when a needle stick occurs. It is a common misperception that causing the wound to bleed will decrease the likelihood of infection. Attempting to determine who placed the needle there and the source of the exposure is unlikely to be successful and should not be considered in determining postexposure care. Taking the rest of the day off might not be a bad idea but should be the last step, not the first.

68. **a.** Regardless of your sexual orientation or previous health history, postexposure prophylaxis should be considered for everyone. Three determining factors decide when and what type of prophylaxis is appropriate: whether there is a presence of antibodies against the agent from either previous exposure or vaccination, whether the source is known and can be tested, and whether the exposure is thought to be significant. A significant needle stick is defined as any wound that results in bleeding.

69. **c.** HIV attaches itself to particular white blood cells called target or T-4 cells and begins to reproduce. Destruction of these cells results in a diminished resistance to infection by opportunistic bacterial and fungal organisms. The nervous system may become infected directly leading to encephalopathy and neuropathies but does not directly infect other organs.

70. **d.** HIV is not excreted in urine, sweat, tears, vomit, or feces in the absence of blood. Transmission only occurs from the transfer of contaminated blood directly through transfusion, through the sharing of needles, or through sexual intercourse from infected semen and vaginal secretions. Body fluids that are not derived from serum such as tears, sweat, and urine will not contain the virus. Vomit, unless it contains blood, is also safe.

71. **b.** False. Once infected with HIV there is an incubation period before detectable levels of HIV antibodies are present. This incubation period can last from 6 to 12 weeks during which time the blood still contains the infectious agent but would appear safe according to testing.

72. **a.** Hepatitis A is a self-limited disease presenting with flulike symptoms consisting of low-grade fever, malaise, and anorexia. Once contracted, the body acquires lifelong immunity and does not result in a chronic infection. Hepatitis B and C can result in a chronic infection of the liver leading to hepatic failure and a chronic carrier state.

73. **c.** Tuberculosis is more prevalent in persons living in close quarters where the transmission of the infected airborne particles can easily spread the disease. Although it is true that HIV-infected persons are more likely to contract TB, the two agents are transmitted by different routes (HIV via blood and TB via airborne spread). The deterioration of the public health system along with the lack of routine screening of immigrants has resulted in a significant increase in the incidence of TB in the United States.

74. **b.** When transporting a patient with a productive or persistent cough who may have other risk factors for TB, a high index of suspicion should lead you to take proper protective measures. These measures would include having the patient wear a surgical mask to reduce the production of airborne particles, donning a HEPA mask to protect you from inhaling any particles, and attempting to ventilate the ambulance to enhance the removal of infected particles. The yearly TB skin test determines whether you have been infected or exposed but does not prevent contraction of the disease.

75. **c.** Meningitis can be caused by a variety of bacteria, viruses, and other microorganisms such as tuberculosis and fungi. Viral causes are the most common and are referred to as aseptic meningitis. However, any patient suspected of

having meningitis should be considered highly infectious and proper protection taken.

76. b. The early symptoms of meningococcal meningitis include upper respiratory congestion, sore throat, and runny nose. The secretions from these areas contain high concentrations of the bacteria that enter the host from transmission to the mucous membranes. The use of a surgical mask by both you and the patient along with routine BSI procedures offers the best personal protection against infection.

77. c. Antibiotic postexposure prophylaxis is only available for meningococcal meningitis and not for any other cause. The use of an antiviral medications such as ZDV is indicated for HIV exposure, immunoglobulin for hepatitis exposure, and INH administration for TB exposure.

BEHAVIORAL AND PSYCHIATRIC DISORDERS

17

1. Which of the following statements regarding mental health problems is true?
   a. One in seven persons will require treatment at some time in his or her life for an emotional disturbance.
   b. It is estimated that as much as 20% of the U.S. population has some form of mental illness.
   c. Mental health problems incapacitate more people in the U.S. than all other health problems combined.
   d. All are true.

2. A 32-year-old woman experiences severe anxiety when crossing bridges and begins to alter her route to work so that she does not cross any bridges while driving her car. This is an example of a:
   a. psychosis
   b. neurosis
   c. phobia
   d. delirium

3. The first step in assessing a behavioral emergency is to:
   a. contain the emotional crisis
   b. evaluate the scene for possible danger
   c. render emergency medical care
   d. survey the scene for medications or signs of substance abuse

4. Because mental illness is a disease process, all EMS responses for behavioral emergencies require a full, detailed, physical exam of the patient.
   a. true
   b. false

5. Effective interviewing techniques for patients with behavioral emergencies include all of the following *EXCEPT*:
   a. active listening to concerns or complaints
   b. being supportive and empathetic
   c. invalidating the patient's intense feelings
   d. respecting a patient's personal space

6. Delirium and dementia may be difficult to differentiate and may occur at the same time.
   a. true
   b. false

7. The treatment of delirium is targeted mainly at:
   a. long-term treatment in an appropriate facility
   b. counseling patients to reorient themselves to their surroundings
   c. correcting the underlying cause
   d. chemical and physical restraint

8. Dementia is a clinical state characterized by loss of cognitive function in several areas. Although it is a slow, progressive process, often resulting from stroke or Alzheimer's disease, there are other medical illnesses such as lupus and alcoholism that can cause dementia.
   a. true
   b. false

9. Which of the following is an appropriate response for the rescuer in the management of paranoid reactions associated with schizophrenia?
   a. speak quietly with family or bystanders so that the patient does not pick up on their concerns
   b. attempt to gain the patient's confidence through kindness and warmth
   c. do not identify yourself as a paramedic because schizophrenic patients do not feel they need medical attention
   d. maintain an attitude that is friendly, yet somewhat distant and neutral

10. Schizophrenia is a complex disorder that affects more than 2 million adult Americans. Which of the following is true?
   a. Suicide is a rare outcome in schizophrenia, occurring in less than 1 in 25 patients.
   b. Schizophrenia occurs in women twice as frequently as in men.
   c. The initial appearance of schizophrenia in men and women is usually in their early teens or late twenties.
   d. None of the above are true.

11. The ambulance is called by a 35-year-old man with chest pain. You find the patient in the office of a busy law firm. He is in the process of obtaining a divorce. He is sitting in a chair, but is restless, holding his chest. His chief complaints are chest discomfort, nausea, and the sense that he is unable to breathe. He reports that he has not been sleeping well and is very anxious. His blood pressure is 170/96, pulse is 112, and respirations are 28. Which of the following would be the appropriate treatment for this patient?
   a. Withhold oxygen, (he is obviously hyperventilating,) be reassuring, and treat the patient with benzodiazepines for anxiety. The patient has no pertinent medical history and is too young for a heart attack.
   b. Place the patient on oxygen and a cardiac monitor, and perform a full assessment of chest discomfort with vital signs. While reassuring the patient that you are there to care for his problem, you are unable to diagnosis this condition and advise him that he will be transported for further evaluation at the hospital. Analgesics and/or sedation may be appropriate.
   c. This patient is obviously having an acute cardiac event. Rapid transport in emergency mode should be used because "time is muscle." Advise the patient that he is at a critical time in his intervention and needs to lie still and be cooperative so that you can care for him.
   d. Sit and calmly discuss the situation with the patient and his co-workers and let them know that anxiety attacks are common, but not life threatening. Advise the patient that he can stay and complete his business, but should really start "taking it easy from now on." These patients do not require ambulance transport and should be advised to see their personal physician soon.

12. Anxiety disorder is just another name for panic disorder.
   a. true
   b. false

13. You and your partner, both 10-year veterans of your service, recently responded to an MVC where a 4-year-old child was found dead on the scene. There were several other patients that required emergent care and were treated and transported by your crew. Your partner has been quiet lately, seems to be going out more frequently after work to the local bar, and states he hasn't been sleeping lately. He denies any problems at home and says that he is just getting a little "burned out." You suspect your partner is most likely suffering from:
   a. problems at home that he isn't willing to talk about
   b. a serious alcohol or drug problem
   c. anxiety disorder
   d. posttraumatic stress

14. Which of the following statements about bipolar disorder is true?
   a. The manic phase may be characterized by irritability or extreme elation.
   b. Compared with the depressive stage, mania occurs and lasts about the same amount of time.
   c. Suicide is not a threat to these patients because of the rapidly changing behaviors.
   d. Women are more likely to suffer from bipolar disorder.

15. All of the following statements about suicide are false *EXCEPT*:
   a. when a person's depression lifts, the danger of suicide is gone
   b. suicidal people are mentally ill
   c. most people plan their suicide, then present clues of their intent
   d. suicidal tendencies are inherited

16. Asking patients if they are suicidal increases the likelihood that they will attempt suicide.
   a. true
   b. false

17. A 26-year-old woman witnessed her 3-year-old daughter being hit by a car. She slumps to the ground and is quiet. While you assess her, she calmly tells you that she is unable to move her arms and legs and is numb from the neck down. You find no apparent injury, and she has no reaction to painful stimuli in any extremity. She is taken to the hospital where a neurologist examines her and can find nothing physically wrong. This is an example of:
   a. somatization disorder
   b. conversion disorder
   c. malingering
   d. acute psychosis

18. A young mother reports that her child has quit breathing. The child is admitted and observed, and no episodes of apnea appear. The child goes home, and the episodes begin again. The child is admitted and observed with a closed-circuit camera. The mother is witnessed smothering the child with a pillow and calling for assistance when she quits breathing. This is an example of a:
   a. conversion disorder
   b. schizophrenia
   c. somatization disorder
   d. factitious disorder

19. A dissociative disorder would best be exemplified by which of the following?
   a. an unrealistic fear of water leading to total avoidance of water in any form
   b. the belief that everyone is listening to their words and is "out to get them"
   c. an adult who regresses to a childlike state when confronted with a stressful situation
   d. the belief that they can hear the thoughts of others in the wind

20. You are called to the home of a 16-year-old girl who has fainted. You find her in the bathroom vomiting. What findings would be consistent with an eating disorder?
   a. scratches on her soft palate
   b. pale skin and mucous membranes
   c. brittle hair
   d. all of the above

21. All of the following are true regarding eating disorders *EXCEPT*:
   a. they are not seen in obese individuals
   b. they affect more than 5 million Americans
   c. their mortality is 12 times greater in anorexic woman
   d. they are characterized by an unrealistic attitude toward personal appearance

22. The condition in which persons ritually count, cross, and uncross their fingers or perform some other uncontrollable task when under stress is consistent with a(n):
   a. personality disorder
   b. obsessive-compulsive disorder
   c. schizophrenia
   d. none of the above

23. The difference between anorexia nervosa and bulimia is:
   a. bulimia is an intense fear of obesity and anorexia nervosa is an insatiable craving for food
   b. anorexia nervosa is less severe and not life threatening
   c. there is no difference
   d. bulimia is more often associated with binge eating

24. When deciding that your patient requires the application of physical restraint, the most important factor to consider is:
   a. using the proper type of restraint material
   b. ensuring you have sufficient numbers of team members to control the patient
   c. obtaining medical control orders before proceeding
   d. having the patient provide informed consent for the procedure

25. When restraining violent patients, which of the following is true?
   a. They should always be placed prone on the cot so that they can clear their own airway should they vomit.
   b. Handcuffs offer the most reliable form of restraint.
   c. Physical restraints should only be applied after all other measures have been attempted to de-escalate their behavior.
   d. The use of pharmacological restraints should never be used because of the possibility of adverse reactions.

26. Which is true regarding psychiatric conditions in children?
   a. Attention deficit disorder is more common in girls.
   b. Depression is usually less severe than in the adult and less likely to result in suicide.
   c. Any threat of violence should be taken seriously.
   d. Separate the child from the parents to reduce tension and facilitate a better interview.

27. Effective interviewing techniques of the psychiatric patient include all of the following *EXCEPT:*
   a. calming the patient by placing a gentle and reassuring hand on the patient's shoulder
   b. being supportive and empathetic
   c. utilizing active listening
   d. limiting interruptions

28. Asking the patient open-ended questions and taking copious notes are examples of active listening techniques used in the interviewing of the mentally ill patient.
   a. true
   b. false

29. Which of the following is *MOST CORRECT* regarding suicide?
   a. Suicide is the third leading cause of death in 15- to 25-year-olds.
   b. The highest rates of suicide occur in elderly women with terminal illnesses.
   c. With changes in lifestyle, women are just as likely as men to commit suicide.
   d. Successful suicides are more often impulsive and spur-of-the-moment decisions.

Questions 30 through 34 refer to the following scenario:

You are called to the home of a distraught and intoxicated man threatening to commit suicide. As you approach the house you see two small children and a woman on the porch and the man screams, "Stop, I'm serious, and I'll take anyone who gets in my way with me." He tells you that he has been on lithium for many years, and it isn't working. He appears very agitated and is pacing back and forth on the porch with a knife in his hand.

30. Family can often be enlisted to assist in calming the patient and should in this case be asked to help because they are closest to him.
   a. true
   b. false

31. Based on the patient's stated medication he most likely suffers from:
   a. dementia
   b. borderline personality disorder
   c. manic-depressive illness
   d. obsessive compulsive disorder

32. This patient will absolutely require maximal physical restraints to safely transport him.
   a. true
   b. false

33. The patient is restrained by law enforcement, and medical control gives you orders to administer pharmacological restraint. All of the following are acceptable medications to use *EXCEPT:*
   a. succinylcholine
   b. thorazine
   c. Haldol
   d. Valium

34. Law enforcement restrains the patient and recovers the knife. They handcuff both hands behind his back and tie his hands and feet together. He is then placed prone in the back of the ambulance. Which of the following is true?
   a. The use of "hog tying" the patient is acceptable if performed by law enforcement who incur any liability for its use.
   b. This form of physical restraint is known to result in a condition called "abdominal strangulation," which can be deadly.
   c. Any restraint method applied by law enforcement must be assessed for appropriateness and adequacy by EMS prior to assuming responsibility of the patient.
   d. All of the above are true.

Questions 35 through 37 refer to the following scenario:

A 47-year-old man with a history of schizophrenia recently had his medications adjusted. He awoke unable to straighten his neck. On assessment you find him awake and alert complaining of severe pain in his neck, which is twisted to his extreme right. His speech is slurred from an inability to control his facial muscles and tongue.

35. This condition is most likely caused by:
   a. cerebral vascular accident
   b. dystonic reaction from his medication
   c. opiate withdrawal
   d. Munchausen syndrome

36. The appropriate treatment for this condition is:
   a. diphenhydramine 25 mg intravenously
   b. thorazine 100 mg intramuscularly
   c. immobilization in a cervical collar to prevent spinal trauma
   d. diazepam 5 mg IM

37. After you administer the proper medication, the patient begins to feel better and declines transport. He is awake and alert, oriented times three, and states that he will follow up with his counselor in the clinic this week. Which of the following is the most appropriate next step?
    a. Enlist the aid of law enforcement to force the patient to seek care.
    b. Contact medical control to explain to the patient that the effects of the treatment medication may wear off and the rigidity return.
    c. Release the patient only if you can confirm the counselor appointment.
    d. Never release such a patient because he is mentally disturbed.

Questions 38 through 40 pertain to the following scenario:

You are called to care for a 40-year-old man who has attempted suicide by cutting his wrists. Blood is spurting from the wounds, and the patient is flailing his arms around as he screams at you, "I just want to die."

38. He states that he is hearing voices that tell him that Satan wants him to kill himself. The best way to deal with his psychosis is to:
    a. tell him clearly and sternly that Satan does not talk to him
    b. tell him to come into the ambulance, which is protected from the cosmic rays on which Satan transmits his messages
    c. tell him that you can sense that he his afraid and frustrated and that you want to help him
    d. ask him why Satan would tell him to kill himself

39. All of the following are appropriate means to control the patient's bleeding wounds *EXCEPT:*
    a. apply the physical restraints over the wounds with sufficient pressure to stop the arterial bleeding
    b. attempt to calm the patient, which will result in lowering his agitation and blood pressure
    c. give the patient some dressings and ask him to apply direct pressure over the wounds
    d. ask the patient to stop flailing his arms

40. Each of the following is true regarding techniques used to successfully transport the patient to the hospital for evaluation *EXCEPT:*
    a. the patient should not be approached until law enforcement arrives
    b. proper BSI for this case would include face shield, mask, gloves, and gowns
    c. an intravenous line must be established to facilitate the administration of pharmacological restraints
    d. despite the apparent severity of the patient's wounds and the emergent necessity to care for them, the use of active listening along with supportive and empathetic approach should always be used

ANSWERS TO CHAPTER 17: BEHAVIORAL AND PSYCHIATRIC DISORDERS

1. d. Mental health problems have a wide range of symptoms and presentations. Abnormal behavior is often defined as deviation from expected societal norms, behaviors that interfere with ability to function or their general well being, and any harmful behavior to self or others.

2. c. The level of fear associated with phobias can disable persons suffering from this disorder. Although psychosocial mental illness may have many causes, direct links to the specific fear or anxiety is sometimes unknown. Psychosis is an illness that involves major distortions of reality. Neurosis is a restricted ability to achieve optimal function in social settings. Delirium is an abrupt disorientation of time and place.

3. b. The rescuers' safety should always be the first step in assessment of any behavioral or medical response. If a dangerous situation is suspected, the EMS crew should not approach the patient until police are present and the potential for danger is controlled. Containing the crisis may mean limiting the number of people around the patient or isolating the patient if necessary. All life-threatening illnesses or injuries should be managed, and as part of the assessment, information should be gathered by surveying the scene for evidence of violence, substance abuse, or suicide attempt.

4. b. In the absence of any life-threatening findings and if the patient demonstrates apprehension or disapproval, a full examination may be deferred. In this case, prehospital management may be limited to maintaining an effective rapport with the patient during transport.

5. c. Respond to the patient's feelings by acknowledging them ("You seem very sad."). This may help validate and legitimize the patient's intense and sometimes overwhelming feelings.

6. a. Both delirium and dementia may cause disorientation and impaired memory, thinking, and judgment. Sometimes the two disorders may occur at the same time, especially in older adults or in people with chronic illnesses.

7. c. Correcting the underlying physical disorder may reduce the anxiety associated with delirium. Sedatives may be required to manage the patient. Some groups in specific age groups or with specific medical issues may be more susceptible to delirium than others.

8. a. There are more than 75 different types of dementia identified. Degenerative diseases, metabolic disorders, trauma, tumors, and autoimmune disorders can all be identified in the origin of dementia.

9. d. Being neutral and unemotional helps to lower the patient's level of suspicion. Attempting to gain the patient's confidence with warmth may actually cause the patient to believe that you have ulterior motives. Speaking with the family in hushed tones or giving the patient the impression of secrecy will only feed the paranoia, which may result in violence against the rescuer or bystanders. Clearly identifying yourself as a paramedic and expressing the intent to provide help is an honest approach and important to obtain consent for treatment.

10. d. Schizophrenia affects men and women with equal frequency. One in 10 people with schizophrenia eventually commits suicide. In men, schizophrenia usually appears in the late teens or early twenties, whereas in women, the illness usually appears in the twenties to early thirties.

11. b. Panic attacks may mimic a number of medical emergencies, including myocardial infarction. Therefore any patient who exhibits the signs and symptoms described should be thoroughly assessed at the scene and transported for physician evaluation. Patients with anxiety disorders should not be left alone. There is no way to make a definitive diagnosis of these patients in the field, even if there is a history of anxiety disorders.

12. b. A certain amount of anxiety is useful in adapting to stress. Anxiety disorder displays a persistent, fearful feeling that is not related to reality. Severe anxiety disorders can develop into panic disorder or panic attack, which interferes with the ability to function normally in society. Anxiety disorders affect more than 16 million adults in the United States. Panic disorder affects approximately 2.4 million adults. Both disorders can be complicated with substance abuse and depression. About one third of people with panic disorder develop agoraphobia, or the fear of being in an open, crowded, or public place.

13. **d.** EMS personnel may be subject to posttraumatic disorders as a result of their work. Even those with years of experience may find a situation unbearable to live with, even if they have been exposed to the same situation in the past. A cumulative level of stress at that time in their life may be what brings this particular situation to the unbearable level. Although all other responses may also be valid, it is important for the well-being of emergency workers to recognize changes in co-workers and attempt to get them involved in intervention or treatment to help recognize and deal with the source of the stress.

14. **a.** The manic phase in bipolar disorder can be characterized by talkativeness, flight of ideas, motor activity, and frequent delusions that center around personal grandeur. However, the patient may also exhibit irritability associated by a single event. The manic stage can be very brief or last weeks to months, but compared with depression is rare. As many as 20% of people with bipolar disorder die by suicide, and men and women are equally likely to develop bipolar disorder.

15. **c.** Many people believe that suicide is a spontaneous activity that occurs without warning. Most people plan their self-destruction and then give clues indicating they have become suicidal. Therefore suicidal threats and attempts should be taken seriously. The greatest danger of suicide exists during the first 3 months after a person recovers from a deep depression. Although suicide does tend to run in families, it is not transmitted genetically. More often it indicates poor coping abilities passed on to other family members. Although many victims of suicide are depressed or distraught, most of them would not be diagnosed as mentally ill.

16. **a.** It is a false assumption that by asking the patient if he/she intends to end his/her life that this type of question will encourage the person to kill himself/herself.

17. **b.** A conversion disorder is a mental illness in which painful emotions are repressed and unconsciously converted into physical symptoms. The patient suffering a conversion disorder should be treated as if the symptoms are real because it may be impossible to determine whether they actually have an organic cause.

18. **d.** Factitious disorders are a group of disorders in which symptoms mimic a true illness but actually have been invented and are under the control of the patient for the purpose of receiving attention. The most common example of this disorder is Munchausen syndrome by proxy, where a guardian creates the circumstances in someone else for which the guardian receives attention.

19. **c.** The dissociative disorder occurs when a particular mental function, identity, in this case, is separated from reality. Multiple personality disorder is one form of dissociative illness.

20. **d.** Persons suffering from eating disorders may appear pale from anemia, and their hair may be brittle from malnutrition. Scratches on her soft palate are from inducing vomiting by sticking her finger down her throat.

21. **a.** Eating disorders can occur regardless of body weight and are related to an unrealistic attitude regarding what the proper body shape should be. It is extremely common and associated with an elevated risk of death usually from fatal dysrhythmias.

22. **b.** Impulse control disorders such as obsessive-compulsive disorder and kleptomania represent a group of psychiatric conditions characterized by the inability to resist an impulse to perform what may be socially unacceptable behavior or ritualistic in nature. An example of an obsessive-compulsive disorder would be to repeatedly wash one's hands to the point of injury because of an "obsession" with cleanliness.

23. **d.** Bulimia and anorexia nervosa are the most common examples of eating disorders. They both share common features such as unrealistic perceptions of their body, but bulimia is an insatiable craving for food with binge eating.

24. **b.** The decision to physically restrain a patient should never be taken lightly and should only be performed when you have sufficient numbers of team members to safely control the patient. Although it is important to clearly inform patients why you are restraining them,

it is not necessary to gain their consent as long as you have legal authority through either medical control or law enforcement.

25. c. The decision to physically restrain a patient should be taken only once all attempts to obtain voluntary consent from the patient for transport have failed. These attempts should include verbal techniques that are used to reduce anxiety and informing the patient that physical restraint will be required. The use of handcuffs should be discouraged unless the EMS personnel have keys to unlock them and are familiar with their use or a law enforcement officer is accompanying the patient in the ambulance. Further, they are more likely to cause neurovascular compromise. The physically restrained patient must be transported supine or in the recovery position to maintain airway patency. The use of sedatives may be required to facilitate physical restraint and should be guided by medical control.

26. c. Mental illness in children is more common in boys than in girls. This is particularly true with attention deficit disorder. Depression and violence are just as severe as that of adults and should always be taken seriously. It is often helpful to enlist the aid of parents and caregivers to alleviate the child's fears during an EMS intervention.

27. a. To obtain the most truthful information and keep the patient calm, use proper interviewing techniques. These include being supportive and empathetic and limiting interruptions. It is vital that respect for the patient's personal space be respected by avoiding physical contact.

28. b. False. Active listening involves structuring the interview to assist patients in giving a coherent account of their concerns. Paying close attention and not appearing distracted encourages honest answers to questions. Active listening also entails being empathetic and asking closed-ended questions, which assist in keeping patients on track.

29. a. Women attempt suicide more often, but men are more often successful. Elderly men over the age of 85 have the highest rate of suicide. Those contemplating suicide often develop elaborate plans that lead to greater likelihood of success.

30. b. Scene safety entails the safety not only of the rescuers and patient but bystanders as well. In this case the patient's family is at risk of becoming victims and should be rapidly removed from the scene to a point of safety.

31. c. Lithium is one of the most common agents used in the treatment of manic-depressive illness and schizophrenia. His agitation may be a presentation of his mania or deep depression. Dementia is a condition affecting cognitive function, whereas the personality disorders are often difficult to deal with and usually involve the use of sedatives and anxiolytics.

32. b. False. If the police and EMS rescuers use active listening techniques, along with an honest and empathetic approach, it is entirely possible to convince the patient to put down his knife and come voluntarily. Active listening techniques should always be used prior to resorting to physical restraints. Once physical restraints are indicated, the least restrictive method that ensures both patient and rescuer safety should be utilized.

33. a. The use of paralytics, such as succinylcholine, is not indicated in the treatment of agitation because they may mask the seizure activity and require endotracheal intubation. Thorazine and Haldol are both phenothiazine antipsychotics with a long history of use in these situations. Valium or any benzodiazepine sedative would be appropriate as well but should be used only if close observation of the patient's level of consciousness and airway can be monitored.

34. c. Placing a patient in the "hog tied" restraint with both arms and legs behind his back and then placing the patient on his stomach can result in death from "positional asphyxia" because the patient's ability to breathe is impaired. It is not acceptable by either law enforcement or EMS and should never be performed. EMS is ultimately responsible for any method or restraint used and must evaluate the patient's ability to breathe freely, as well as the presence of any neurovascular compromise. If the patient is delivered to you in restraints with which you are unfamiliar or are not consistent with your protocol, you must ask law enforcement to assist you in placing the patient into more appropriate restraints.

35. b. Tardive dyskinesia is a condition caused by phenothiazine antiphsychotics and presents rather dramatically with upper extremity contractures and facial grimaces. Opiate withdrawal usually presents with agitation and restlessness along with nausea and vomiting. The cerebrovascular accident usually presents with weakness rather than rigidity.

36. a. The administration of intravenous diphenhydramine reverses the muscular rigidity and works quickly with minimal side effects. Thorazine administration would only worsen the condition because it is a phenothiazine and the application of physical restraints would cause pain and possibly injury. Benzodiazepines would be ineffectual.

37. b. The patient is coherent and appears aware of his surroundings. It is unlikely that law enforcement will have grounds to force him to comply. The effects of the diphenhydramine are likely to fade over 1 to 2 hours, and the effects of the longer-acting antipsychotic will return. Having the patient speak to medical control has a better than 50% chance of convincing him to go to the hospital.

38. c. It is counterproductive to feed into the patient's psychosis by encouraging abnormal thoughts.

This can backfire on you with surprising consequences. Regardless of the circumstances you do not want to become a focus of his paranoia or fear. Your goal is to get him to trust you, and this is best accomplished through empathetic comments.

39. a. The application of physical restraints should never obscure an injury that must be monitored. Because this patient has an arterial bleed he will require a pressure dressing and possibly a tourniquet, and the presence of physical restraints will inhibit your usual and customary care for this injury.

40. c. The blood from this patient should be considered as lethal a weapon as a knife or gun because the patient may have HIV or hepatitis. Regardless of the nature of the call appropriate BSI should be used. Law enforcement will more than likely be required because of the patient's mental illness and his overt actions. An IV is not necessary for the administration of common medications used as pharmacological restraints, which are usually given IM. As always, the use of proper de-escalation techniques will increase the likelihood of a successful patient encounter.

OBSTETRICS AND GYNECOLOGY

1. The term that refers to the total number of all the woman's current and past pregnancies is:
   a. para
   b. antepartum
   c. nullipara
   d. gravida

2. The structure in which the fetus grows and develops is the:
   a. fallopian tube
   b. vagina
   c. uterus
   d. ovary

3. The bag of water that protects the baby is called the:
   a. afterbirth
   b. pericardial sac
   c. meninges
   d. amniotic sac

4. The placenta:
   a. mixes the baby's blood with the mother's blood and filters waste products
   b. exchanges oxygen, nutrients, and waste products between the mother and fetus
   c. is used by the fetus for food
   d. is normally positioned in the uterus over the cervix

5. Fetal circulation occurs as blood flows from the fetus through:
   a. two umbilical arteries carrying deoxygenated blood and oxygenated blood returns to the fetus through one umbilical vein
   b. two umbilical arteries carrying oxygenated blood and deoxygenated blood returns to the fetus through one umbilical vein
   c. one umbilical artery carrying deoxygenated blood and oxygenated blood returns to the fetus through two umbilical veins
   d. one umbilical artery carrying oxygenated blood and deoxygenated blood returns to the fetus through two umbilical veins

6. The cervix is the:
   a. dense outer portion of the ovary
   b. neck of the uterus
   c. fringed end of the fallopian tube
   d. distal end of the perineum

7. The area of skin between the vagina and the anus that can tear during delivery of a baby is the:
   a. perineum
   b. periosteum
   c. peritoneum
   d. pericardium

8. When taking the vital signs of a pregnant patient in the second trimester of pregnancy, it is normal for the:
   a. heart rate to be faster and blood pressure lower
   b. heart rate to be slower and blood pressure higher
   c. heart rate to be slower and blood pressure lower
   d. heart rate to be faster and blood pressure higher

9. A pregnant patient should be asked:
   a. when the baby is due
   b. whether she is experiencing any pains or contractions
   c. whether there is any bleeding or discharge and when it began
   d. all of the above

10. Questions about labor would normally include all of the following *EXCEPT*:
    a. when labor began
    b. how far apart the contractions are
    c. whether the patient has taken any medications for the pain
    d. the duration of the contractions

11. The most appropriate personal protective equipment to wear when delivering a baby is:
    a. gloves and mask
    b. gloves, gown, eye protection, and mask
    c. gown and mask
    d. eye protection, mask, and gloves

12. The first stage of labor covers the period from:
    a. when EMS is called until EMS arrives at the scene
    b. when regular contractions begin until the cervix is fully dilated
    c. the patient's first contractions to the delivery of the baby's head
    d. dilation of the cervix to the birth of the baby

13. The second stage of labor covers the period from:
    a. delivery of the baby's head to the delivery of the placenta
    b. arrival of the ambulance to the start of transport
    c. complete dilation of the cervix to the birth of the baby
    d. the end of contractions to the presentation of the baby's head

14. The third stage of labor covers the period:
    a. from dilation of the cervix to delivery of the placenta
    b. from the arrival at the hospital to transfer to the obstetrics ward
    c. following the birth of the baby through delivery of the placenta
    d. following delivery of the baby to arrival at the hospital

15. Delivery should be considered imminent when:
    a. contractions are less than 2 minutes apart
    b. contractions last longer than 20 seconds
    c. it is the mother's first pregnancy and contractions are 5 minutes apart
    d. the patient is experiencing lower abdominal pain with no back pain

16. The baby's head bulging against the vaginal opening is known as:
    a. presenting
    b. crowning
    c. birthing
    d. showing

17. During delivery, rotation of the baby's head normally occurs:
    a. when the patient is crowning
    b. after the shoulders deliver
    c. prior to crowning
    d. once the head is delivered

18. The rescuer may insert his or her fingers into a pregnant patient's vagina:
    a. to support the baby's head during delivery
    b. only in the case of a breech delivery or prolapsed cord
    c. to assist in delivery of the baby's shoulders
    d. to check the baby's pulse in the case of a limb presentation

19. The soft areas in a baby's head where the fusion of the bones of the skull is not complete are known as:
    a. fontanelles
    b. varices
    c. follicles
    d. parietes

20. Immediately following delivery of the baby's head, all of the following should be done *EXCEPT*:
    a. stimulating breathing
    b. checking if the umbilical cord is around the baby's neck
    c. checking to be sure the amniotic sac is not covering the baby's mouth and nostrils
    d. suctioning the mouth and nostrils

21. When suctioning a newborn:
    a. wait until delivery is complete to begin suctioning
    b. squeeze the bulb syringe after inserting it
    c. insert the tip of the bulb syringe 2 to 3 inches into the mouth and each nostril
    d. squeeze the bulb syringe before inserting it

22. The first place to suction the newborn is:
    a. the right nostril
    b. the left nostril
    c. the mouth
    d. both nostrils, then the mouth

23. A major concern when caring for newborns is:
    a. starting the mother-infant bonding process
    b. wrapping the newborn in moist towels
    c. guarding against heat loss
    d. a respiratory rate greater than 30

24. To stimulate the newborn to breathe:
    a. hold the baby upside down by the feet and ankles
    b. gently rub the baby's back or flick the soles of the feet
    c. slap the baby sharply on the buttocks
    d. ventilate the baby with an oxygen-powered resuscitator

25. After delivery is completed but before the cord is cut, the baby should be positioned:
    a. at the same level as the mother's vagina
    b. higher than the mother
    c. with its head slightly elevated
    d. lower than the mother

26. The generally recommended time to cut the umbilical cord is:
    a. after delivery of the placenta
    b. 10 to 15 minutes after delivery
    c. before the infant starts to breathe
    d. after pulsations in the cord cease

27. When the decision is made to cut the umbilical cord, the first clamp should be placed:
    a. about 4 inches away from the baby
    b. about 4 inches away from the mother
    c. 10 inches from the baby
    d. 10 inches from the mother

28. After cutting the cord, the baby should be positioned:
    a. on the right side
    b. with the head slightly higher than its trunk
    c. in a prone position
    d. with the head slightly lower than the trunk

29. If the newborn is breathing but his or her heart rate is below 100:
    a. flick the soles of the feet
    b. start chest compressions only
    c. start artificial ventilations
    d. perform CPR

30. An assessment of the APGAR score should be made:
    a. immediately following delivery and upon reaching the hospital
    b. 1 and 5 minutes after birth
    c. 5 and 10 minutes after birth
    d. immediately following delivery and 10 minutes later

For questions 31 and 32 refer to the APGAR scale in Table 18-1.

31. A newborn presents with some pink skin color but bluish hands and feet, a pulse rate of 140, a weak cry, good muscle tone, and a breathing rate of 36. The APGAR score is:
    a. 6
    b. 7
    c. 8
    d. 9

32. A baby was delivered by his father 3 minutes prior to your unit's arrival. He is cyanotic, has a pulse rate of 106, a weak cry, no muscle tone, and a breathing rate of 18. The APGAR score is:
    a. 3
    b. 4
    c. 5
    d. 6

Table 18-1   THE APGAR SCALE

Sign	0	1	2
Appearance (skin color)	Bluish or pale	Pink or typical newborn color; hands and feet are blue	Pink or typical newborn color; entire body
Pulse (heart rate)	Absent	Below	Over 100
Grimace (irritability)	No response	Crying; some motion	Crying; vigorous
Activity (muscle tone)	Limp	Some flexion—extremities	Active; good motion in extremities
Respiratory effort	Absent	Slow and irregular	Normal; crying

33. The placenta usually delivers:
    a. 30 to 45 minutes after birth
    b. immediately after the cord is cut
    c. 1 hour after birth
    d. within 20 minutes of birth

34. After the placenta has been delivered:
    a. wrap it in a towel, place it in a plastic bag, and take it to the hospital with the mother
    b. discard it
    c. have the mother walk to induce uterine contraction
    d. sit the mother in an upright position

35. Postpartum hemorrhage is defined as:
    a. more than 500 mL of blood loss after delivery of the newborn
    b. bleeding that occurs 24 hours or later following delivery of the newborn
    c. any bleeding associated with delivery of the newborn
    d. hemorrhage that occurs in the third trimester of pregnancy

36. Excessive maternal bleeding after delivery may be managed in all of the following ways *EXCEPT*:
    a. massaging the mother's lower abdomen
    b. packing the vagina with a sterile dressing
    c. having the baby nurse
    d. placing a sterile pad over the vaginal opening

37. Pharmacological management of postpartum hemorrhage may include administering:
    a. magnesium sulfate
    b. amiodarone
    c. procainamide
    d. oxytocin

38. A newborn is considered premature if he or she:
    a. is born before the ninth month of pregnancy
    b. weighs more than 6 pounds
    c. delivers before 37 weeks (8 months) of gestation
    d. delivers before the expected due date

39. A correct statement regarding premature infants is:
    a. do not give oxygen because it will cause blindness
    b. the head is smaller in proportion to the rest of the body
    c. do not suction the mouth or nose because it can cause excessive drying of the mucous membranes
    d. they are at risk for hypothermia

40. The most common traumatic cause of fetal death is:
    a. maternal death
    b. drug abuse by the mother
    c. strangulation by the umbilical cord
    d. suffocation by the amniotic sac

41. When caring for an injured pregnant patient, the general rule is:
    a. do not waste time providing spinal immobilization if delivery is imminent
    b. the life of the unborn child takes precedence over the life of the mother
    c. the life of the mother takes precedence over the life of the unborn child
    d. there is little concern unless the patient is near term

42. Breech presentation refers to an abnormal delivery in which the:
    a. baby's shoulders have difficulty passing through the birth canal
    b. amniotic sac fails to rupture
    c. baby's buttocks deliver first
    d. umbilical cord is wrapped around the baby's neck

43. Management of a breech delivery may include:
    a. pulling on the baby to assist with delivery
    b. placing two gloved fingers in the vagina to form an airway for the baby
    c. having the mother cross her legs to delay delivery
    d. placing one hand over the vaginal orifice to prevent delivery

44. In a situation involving a prolapsed cord, breech presentation, or limb presentation, the mother may be placed:
    a. in a head-down position with her pelvis elevated
    b. on her right side with her legs squeezed together
    c. in a prone position
    d. on her back with her head higher than her feet

45. When examining a patient in labor, if a prolapsed cord is discovered:
    a. do not allow anything to touch the cord
    b. attempt to push the cord back into the vagina and uterus
    c. insert several gloved fingers into the vagina and gently push on the baby's head to take pressure off the cord
    d. pull on the cord to induce delivery

46. If a delivery involving a limb presentation is encountered:
    a. attempt to push the limb back into the uterus
    b. encourage the mother to push
    c. pull on the limb to assist delivery
    d. immediately transport the patient to the hospital

47. When a pregnant patient with a spinal injury is transported on a backboard, the backboard should be:
    a. elevated at the head
    b. tilted on its right side
    c. tilted on its left side
    d. completely flat

48. Third-trimester bleeding is usually a result of all of the following medical conditions *EXCEPT*:
    a. abruptio placentae
    b. ruptured ovarian cyst
    c. uterine rupture
    d. placenta previa

49. Placenta previa refers to a condition in which the:
    a. placenta separates prematurely from the wall of the uterus
    b. fetus is not connected to the placenta with an umbilical cord
    c. placenta develops in an abnormal location low in the uterus
    d. placenta does not deliver in one piece

50. When a patient suffers from abruptio placentae, the placenta:
    a. delivers at the same time as the infant
    b. is torn during delivery
    c. delivers in an abrupt, rapid manner
    d. has separated prematurely from the wall of the uterus

51. The abnormal condition that may occur in the last 3 months of pregnancy that most often is characterized by sudden, severe, low abdominal pain with or without vaginal bleeding is:
    a. abruptio placentae
    b. uterine inversion
    c. placenta previa
    d. eclampsia

52. When a fertilized egg starts to develop in an area outside the uterus, this is known as:
    a. pelvic inflammatory disease
    b. a spontaneous abortion
    c. an ectopic pregnancy
    d. uterine inversion

53. Abnormally low blood pressure in a pregnant patient may be caused by:
    a. toxemia of pregnancy
    b. compression of the aorta by the baby
    c. premature uterine contractions
    d. compression of the vena cava by the growing uterus

54. EMS personnel should be alert for the possibility of seizures when a pregnant patient presents with:
    a. swelling of the face, hands, and feet
    b. abnormally low blood pressure
    c. sudden loss of weight
    d. severe lower abdominal pain

55. After seizures are experienced by a pregnant patient, the patient should be transported:
    a. in a supine position
    b. rapidly using red lights and siren
    c. with her legs and feet elevated
    d. with her shoulders and head elevated

56. Management of seizure activity in an eclamptic obstetric patient may include administering:
    a. diazepam and diphenhydramine
    b. naloxone and diphenhydramine
    c. magnesium sulfate and diazepam
    d. lidocaine and magnesium sulfate

57. Spontaneous abortion refers to:
    a. a miscarriage that usually occurs before the twelfth week
    b. self-induced termination of pregnancy
    c. bleeding that occurs before the thirty-seventh week of pregnancy
    d. incorrect placement of the placenta on the wall of the uterus

58. An important part of managing a miscarriage includes:
    a. discarding of fetal tissues to avoid disturbing the mother
    b. advising the patient to make an appointment with her obstetrician
    c. rendering emotional support to the mother and father
    d. transporting the patient on her left side with her head elevated if she is in shock

59. The main purpose of the prehospital physical exam of the sexual assault patient is to:
    a. attempt to ascertain who may have committed the assault
    b. identify any physical trauma for which the patient needs immediate attention
    c. find and collect physical evidence
    d. provide a basis for prosecuting the perpetrator of the crime

60. When managing a sexual assault patient:
    a. tell the patient how the assault could have been avoided
    b. reassure the patient she is now safe
    c. tell the patient everything will be all right
    d. avoid any physical examination of the patient

61. Appropriate care for a sexual assault patient should include:
    a. being careful to preserve any evidence
    b. encouraging the patient to wash and change clothes
    c. getting as much information as possible about the incident
    d. wearing a gown and mask to avoid possible exposure to a sexually transmitted disease

62. Documentation regarding a sexual assault that should be included on an EMS report includes:
    a. the rescuer's personal opinions about the incident
    b. what the patient said and things that are directly observed
    c. theories regarding who the rescuer thinks may be involved in the incident
    d. all of the above

63. Pelvic inflammatory disease:
    a. may result in significant internal hemorrhage
    b. is characterized by pain that is usually relieved by walking
    c. has symptoms that generally start about a week before patient's menstrual period
    d. usually has a gradual onset

64. A ruptured ovarian cyst:
    a. is characterized by a slow onset of pain with the discomfort gradually getting worse
    b. is initially accompanied by diffuse abdominal pain
    c. often occurs about a week before onset of menstrual bleeding
    d. presents no danger of internal hemorrhage

ANSWERS TO CHAPTER 18: OBSTETRICS AND GYNECOLOGY

1. d. The term *gravida* refers to the number of all the woman's current and past pregnancies. *Para* refers only to the number of the woman's past pregnancies that have remained viable to delivery. *Antepartum* refers to the maternal period before delivery, and *nullipara* refers to a woman who has never delivered a live birth.

2. c. The uterus is a muscular organ in which the fetus grows and develops. The ovaries produce sex hormones and ova. Ova are carried from the ovaries to the uterus by the fallopian tubes. The vagina is the lower part of the birth canal.

3. d. The amniotic sac protects the infant in the uterus. *Afterbirth* is another term for the placenta. The pericardial sac encloses the heart, and the meninges are membranes that surround the brain and spinal cord.

4. b. The placenta exchanges oxygen, nutrients, and waste products between the mother and the fetus. It is normally positioned high in the uterus and does not allow mixing of the baby's with the mother's blood.

5. a. Fetal circulation occurs as blood flows from the fetus through two umbilical arteries carrying deoxygenated blood and oxygenated blood returns to the fetus through one umbilical vein.

6. b. The cervix is the neck of the uterus. The dense outer portion of the ovary is the cortex. The fimbriae are the fringelike structures located at the ends of the fallopian tubes.

7. a. The perineum is the area of skin between the vagina and anus. During delivery, the skin in this area may tear because of the pressure exerted by the fetus as it passes through the birth canal. The periosteum is a fiberlike covering of the bones, the pericardium is the sac around the heart, and the peritoneum is the membrane lining the abdominal cavity.

8. a. When taking the vital signs of a pregnant patient, it is common for the heart rate to be faster because of a need for increased cardiac output. Also, the blood pressure decreases during the second trimester because of the reduction in peripheral resistance.

9. d. All of the above. An obstetric patient should be questioned concerning when the baby is due and if the patient is experiencing any pains or contractions. Ask if she has been experiencing any bleeding or discharge, if the water has broken, and if so, when.

10. c. Question the patient concerning how far apart her labor pains are and the duration of the pain. It is also helpful to know when the pain started.

11. b. When delivering a baby, it is recommended that the caregiver wear gloves and a gown because of the amount of blood and fluids present, as well as a mask and protective eyewear. Because there is generally time to prepare for delivery, EMS personnel should be more cognizant of taking the proper personal protective precautions.

12. b. The first stage of labor covers the time period from the beginning of regular contractions until the cervix is fully dilated. It is also known as the *dilation stage*. The average time for this stage is 12.5 hours in primipara, 7 hours in multipara.

13. c. The second stage of labor covers the time period from complete dilation of the cervix to the birth of the baby. It is also known as the *expulsion stage*. The average time for this stage is 80 minutes in primipara, 30 minutes in multipara.

14. c. The third stage of labor covers the time period following the birth of the baby through the delivery of the placenta. It is also known as the *placental stage*. The average time for this stage is 5 to 20 minutes.

15. a. Consider delivery imminent if contractions are less than 2 minutes apart or if the patient is crowning. Labor during a first delivery will take longer than subsequent deliveries. Transport unless delivery is expected within 5 minutes. Remember, there are worse places to have a baby than in the back of an ambulance, so don't be afraid to transport.

16. b. Crowning is the term used for when the baby's head bulges against the vaginal opening.

17. d. Rotation of the baby's head normally occurs once the head is delivered to facilitate delivery of the shoulders.

18. b. There are only two cases in which a rescuer should insert fingers into a pregnant patient's vagina: (1) in the case of a breach birth to form an airway for the baby and (2) in the case of a prolapsed cord to relieve pressure on the cord. Always wear sterile gloves to diminish the risk of infecting the mother.

19. a. The fontanelles are soft areas in a baby's head where the cranial bones have not fused. Care must be exercised to avoid pushing on these areas while managing the infant's head during normal or abnormal delivery. Varices are dilated and tortuous blood vessels. Follicles are masses of cells usually containing a cavity, and parietes are walls of a body cavity.

20. a. Immediately following delivery of the baby's head is not the time to stimulate breathing. It is the time to check for the umbilical cord around the baby's neck, to check to ensure that the amniotic sac is not in place over the baby's head and face, and to suction the mouth and nose. If the amniotic sac is not broken, puncture it and push it away from the newborn's head and mouth.

21. d. As soon as the baby's head delivers, suction should be applied immediately. Always squeeze the bulb before inserting, and insert it only 1 to 1½ inches into the mouth and nostrils.

22. c. Despite the fact that newborns are obligatory nose breathers, the mouth of the newborn should be suctioned first, then the nostrils. This prevents aspiration of matter in the mouth in the event that spontaneous breathing is stimulated by suctioning the nostrils.

23. c. After delivery, guard against heat loss in a newborn. Quickly dry the infant and wrap him in a warm blanket. Because the infant's head is so large, a covering (such as a stockinette) should always be placed over the head to diminish heat loss. Respiratory rates greater than 30 breaths a minute are normal for a newborn.

24. b. Breathing may be stimulated by gently rubbing the baby's back or tapping the soles of the feet. Do not hold the baby upside down, slap the baby, or use an oxygen-powered breathing device.

25. a. Following delivery, the baby should be kept level with the mother's vagina until the cord is clamped and cut. Positioning the baby too high may cause hypovolemia, because blood is siphoned back into the placenta. Placing the baby too low may cause fluid overload.

26. d. After pulsations in the umbilical cord cease, it may safely be clamped and cut.

27. a. The first umbilical clamp should be placed about 4 inches or 4 adult finger widths away from the baby. The second clamp is then placed about 2 inches farther away from the first clamp, toward the placenta. Cut between the clamps.

28. d. After the cord is cut, position the baby with his head slightly lower than the trunk to facilitate the drainage of fluids from the mouth and nose.

29. c. Start artificial ventilations if the newborn's heart rate drops below 100. Low heart rates are often a result of low oxygenation, so good ventilation can actually increase the infant's heart rate. If the heart rate remains less than 60 to 80 beats per minute and does not increase despite 30 seconds of adequate assisted ventilations with 100% oxygen, start chest compressions.

30. b. An assessment of the APGAR score should be made 1 minute and 5 minutes after birth. APGAR is an acronym for *Appearance, Pulse, Grimace, Activity, Respiratory* effort.

For questions 31 and 32 refer to the APGAR scale in Table 18-1.

31. c. The patient's APGAR score is 8: Appearance = 1, Pulse = 2, Grimace = 1, Activity = 2, Respiratory effort = 2.

32. b. The patient's APGAR score is 4: Appearance = 0, Pulse = 2, Grimace = 1, Activity = 0, Respiratory effort = 1.

33. d. The placenta should normally deliver in about 20 minutes but may take up to 30 minutes.

34. a. The placenta should be wrapped in a towel, then placed in a plastic bag and taken to the hospital for examination. Do not have the patient squeeze her legs together or walk around.

35. a. Postpartum hemorrhage is defined as more than 500 mL of blood loss following delivery of the newborn. It frequently occurs within the first few hours after delivery.

36. b. Maternal bleeding may be managed by massaging the patient's abdomen, having the baby suckle, or placing the patient in the shock position with a sterile pad over the vaginal opening. Never pack the vagina.

37. d. Oxytocin may be administered to a patient to help control postpartum hemorrhage.

38. c. A baby born before 37 weeks (8 months) of gestation or one that weighs less than $5\frac{1}{2}$ pounds is considered premature. Term newborns weigh about 7 pounds.

39. d. Premature babies are very susceptible to hypothermia. If oxygen is given over a short period of time, it should not cause complications. The head is usually larger, and suctioning may need to be repeated frequently because the airways can easily become obstructed.

40. a. Maternal death is the most common traumatic cause of fetal death. If the mother dies of trauma, perform CPR and transport her to a hospital. A physician may be able to perform an emergency cesarean section and save the infant.

41. c. The general rule is that the life of the mother takes precedence over the life of the unborn child. Spinal immobilization should still be accomplished.

42. c. A breech presentation occurs when the baby's buttocks or lower extremities are low in the uterus and deliver first. Shoulder dystocia occurs when the fetal shoulders lodge against the maternal symphysis pubis and the sacrum, blocking shoulder delivery.

43. b. It may be necessary to place two gloved fingers in the mother's vagina to form an airway for the baby. Do not pull on the baby or in any way attempt to delay or speed delivery.

44. a. Patients may be placed in a head-down position with the hips elevated when such obstetric emergencies as breech or limb presentation or a prolapsed cord are encountered. This may relieve pressure on the cord.

45. c. Management of a prolapsed umbilical cord may include inserting several gloved fingers into the vagina and gently pushing on the baby's head to relieve the pressure on the cord. Do not attempt to push the cord back into the vagina. Any exposed portion of cord should be covered with moist, sterile dressings.

46. d. In the case of a limb presentation, immediate transportation is of utmost importance. Do not attempt to push the limb back into the

Table 18-1 THE APGAR SCALE

Sign	0	1	2
Appearance (skin color)	Bluish or pale	Pink or typical newborn color; hands and feet are blue	Pink or typical newborn color; entire body
Pulse (heart rate)	Absent	Below	Over 100
Grimace (irritability)	No response	Crying; some motion	Crying; vigorous
Activity (muscle tone)	Limp	Some flexion—extremities	Active; good motion in extremities
Respiratory effort	Absent	Slow and irregular	Normal; crying

uterus or pull on the limb to assist delivery. When a limb presentation occurs, the infant needs to be delivered by cesarean section.

47. **c.** When transporting an injured pregnant female on a backboard, the backboard should be tilted on its left side. This relieves the pressure that the fetus may place on the vena cava, which is a major blood vessel in the abdomen.

48. **b.** Third trimester bleeding is usually a result of abruptio placentae, uterine rupture, or placenta previa. Ruptured ovarian cyst is not a cause of third-trimester bleeding because it does not result in vaginal bleeding.

49. **c.** In placenta previa, the placenta develops in an abnormal location low in the uterus and close to or over the cervix. This can interfere with normal delivery. Also, as the cervix dilates, the placenta tears and bleeding occurs.

50. **d.** In abruptio placentae (also called *placenta abruptio*), the placenta partially or completely separates from the wall of the uterus.

51. **a.** Abruptio placentae is most often characterized by sudden, severe, low abdominal pain. It may or may not be accompanied by bleeding. Placenta previa generally presents with bright red bleeding but may be painless. Uterine inversion is a rare emergency in which the uterus turns inside out after delivery and extends through the cervix. Uterine inversion usually results from pulling on the umbilical cord and is accompanied by severe blood loss.

52. **c.** In an ectopic pregnancy, the fertilized egg starts to develop in an area outside of the uterus, often within a fallopian tube. The fallopian tube is not large enough to support the growth of the fetus and will eventually rupture. When this occurs, it produces abdominal pain and, more important, massive bleeding, which may be fatal if not corrected quickly.

53. **d.** Compression of the mother's vena cava (the vein that returns blood from the lower body to the heart) by the baby in the uterus can cause abnormally low blood pressure. If this is suspected, transport the patient on her left side to take pressure off the vessel.

54. **a.** Swelling of the face, hands, and feet of a pregnant patient are signs of preeclampsia and EMS personnel should be alert to the possibility of the patient having a seizure. Also, the patient may have an elevated blood pressure and a recent history of sudden weight gain.

55. **d.** After a pregnant patient has experienced seizures, the patient should be transported with the shoulders and head elevated. Use of the ambulance siren should be avoided as it may precipitate additional seizures.

56. **c.** The two primary medications used to manage seizure activity related to eclampsia are magnesium sulfate and diazepam. Closely monitor the patient's vital signs because diazepam may precipitate a fall in blood pressure and can also jeopardize fetal circulation.

57. **a.** Spontaneous abortion is an abortion that usually occurs before the twelfth week of gestation. The lay term is *miscarriage.* The cause is often unknown, but predisposing factors include acute or chronic illness in the mother, abnormalities in the fetus, and abnormal attachment of the placenta. Self-induced termination of pregnancy under any condition not allowed by law is criminal abortion. Placenta previa involves an incorrect placement of the placenta on the wall of the uterus. Bleeding that occurs before the thirty-seventh week of pregnancy may be related to number of problems and should be assessed by a physician.

58. **c.** An important part of managing a miscarriage includes providing emotional support to the parents. Tissues should be taken to the hospital for examination. Because the EMS personnel cannot adequately assess the patient's uterus, the patient should be evaluated at a hospital. If the patient displays signs of shock, transport her on her back with her legs elevated and treat for shock per local protocols.

59. **b.** The main purpose of the prehospital physical exam of sexual assault patient is to identify any physical trauma, primarily outside of the pelvic area for which the patient needs immediate attention. Although EMS personnel want to avoid disturbing evidence or a crime scene as much as possible, it is not their place unless specially trained to collect evidence or investigate the crime.

60. b. Always act in a professional, reassuring manner, and reassure the patient she is now safe. Do not tell the patient how the assault could have been avoided or that everything will be all right. The patient should be examined, but the exam may have to be altered to fit the situation.

61. a. Be careful to preserve evidence at the scene and on the patient. Although EMS personnel cannot prohibit it, the patient should be discouraged from changing clothes, washing, or using the bathroom. EMS personnel are usually not police officers and should not question the patient about specifics relating to the assault.

62. b. Only facts should be noted on the EMS report. This could include what the patient said as well as what can be directly observed. This document will probably be used in court, so avoid including personal opinions or theories.

63. d. Pelvic inflammatory disease usually has a gradual onset. It is characterized by diffuse pain often described as a steady ache. The patient may also find it painful to walk. The inflammation frequently occurs within 7 to 10 days following the menstrual period. PID is infection related, not associated with internal hemorrhage.

64. c. A ruptured ovarian cyst is usually characterized by a sudden onset of pain that often occurs about a week before onset of menstrual bleeding. In the acute stage, the pain is often unilateral. Although rare, a ruptured ovarian cyst can result in significant internal hemorrhage.

Neonatology and Pediatrics

Neonatology

1. The three major physiological adaptations necessary for survival of the neonate include all of the following *EXCEPT*:
   a. emptying fluids from the lungs and beginning ventilation
   b. switching from anaerobic to aerobic metabolism
   c. changing the circulatory pattern
   d. maintaining body temperature

2. Intrapartum risk factors associated with the need for resuscitation of the newborn include:
   a. maternal hypertension or postterm gestation
   b. rupture of membranes greater than 24 hours before delivery or meconium-stained amniotic fluid
   c. toxemia of pregnancy or diabetes
   d. mother's age greater than 35 or multiple gestation

3. Administration of naloxone to a neonate would most likely be considered if:
   a. pulse rate is less than 100 and does not increase despite 30 seconds of ventilation with 100% oxygen
   b. the mother is addicted to narcotics
   c. benzodiazepines were administered to the mother during delivery
   d. the mother received narcotics within 4 hours of delivery

4. When naloxone is indicated for a neonate with respiratory depression, the recommended dose is:
   a. 0.5 mg/kg
   b. 0.01 mg/kg
   c. 0.1 mg/kg
   d. 1 mg/kg

5. Concerning umbilical circulation, all of the statements are true *EXCEPT*:
   a. an umbilical artery carries deoxygenated blood
   b. an umbilical vein carries oxygenated blood
   c. there are two umbilical arteries and one umbilical vein
   d. there are two umbilical veins and one artery

6. An important consideration when caring for newborns is that they:
   a. breathe primarily through their mouth
   b. breathe primarily through their nose
   c. breathe through both the mouth and nose
   d. breathe slower than adults

7. Secondary apnea in the neonate describes:
   a. a self-limited condition controlled by P_{CO_2} levels that is common immediately after birth
   b. absence of respirations associated with intrauterine asphyxia
   c. respirations that are absent and do not begin again spontaneously
   d. absence of respirations caused by a slow heart rate

8. When considering supplemental oxygen administration to a neonate:
   a. administer oxygen at 5 L/min if central cyanosis is present in an infant with spontaneous respirations and an adequate heart rate
   b. administer oxygen if the infant presents with acrocyanosis (peripheral cyanosis) immediately following delivery
   c. avoid oxygen administration if possible as it will likely cause blindness
   d. use oxygen only if the neonate is in cardiac arrest

9. If the newborn is breathing but his or her heart rate is below 100:
   a. begin chest compressions
   b. intubate the newborn
   c. begin ventilating the infant with 100% oxygen
   d. administer oxygen by nonrebreather mask

10. Endotracheal intubation is indicated when resuscitating the neonate if:
    a. the patient is showing signs of severe hypoxia or respirations are absent
    b. increasing intracranial pressure is suspected or the patient has signs of peripheral cyanosis
    c. the child's oxygen saturation is less than 90%
    d. bag-valve-mask ventilation is ineffective or prolonged positive-pressure ventilation is necessary

11. If signs of hypovolemia are present in a neonate, appropriate fluid resuscitation would include:
    a. a fluid bolus of 10 mL/kg of isotonic crystalloid solution followed by a second bolus of 10 mL/kg if signs of shock persist
    b. a single fluid bolus of 20 mL/kg of isotonic colloid solution followed by a continuous infusion of crystalloid solution
    c. a 50-mL bolus of colloid solution followed by an IV drip of vasopressor agents to maintain blood pressure
    d. a 100-mL bolus of hypertonic crystalloid solution followed by a continuous infusion of crystalloids if signs of shock persist

12. If hypoglycemia is suspected in the neonate, appropriate therapy may include administration of:
    a. 2 to 5 mL/kg of dextrose 50% solution given over 10 minutes
    b. 4 to 6 mL/kg of dextrose 5% solution given over 15 minutes
    c. 5 to 10 mL/kg of dextrose 10% solution given over 20 minutes
    d. 10 to 15 mL/kg of dextrose 25% solution given rapid IV push

13. The neonate is considered bradycardic once the heart rate drops below:
    a. 60
    b. 80
    c. 100
    d. 120

14. Two likely causes of persistent vomiting in the first 24 hours of life of the neonate are:
    a. a viral infection and narcotics withdrawal
    b. delivery-induced hypoglycemia and a bacterial infection
    c. acute neonatal hypothyroidism and chronic metabolic acidosis
    d. an obstruction in the upper digestive tract and increased intracranial pressure

15. Bradycardia and cardiac arrest in the neonate are usually the result of:
    a. metabolic disturbances
    b. hypoxia
    c. congenital heart defects
    d. intracranial hemorrhage

16. The presence of meconium indicates:
    a. a lack of lubricating fluid in the birth canal
    b. possible fetal distress during labor
    c. an abnormal passage of the baby through the birth canal
    d. the probability of a breech presentation

17. The primary problems for the neonate associated with a meconium emergency are:
    a. cardiac complications
    b. neurological complications
    c. respiratory complications
    d. intestinal complications

18. Management of the neonate with a serious meconium emergency includes:
    a. inserting an endotracheal tube, hyperventilating the patient for 3 minutes, then performing endotracheal suctioning with the appropriate-size suction catheter
    b. avoiding placement of a gastric tube to avoid stimulating the neonate's gag reflex
    c. administering 100% oxygen using a blow-by method and intubating only if bradycardia develops
    d. performing direct endotracheal suctioning using the ET tube as a suction catheter

Pediatrics

19. The three primary components of the Pediatric Assessment Triangle are:
    a. airway, breathing, mental status
    b. respiratory effort, mental status, muscle tone
    c. circulation, respiratory rate, skin color
    d. appearance, work of breathing, circulation

20. Managing infants and children is different from managing adults because younger patients:
    a. are more trustful and less fearful
    b. like to ride in ambulances
    c. tend to be more fearful and may have difficulty communicating
    d. have less difficulty communicating

21. When an infant or child with a non–life-threatening problem is encountered:
    a. take a little more time to perform the examination
    b. treat the infant or child like a small adult
    c. it is not necessary to perform an assessment
    d. perform the examination the same way it would be performed on an adult

22. If a procedure must be performed that may cause pain:
    a. restrain the child before proceeding
    b. tell the child it will not hurt
    c. tell the child in advance it will hurt
    d. have the parents leave the room

23. When caring for a sick or injured child:
    a. never allow parents to be present
    b. allow parents to be present only if absolutely necessary
    c. allow only one parent to be present at any time
    d. make judicious use of the parents for assistance

24. The first priority when assessing an infant or child is evaluating:
    a. airway and breathing
    b. pulse and blood pressure
    c. amount of movement
    d. response to external stimuli

25. An important consideration when managing a sick or injured infant or child is:
    a. the rescuer's general impression of the child
    b. whether the child has a good blood pressure
    c. when the child last took a nap
    d. that both parents are present before care is begun

26. When performing a detailed physical exam on a newborn or infant, first examine the:
    a. head
    b. neck
    c. abdomen
    d. heart and lungs

27. When performing a detailed physical exam on a toddler:
    a. start with vital signs
    b. use a trunk-to-head approach
    c. examine only exposed areas
    d. use a head-to-toe approach

28. When assessing an infant, increasing intracranial pressure should be suspected if the infant displays:
    a. fever accompanied by a rash
    b. bulging fontanelles
    c. a heart rate above 140
    d. vigorous crying with little or no tearing

29. The number one cause of death among infants and children is:
    a. traumatic injury
    b. poisoning
    c. drowning
    d. child abuse

30. The pulse of infants and children is normally:
    a. slower than an adult's
    b. faster than an adult's
    c. the same as an adult's
    d. weak and thready

31. Generally, when assessing pediatric patients, blood pressure is assessed:
    a. only on children younger than 6 years
    b. on all infants and children
    c. only on children older than 3 years
    d. on all children who have sustained trauma

32. The single most important factor in accurately obtaining a child's blood pressure is the:
    a. child's emotional state
    b. limb used
    c. age of the patient
    d. size of the blood pressure cuff

33. When opening the airway of an infant or child:
    a. tilt the head forward
    b. keep the neck totally neutral
    c. tilt the head as far back as possible
    d. do not hyperextend the neck

34. If a child is breathing rapidly and exhibits signs of increased breathing effort:
    a. respiratory or general fatigue may rapidly develop
    b. the child is likely reacting normally to a stressful situation
    c. immediate administration of bronchodilators is indicated
    d. use caution administering oxygen, because it can cause respiratory arrest

35. Primary differences between adult and pediatric airway anatomy include:
    a. the epiglottis is narrower and longer in children than adults
    b. pediatric patients tend to have larger airways and smaller tongues
    c. the vocal cords of an infant slope from front to back
    d. the cricoid cartilage is the widest part of the airway in the infant and young child and the vocal cords are the narrowest part

36. When an oropharyngeal airway is used to maintain the airway of a pediatric patient:
    a. insert the airway right side up without using the rotating maneuver that would be used for an adult
    b. ascertain what size airway would reach from the corner of the mouth to the earlobe, then insert the next smaller size airway
    c. insert the airway upside down and rotate it once in the proper position
    d. visualize the oropharynx first with a laryngoscope to check for obstructions

37. When using a rigid suction catheter to suction an infant or a young child, a key concern is that suctioning may cause:
    a. hypertension
    b. tachycardia
    c. decreased carbon dioxide levels in the blood
    d. bradycardia

38. If a seriously ill or injured infant or child will not tolerate an oxygen mask:
    a. restrain the child and force him or her to wear the mask
    b. use a blow-by technique to enrich the surrounding air
    c. wait for the child to calm down, then administer oxygen
    d. refrain from using oxygen because the stress can worsen the medical problem

39. The best way to determine the breathing rate of a newborn or infant is to:
    a. watch the chest rise from a distance
    b. listen with a stethoscope
    c. place one hand on the patient's chest
    d. place one hand on the patient's abdomen

40. Regarding respiratory distress in infants and children, all of the following statements are correct *EXCEPT*:
    a. nasal flaring in children is a sign of increased respiratory effort
    b. infants and children have a relatively large respiratory reserve
    c. "see-saw" breathing is more commonly seen in infants than adults
    d. infants and children often use accessory muscles to enhance respiratory effort

41. The best place to look for cyanosis in an infant or child is the:
    a. oral mucosa
    b. abdomen
    c. hands
    d. feet

42. Two illnesses most often characterized by wheezing in children are:
    a. epiglottitis and croup
    b. pneumonia and asthma
    c. bronchiolitis and epiglottitis
    d. asthma and bronchiolitis

43. When administering nebulized albuterol to a pediatric patient, the recommended dose is:
    a. 0.01 mL/kg diluted in 0.3 mL of normal saline and administered over 5 to 10 minutes
    b. 1 to 2 mg/kg diluted in 10 mL of normal saline and administered over 20 minutes
    c. 0.01 to 0.03 mL/kg (0.05 to 0.15 mg/kg) to a maximum dose of 0.5 mL diluted in 2 mL of normal saline and administered over 5 to 15 minutes
    d. 5 mL of a 5% solution administered over 10 minutes

44. A sign of an upper airway obstruction is:
    a. stridor on inspiration
    b. wheezing on expiration
    c. rhonchi
    d. rales

45. Lower airway disease should be suspected if:
    a. stridor is heard on inspiration
    b. wheezing is heard on expiration
    c. the patient has a slow breathing rate
    d. the patient presents with a sore throat and drooling

46. The point at which an infant or child is considered to be in respiratory arrest is when the respiratory rate drops below:
    a. 8 breaths per minute
    b. 10 breaths per minute
    c. 12 breaths per minute
    d. 14 breaths per minute

47. Oxygen should be given to infants and children:
    a. only if trauma is present
    b. only if the child will tolerate it
    c. any time a respiratory emergency is present
    d. whenever a child has a breathing rate over 16

48. Two serious upper respiratory infections in children that EMS personnel may encounter are:
    a. croup and epiglottitis
    b. asthma and bronchitis
    c. epiglottitis and asthma
    d. bronchiolitis and emphysema

49. Status asthmaticus is best described as:
    a. a severe asthma attack that responds only to subcutaneous epinephrine
    b. an asthma attack accompanied by signs of anaphylactic shock
    c. an asthma attack that requires the patient to use a metered-dose inhaler multiple times in a short period
    d. a severe, prolonged asthma attack that cannot be broken by aggressive pharmacological interventions

50. A pediatric patient suffering from croup and presenting with stridor but not wheezing will benefit the most from receiving:
    a. subcutaneous epinephrine
    b. cool mist or humidified oxygen
    c. metaproterenol by metered dose inhaler
    d. nebulized albuterol

51. A child who presents with a high fever, very sore throat, pain when swallowing, and drooling should be suspected of having:
    a. croup
    b. bronchitis
    c. epiglottitis
    d. asthma

52. A respiratory disease that gets worse at night and is characterized by a loud "seal bark" cough is:
    a. epiglottitis
    b. croup
    c. tonsillitis
    d. asthma

53. Febrile seizures:
    a. seldom need evaluation at a hospital
    b. occur in most infants with fevers
    c. signify serious brain disorders
    d. occur because of a rapid rise in temperature

54. Status epilepticus is best described as:
    a. recurrent seizures without an intervening period of consciousness
    b. new onset of seizures experienced by a child with no history of seizure activity
    c. seizures that were preceded by recent complaints of headache and/or stiff neck
    d. three or more seizures within a 5-hour period

55. For a pediatric patient over 5 years of age, the recommended IV or IO dose for diazepam for seizures is:
    a. a single-dose slow IV push of 5 mg
    b. 0.2 mg slow IV push every 3 minutes up to a maximum of 2 mg
    c. 1 mg slow IV push every 2 to 5 minutes up to a maximum of 10 mg
    d. 1 mg/kg every 5 minutes until the seizure abates

56. If an IV or IO route cannot be established in a seizure patient, diazepam may be administered:
    a. orally
    b. sublingually
    c. subcutaneously
    d. rectally

57. In a cardiac arrest situation, the recommended IV/IO pediatric dose for epinephrine is:
    a. a first dose of 0.01 mg/kg of 1:10,000 and subsequent doses of 0.01 mg/kg of 1:10,000 every 3 to 5 minutes
    b. the first three doses of 0.1 mg/kg of 1:10,000 and subsequent doses of 0.02 mg/kg of 1:1,000 every 5 to 10 minutes
    c. a first dose of 0.2 mg/kg of 1:10,000 and subsequent doses of 0.1 mg/kg of 1:1,000 every 3 to 5 minutes
    d. 0.2 mg/kg of 1:10,000 solution administered every 3 to 5 minutes

58. The recommended IV/IO pediatric dose for atropine is:
    a. 0.02 mg/kg with a maximum single dose of 0.5 mg in a child and 1.0 mg in an adolescent
    b. 0.1 mg/kg with a minimum dose of 1.0 mg
    c. 0.2 mg/kg for a child and 0.4 mg/kg for an adolescent
    d. 1 mg for a child and 2 mg for an adolescent

59. The recommended IV pediatric dose for adenosine is:
    a. 0.05 mg/kg rapid IV push with a minimum dose of 6 mg
    b. 0.1 mg/kg rapid IV push for the first dose with a maximum dose of 6 mg
    c. 6 mg slow IV push given over 5 minutes
    d. 60 mg mixed in 100 mL of IV fluid and administered over 20 minutes

60. Pharmacological intervention for a pediatric patient with hemodynamically unstable bradycardia would normally consist of:
    a. administering atropine first, followed by epinephrine if no improvement results
    b. administering atropine, followed by dopamine if there is no improvement after the second dose
    c. administering epinephrine first, followed by atropine if no improvement results
    d. administering epinephrine first, followed by pacing if there is no improvement after 10 minutes

61. If a pediatric patient needs to be defibrillated, the recommended energy levels are:
    a. the first three defibrillations at 2 J/kg, 4 J/kg, 4 J/kg and subsequent defibrillations at 4 J/kg
    b. the first three defibrillations at 5 J/kg and subsequent defibrillations at 10 J/kg
    c. the first three defibrillations at 20 J and subsequent defibrillations at 40 J
    d. the first three defibrillations at 20 J, 40 J, 60 J and subsequent defibrillations at 60 J

62. Dysrhythmias in pediatric patients are most often due to:
    a. metabolic or endocrine disorders
    b. congenital heart defects or atherosclerosis
    c. respiratory infections or kidney disorders
    d. hypoxia or structural heart disease

63. The most common type of trauma in children is:
    a. open injury
    b. penetrating injury
    c. open fractures
    d. blunt injury

64. When assessing a child who was in a motor vehicle crash and was restrained only with a lap belt, suspect:
    a. abdominal and lower spine injuries
    b. head injuries
    c. chest and arm injuries
    d. leg injuries

65. An area that commonly needs to be padded when a child is affixed to a backboard is:
    a. under the shoulders
    b. under the head
    c. under the lower back
    d. under the occiput

66. A correct statement concerning PASG use on children is that it should be used:
    a. if the patient can be placed in a leg of the garment
    b. any time hypovolemic shock is present
    c. only if the child fits properly in the garment
    d. any time the blood pressure is below 90 systolic

67. When using the PASG on children, inflate the:
    a. legs and then the abdominal compartment
    b. abdominal compartment and then the legs
    c. abdominal compartment only
    d. legs only

68. Secondary drowning syndrome refers to:
    a. drowning after being injured in the water
    b. drowning after developing respiratory arrest
    c. a medical condition wherein the patient drowns from fluid in the lungs
    d. deterioration that occurs following a near-drowning event and after the patient has resumed normal breathing

69. The most accurate indicator of early shock in an infant or young child with trauma is:
    a. blood pressure
    b. pale, cool, and clammy skin
    c. a pulse rate greater than 120 beats per minute
    d. capillary refill time

70. A pediatric patient in hemorrhagic shock displaying significant tachycardia, thready peripheral pulses and hypotension, and prolonged capillary refill would be classified as suffering from:
    a. very mild hemorrhage
    b. mild hemorrhage
    c. moderate hemorrhage
    d. severe hemorrhage

71. Vomiting and diarrhea may be of special concern in children because:
    a. children can dehydrate rapidly
    b. these signs indicate an underlying serious abdominal problem
    c. there is a high likelihood the patient will have a febrile seizure
    d. they indicate a serious underlying infection

72. A sign of shock in infants would be:
    a. copious amounts of tears when crying
    b. decreased urine output
    c. frequent urination
    d. flushed skin

73. If a pediatric patient shows signs of significant hypovolemia, appropriate fluid resuscitation should be initiated by administering a:
    a. single fluid bolus of 20 mL/kg of isotonic colloid solution followed by a continuous infusion of crystalloid solution
    b. fluid bolus of 20 mL/kg of isotonic crystalloid solution followed by additional boluses of 20 mL/kg until systemic perfusion improves
    c. rapid 50 mL bolus of colloid solution followed by an IV drip of vasopressor agents to maintain blood pressure
    d. 100 mL bolus of hypertonic crystalloid solution followed by a continuous infusion of crystalloids if signs of shock persist

74. A fever is of particular concern if the child also:
    a. complains of an earache
    b. has a rash
    c. feels achy
    d. cries when being examined

75. The primary cause of sudden infant death syndrome (SIDS) is:
    a. external suffocation
    b. unknown
    c. choking
    d. parental neglect

76. When a SIDS situation is encountered:
    a. question the parents regarding what they may have done to contribute to the death
    b. never institute CPR because this may compromise the police investigation of the death
    c. think of the parents or other caregivers and loved ones as patients also
    d. try to forget about the situation and do not discuss it with other crew members

77. Physical abuse may be defined as:
    a. giving insufficient attention to a child
    b. improper or excessive action that injures or causes harm
    c. striking a child as a form of discipline
    d. all of the above

78. Suspect child abuse if:
    a. an isolated bruise in the process of healing is noted
    b. an isolated scar from a burn is found while examining the patient
    c. the parents tell the same story about how the injury occurred
    d. an injury is inconsistent with its described mechanism

79. If child abuse is suspected:
    a. privately report suspicions to the emergency department staff
    b. attempt to get the parents to confess to child abuse
    c. advise the parents you are going to have them investigated for child abuse
    d. take the child to the hospital without parental consent

80. When a child connected to a malfunctioning home ventilator is encountered:
    a. refer to the instruction manual to determine how to operate the unit and adjust the machine's settings
    b. remove the patient from the ventilator and use a nonrebreather mask at 15 lpm
    c. treat the patient and do not try to correct the malfunction
    d. start CPR and transport

81. If bleeding is noted in the area where a central IV line enters the skin:
    a. soak up the blood with loose, bulky dressings
    b. apply ice to the area
    c. clamp off the IV tubing
    d. control the bleeding by applying pressure

82. A gastrostomy tube:
    a. hooks directly into a major blood vessel
    b. is placed directly into the brain to relieve intracranial pressure
    c. is placed directly into the trachea through a hole in the neck
    d. is placed directly into the stomach for feeding

83. Two positions in which an infant or child with a gastrostomy tube may be transported are:
    a. lying on the back or lying on the left side with the head lower than the trunk
    b. sitting or lying on the right side with the head elevated
    c. in a position of comfort or prone with the head lower than the trunk
    d. supine or prone with the head elevated

84. A ventriculoperitoneal shunt runs from the:
    a. brain to the abdomen to drain excess cerebrospinal fluid
    b. heart to the lungs to reoxygenate blood
    c. ears to the throat to relieve pressure behind the eardrum
    d. kidneys to the bladder to drain excess urine

85. Infants or children with shunts are particularly prone to:
    a. high fevers
    b. rapid heart rates
    c. respiratory arrest
    d. hypoperfusion

86. A 5-year-old child who has a shunt is complaining of a headache accompanied by nausea. Parents say the child has also been vomiting. You suspect:
    a. a viral illness
    b. an excess of cerebrospinal fluid in the stomach causing nausea
    c. the child has accidentally ingested a poison
    d. increasing intracranial pressure

87. Your unit responds to a call for a pediatric cardiac arrest. On arrival you find a 6-year-old patient with a history of congenital heart disease. You are surprised to see ventricular fibrillation when the child is placed on the cardiac monitor. The child weighs approximately 55 pounds. Your initial three defibrillations would be:
    a. 50 J, 100 J, 100 J
    b. 55 J, 110 J, 165 J
    c. 100 J, 150 J, 200 J
    d. 200 J, 300 J, 360 J

88. An IV is rapidly established and your partner gets ready to administer the first dose of epinephrine. The correct dose would be:
    a. 0.2 mg of 1:1000 solution
    b. 0.25 mg of 1:10,000 solution
    c. 0.5 mg of 1:1,000 solution
    d. 1 mg of 1:10,000 solution

89. A mother calls your unit to check her 7-year-old son who suddenly developed shortness of breath and chest pain. Upon your arrival, the patient also has an altered level of consciousness. During the patient assessment, you notice that the patient has a central venous line in place and the line appears to be torn and leaking about 5 inches away from the insertion site. A cause of this patient's dyspnea and altered level of consciousness that must especially be considered in this case is:
    a. hypoglycemia
    b. increasing intracranial pressure
    c. septic shock
    d. air embolism

90. Management of the patient with a torn or leaking central venous catheter would include:
    a. attempting to flush the IV line to clear blood clots that could disrupt flow of medication
    b. removing the catheter and applying direct pressure to the insertion site
    c. clamping the line between the tear and the patient
    d. positioning the patient on his or her back with the head slightly elevated

91. A young mother has called 9-1-1 because she thinks her 3-year-old child may have accidentally ingested something. She noticed about 15 minutes ago that the child seemed to have abdominal pain. On your arrival, you also note the child is lethargic, tachypneic, and hyperthermic. You suspect the child has ingested:
    a. acetaminophen
    b. hydrocarbons
    c. salicylates
    d. tricyclic antidepressants

ANSWERS TO CHAPTER 19: NEONATOLOGY AND PEDIATRICS

Neonatology

1. **b.** At birth, neonates make three major physiological adaptations necessary for survival. These are emptying fluids from their lungs and beginning ventilation, changing their circulatory pattern, and maintaining body temperature. Although the infant was not breathing while in the uterus, oxygen was being supplied by the mother, which allowed normal aerobic metabolism to occur.

2. **b.** Intrapartum refers to during labor and delivery. Rupture of membranes more than 24 hours before delivery, meconium-stained amniotic fluid, premature labor, abnormal presentation, and prolapsed cord are a few intrapartum risk factors. Antepartum refers to before labor and delivery. Antepartum risk factors include multiple gestation, postterm gestation, toxemia, hypertension, diabetes, and age factors, to name a few.

3. **d.** Administration of naloxone to a neonate may be considered if the mother received narcotics within 4 hours of delivery and the infant shows signs of respiratory depression. Because naloxone may induce a withdrawal reaction in an infant born to a mother addicted to narcotics, medical direction may advise against administering naloxone and may recommend prolonged ventilatory support instead.

4. **c.** When naloxone is indicated for a neonate with respiratory depression, the recommended dose is 0.1 mg/kg.

5. **d.** There are two umbilical arteries and one umbilical vein. Umbilical arteries carry deoxygenated blood from the fetus to the placenta. The umbilical vein carries oxygenated blood from the placenta to the fetus.

6. **b.** Newborns are obligate nose breathers. In many cases, suctioning the secretions from an infant's nasopharynx can improve breathing problems.

7. **c.** Secondary apnea describes respirations that are absent and do not begin again spontaneously. Primary apnea is a self-limited condition controlled by P_{CO_2} levels that is common immediately after birth.

8. **a.** Administer oxygen at 5 L/min if central cyanosis is present in an infant with spontaneous respirations and an adequate heart rate. Acrocyanosis (peripheral cyanosis) is common in the first few minutes of life and is not indicative of hypoxemia. Oxygen administration can usually be instituted in the prehospital setting without concern for potential long-term hazards such as retinopathy. In most cases, oxygen can be carefully administered via a nonrebreather mask or through use of a blow-by method where appropriate. Avoid directing the oxygen at the infant's face because this can irritate the trigeminal nerve and cause the baby to stop breathing. This situation can be minimized by using warm oxygen and directing the flow to one side of the baby's nose.

9. **c.** Start artificial ventilations if the newborn's heart rate drops below 100. Low heart rates are often a result of low oxygenation, so good ventilation can actually increase the infant's heart rate. Any time a newborn infant's heart rate is below 60 beats per minute despite effective positive-pressure ventilation with 100% oxygen for approximately 30 seconds, chest compressions should be started.

10. **d.** In many cases, the neonate can be adequately ventilated with a bag-valve-mask without the need for endotracheal intubation. However, intubation is indicated if bag-valve-mask ventilation is ineffective or prolonged positive-pressure ventilation is necessary.

11. **a.** If signs of hypovolemia are present in a neonate, appropriate fluid resuscitation would include a fluid bolus of 10 mL/kg of isotonic crystalloid solution followed by a second bolus of 10 mL/kg if signs of shock persists. Always follow local protocols regarding fluid resuscitation.

12. **c.** If hypoglycemia is suspected in the neonate 5 to 10 mL/kg of dextrose 10% solution may be administered over 20 minutes or 2 to 4 mL/kg of $D_{25}W$.

13. **c.** The neonate is considered bradycardic once the heart rate drops below 100. Bradycardia is most frequently caused by hypoxia.

14. **d.** Persistent vomiting in the first 24 hours of life suggests the neonate may most likely be suffering from an obstruction in the upper digestive

tract or increased intracranial pressure. If the vomitus contains dark blood, it is usually a sign of life-threatening illness.

15. b. Bradycardia and cardiac arrest in the neonate are usually the result of hypoxia. Prehospital care personnel should aggressively manage the airway and provide supplemental oxygen to the neonate as necessary.

16. b. The presence of meconium (the dark-green contents of the intestines of the fetus) in the amniotic fluid indicates possible fetal distress during labor. The amniotic fluid resembles thick pea soup. If meconium is present, a sample can be used to test for maternal drug use. Therefore a specimen should be collected and transported with the neonate to the emergency department.

17. c. The presence of meconium in the amniotic fluid denotes a true emergency. If the infant aspirates meconium, breathing complications may be serious to fatal. If a meconium emergency exists, rapid transportation to a hospital is warranted. Take extra care to thoroughly suction the infant.

18. d. If the neonate is depressed or the meconium is thick or particulate, direct endotracheal suctioning should be performed using the ET tube as a suction catheter. This should be done quickly and preferably before the neonate has taken his or her first breath. Quickly intubate the trachea and apply suction to the tube while withdrawing it. Repeat the intubation-suction-extubation cycle until no further meconium is obtained, then continue resuscitative measures as needed. If possible, do not ventilate via the ET tube between intubations. However, if bradycardia develops, the infant may need to be ventilated using a bag-valve-mask device after suctioning to prevent persistent bradycardia and hypoxia. Also, a gastric tube may be placed to prevent aspiration of gastric contents.

Pediatrics

19. d. The three components of the Pediatric Assessment Triangle are appearance, work of breathing, and circulation. When assessing appearance, consider the patient's mental status and muscle tone. To assess work of breathing, consider respiratory rate and respiratory effort. Circulation assessment includes looking at the patient's skin signs and skin color.

20. c. Infants and children tend to be more fearful than adults and may have difficulty communicating. The ambulance may present a frightening environment for a child.

21. a. Unless a serious emergency exists, take a little more time when dealing with a child to explain and perform the examination. This will help put the child at ease. Alter the exam to fit the circumstances but do not skip the assessment. Infants and children should not be thought of as "little adults."

22. c. Tell a child in advance if a procedure will hurt. If a child is lied to or surprised, he or she may not trust the caregiver for the remainder of the care period. Parents can be used to lend support provided they can handle the situation. Do not restrain a child unless absolutely necessary.

23. d. Make judicious use of the parents to assist in examining and caring for infants and children. Parents can be used to calm the child. If a parent is agitated, however, this will agitate the child.

24. a. When assessing a child, the first concern is the patient's airway and breathing status. This is especially important with young children and infants because cardiac arrest is normally secondary to respiratory arrest. Aggressive airway management can make a difference.

25. a. The rescuer's general impression of the child's well-being is an important consideration. Physical signs may not always be as valuable as the rescuer's impression of how serious the child's injuries are. Although it is best to have the permission of a parent to institute care, care can be rendered under implied consent if no parents are present.

26. d. When performing a detailed physical exam on a newborn or infant, examine the heart and lungs first and the head last. It is best to obtain heart and lung sounds before the child becomes agitated by the rest of the exam.

27. b. When performing a detailed physical exam on a toddler, use a trunk-to-head approach. This approach is used to build confidence and should be taken before the child becomes agitated. Airway, breathing, and circulation still take priority over vital signs.

28. b. As intracranial pressure increases, the fontanelle may become tight and bulging.

29. a. Traumatic injury is the number one cause of death among infants and children. Most pediatric deaths are preventable.

30. b. The pulse rate of infants and children is normally faster than that of adults because of their faster metabolic rate.

31. c. Generally, when assessing pediatric patients, blood pressure is assessed on children older than 3 years.

32. d. The single most important factor in accurately obtaining a child's blood pressure is the size of the cuff. The cuff should be two thirds the width of the upper arm.

33. d. When opening the airway of an infant or child, do not hyperextend the neck. Hyperextending the neck can cause airway obstruction.

34. a. A child who is breathing rapidly and displaying signs of increased breathing effort is compensating. The child's condition may deteriorate rapidly because of rapid respiratory muscle fatigue or general fatigue.

35. a. There are a number of differences between adult and pediatric airway anatomy that must be taken into consideration, especially when performing endotracheal intubation. For one thing, the epiglottis is narrower and longer in children than adults and therefore more difficult to control with a laryngoscope blade. Additionally, the cricoid cartilage is the narrowest part of the airway in the infant and young child. As the child reaches 8 to 10 years of age, the vocal cords become the narrowest part, like in adults. Also, pediatric patients, especially infants, tend to have a relatively small upper airway and the tongue is disproportionately large and the vocal cords of an infant slope from back to front, frequently causing an ET tube to hang up in the angle caused by the cords.

36. a. Oral airways are inserted differently in children than in adults. Because of loose teeth and soft

tissue, the airway should be inserted right side up and not upside down and rotated. A tongue blade should be used to assist in placement.

37. d. When suctioning an infant or young child, continually monitor the child's heart rate. Suctioning can stimulate nerves in the throat and cause the child's heart rate to slow.

38. b. If a seriously ill or injured infant or child will not tolerate an oxygen mask, use a blow-by technique. This can be accomplished using a variety of methods. Oxygen tubing can be held about 2 inches from the patient's face, or it may be inserted into a paper cup held near the child's face. As an alternative, an oxygen mask may be held near the child's face. The objective is to increase the concentration of oxygen in the surrounding air. A good indication of the child's need for oxygen is whether he or she will accept it. Seriously ill or injured infants or children do not usually fight the oxygen mask.

39. a. The best way to determine the breathing rate of a newborn or infant is to watch the chest rise from a distance. Touching the child can cause agitation that will affect the breathing rate.

40. b. Infants and children have relatively small respiratory reserves and may deteriorate quickly. Signs of respiratory distress include nasal flaring, use of accessory muscles, and "see-saw" breathing, that is, the abdomen and chest move in opposite directions with each respiration.

41. a. The best place to check for cyanosis in an infant or child is the oral mucosa, lips, or the tongue. Use caution if checking the nail beds of an infant, even when they appear cyanotic; they still may not be an accurate indicator of central circulation status.

42. d. Asthma and bronchiolitis are the two illnesses most often characterized by wheezing in children.

43. c. When administering nebulized albuterol to a pediatric patient, the recommended dose is 0.01 to 0.03 mL/kg (0.05 to 0.15 mg/kg) to a maximum dose of 0.5 mL diluted in 2 mL of normal saline and administered over 5 to 15 minutes.

44. a. Stridor is heard on inspiration and is a sign of upper airway obstruction.

45. b. If wheezing is noted on expiration, lower airway disease should be suspected. Wheezes are high pitched, musical noises caused by high-velocity air traveling through narrowed airways.

46. b. An infant or child is considered to be in respiratory arrest when the respiratory rate drops below 10 breaths per minute. The patient may also exhibit limp muscle tone, unconsciousness, slow or absent heart rate, and weak or absent distal pulses. Artificial ventilations should be started immediately.

47. c. Any time a respiratory emergency is present, administer oxygen. Hypoxia in children is the leading cause of cardiac arrest.

48. a. Croup and epiglottitis are two serious upper respiratory infections that EMS personnel may encounter when managing a child with respiratory difficulty. Bronchiolitis is a lower respiratory disease frequently caused by RSV (respiratory syncytial virus) infection. Although generally benign and self-limiting, severe bronchiolitis can be life threatening. RSV is the leading cause of lower respiratory tract disease in infants and young children. RSV infection symptoms range from those of a bad cold to severe bronchiolitis or pneumonia.

49. d. Status asthmaticus is best described as a severe prolonged asthma attack that cannot be broken by aggressive pharmacological interventions. This is a serious medical emergency that warrants prompt transport with aggressive treatment continued en route to the hospital.

50. b. A pediatric patient suffering from croup and presenting with stridor but not wheezing will benefit the most from receiving cool mist, humidified, or nebulized oxygen. The patient's primary problem is related to upper airway problems, primarily subglottic edema, as opposed to lower airway constriction.

51. c. Children who complain of a very sore throat and pain when swallowing that begins suddenly and that may be accompanied by a fever and drooling should be suspected of having epiglottitis. Epiglottitis is a bacterial illness and is a true emergency because the patient is in danger of developing a complete airway obstruction because of swelling of the epiglottis and supraglottic structures. Allow the child to remain in whatever position makes it easiest to breathe. No attempt to visualize the airway should be made if the child is still ventilating adequately. The receiving hospital should be notified prior to EMS arrival so that they may prepare for what may be a very difficult patient management scenario.

52. b. Croup is a viral illness that results in inflammation of the larynx, trachea, and bronchi. The child will normally display mild symptoms including fever and respiratory difficulty during the day, but at night the child's condition will worsen. A loud "seal bark" cough is characteristic of the illness.

53. d. The occurrence of febrile seizures is linked to a rapid rise in temperature and not the final degree of the fever. They usually occur in children 6 months to 5 years old and are generalized seizures. Approximately 5% of children with fevers develop febrile seizures, but most never have a repeat episode. The child should be evaluated at a hospital.

54. a. Status epilepticus is best described as recurrent seizures without an intervening period of consciousness, or continuous seizure activity lasting 30 minutes or longer. Status epilepticus is a true emergency that can lead to hypotension and cardiovascular, respiratory, and renal failure. It can also lead to permanent brain damage.

55. c. For a pediatric patient older than 5 years, the recommended IV or IO dose for diazepam for seizures is 1 mg slow IV push every 2 to 5 minutes up to a maximum of 10 mg.

56. d. If an IV or IO route cannot be established in a seizure patient, diazepam may be administered rectally. A higher dose of 0.5 mg/kg is generally required because absorption is incomplete.

57. a. In a cardiac arrest situation, the recommended IV/IO pediatric dose for epinephrine is a first dose of 0.01 mg/kg of 1:10,000 and subsequent doses of 0.01 mg/kg of 1:10,000 every 3 to 5 minutes. The endotracheal dose is 0.1 mg/kg of 1:1000.

58. a. The recommended IV/IO pediatric dose for atropine is 0.02 mg/kg with a minimum dose of 0.1 mg and a maximum single dose of 0.5 mg in a child and 1.0 mg in an adolescent.

It may be repeated once in 5 minutes for a maximum child total dose of 1.0 mg and a maximum adolescent total dose of 2.0 mg.

59. b. The recommended IV pediatric dose for adenosine is 0.1 for the first dose (with a maximum dose of 6.0 mg) and 0.2 mg/kg for the second dose (with a maximum dose of 12.0 mg). It is given rapid IV push.

60. c. Pharmacological intervention for a pediatric patient with hemodynamically unstable bradycardia would normally consist of administering epinephrine first, followed by atropine if no improvement results.

61. a. Pediatric patients seldom need to be defibrillated. However, in the event defibrillation is indicated, the first three defibrillations should be 2 J/kg, 4 J/kg, 4 J/kg, with subsequent defibrillations at 4 J/kg administered 30 to 60 seconds after each medication.

62. d. Dysrhythmias in pediatric patients are most often due to hypoxia or structural heart disease. The most common dysrhythmias seen in pediatric patients are sinus tachycardia, SVT, bradycardia, and asystole.

63. d. Blunt injury is the leading cause of traumatic death in children.

64. a. When a child who was restrained only with a lap belt is involved in a motor vehicle crash, suspect abdominal and lower spine injuries. With children, lap belts are often improperly positioned with the lap belt above the pelvis. In a crash, compression injuries to the soft abdominal organs can occur. If the child is not wearing a diagonal shoulder strap, the uncontrolled forward movement of the upper body can cause spinal injuries.

65. a. Because children have larger heads than adults, it is often necessary to pad under the shoulders and/or upper torso to keep the spine in a neutral, in-line position. Padding under the head or occiput (the posterior part of the skull) is inappropriate because it will tilt the head even further forward.

66. c. Use the PASG on children only if the child fits properly in the garment. Do not place the child in one leg of the garment. The device may be used in cases of trauma with signs of severe hypotension and pelvic instability. Follow local protocols on indications for use.

67. d. When using the PASG on children, inflate the legs only; do not inflate the abdominal compartment because children use their abdominal muscles for breathing. The younger the child, the more he or she uses these muscles to breathe. Inflation of the abdominal compartment can greatly interfere with the child's breathing. Consult local protocols for precise guidelines on inflating the PASG for children.

68. d. Secondary drowning syndrome refers to deterioration that occurs following a near drowning event and after the patient resumes normal breathing. This syndrome may occur minutes to hours later.

69. d. Delayed capillary refill time is the most accurate indicator of shock in infants and children. Adequate blood pressure in children can often be maintained until the end and tends to drop only immediately before death.

70. c. A pediatric patient in hemorrhagic shock displaying significant tachycardia, thready peripheral pulses and hypotension, and prolonged capillary refill would be classified as suffering from moderate hemorrhage. The patient has at this point experienced a blood volume loss of about 25%.

71. a. In infants and children, vomiting and diarrhea can cause rapid dehydration, and profound fluid and electrolyte imbalance can occur. Dehydration compromises cardiac output and systemic perfusion. These signs do not always indicate serious illness or infection. Gastrointestinal upset exhibited as vomiting and diarrhea may even accompany a minor ear infection.

72. b. Decreased urine output is a sign of shock in infants. To determine if this sign is present, ask parents about diaper wetting. The patient will be pale, and tears will be absent even when the child is crying.

73. b. If a pediatric patient shows signs of significant hypovolemia, appropriate fluid resuscitation should be initiated by administering a fluid bolus of 20 mL/kg of isotonic crystalloid solution followed by additional boluses of 20 mL/kg until systemic perfusion improves.

Always follow local protocols regarding fluid resuscitation.

74. b. Fever accompanied by a rash may signify a serious medical condition is present.

75. b. The cause of sudden infant death syndrome (SIDS) is largely unknown. All other causes including suffocation, choking, and neglect must be ruled out to make the diagnosis.

76. c. Parents or other caregivers and loved ones of SIDS babies should be viewed as patients also and given emotional support. Do not question them on what they may have done to contribute to the death because there are usually no external factors involved. They will already feel guilty, and questioning will add to the guilt. CPR may be initiated and the child transported if the infant is potentially or questionably viable. The situation will be very stressful to EMS personnel as well and should be discussed if the crew wishes. CISM is a valuable resource in these cases.

77. b. Physical abuse is improper or excessive action that injures or causes harm to a child. Giving insufficient attention to a child is considered neglect. Physical abuse and neglect are the two forms of child abuse EMS providers are likely to encounter.

78. d. Suspect child abuse if the injury is inconsistent with its described mechanism or if parents cannot account for all the child's injuries. If the child displays different injuries, such as burns or bruises in various stages of healing, this should also alert the rescuer to the possibility of child abuse. Repeated calls to the same residence or for the same child to provide care for various injuries may also be a clue. An isolated injury or burn does not necessarily signal abuse.

79. a. If child abuse is suspected, report it privately to the emergency department staff. It should also be reported to the appropriate authorities as specified by state and local laws. Do not discuss it with the parents. Parental consent normally must still be obtained before the child can be transported.

80. c. There are numerous types of artificial ventilators and they operate differently. Therefore, in general, EMS personnel should not try to troubleshoot a ventilator problem or adjust the machine's settings. In some cases the parents or another caregiver may be able to assist in managing the patient because they should be familiar with the operation of the ventilator. However, EMS personnel should always treat the patient, meaning attention should be given to improving airway patency, ventilation, and oxygenation. Do not remove the patient from the ventilator because it is breathing for the patient unless the machine is not adequately ventilating the patient, in which case perform manual ventilations.

81. d. If bleeding is noted in the area where a central IV line enters the skin, control the bleeding by applying pressure. Do not clamp off the IV tubing unless blood is flowing from the tubing and do not apply ice to the area.

82. d. A gastrostomy tube is placed directly into the stomach for feeding.

83. b. Two positions in which an infant or child with a gastrostomy tube may be transported are sitting or lying on the right side with the head elevated. This reduces the risk of aspiration.

84. a. A ventriculoperitoneal shunt runs from the brain to the abdomen to drain excess cerebrospinal fluid.

85. c. Infants and children with shunts are particularly prone to respiratory arrest. If signs of increased intracranial pressure are present, medical direction may recommend endotracheal intubation and hyperventilation.

86. d. When a patient with a shunt is complaining of a headache accompanied by nausea, suspect the patient has increasing intracranial pressure until proven otherwise.

87. a. The initial energy levels for pediatric defibrillation is 2 J/kg, 4 J/kg, 4 J/kg. The patient weighs approximately 25 kg. Therefore the initial three shocks would be delivered at 50 J, 100 J, 100 J. Subsequent shocks would also be delivered at 4 J/kg.

88. b. The initial pediatric IV/IO dose for epinephrine in cardiac arrest is 0.01 mg/kg of 1:10,000 solution. Because the patient weighs 25 kg, the initial dose should be 0.25 mg.

89. d. A torn or leaking catheter (cracked line) may allow air to enter the tubing and lead to an air embolism. The shortness of breath, chest pain, and altered level of consciousness should alert EMS personnel to the possibility that an air embolism has occurred. Although other causes should be considered, in this case the possibility that an air embolism has occurred especially needs to be taken into consideration because it will have an effect on patient management.

90. c. A torn or leaking central venous catheter should be clamped between the tear and the patient. Position the patient on his or her left side with the head slightly lowered to help prevent the embolism from traveling to the brain or lungs.

91. c. The child is displaying classic signs and symptoms of salicylate poisoning. These initially include lethargy and confusion, abdominal pain and vomiting, tachypnea, and hyperthermia, and eventually respiratory and cardiac failure.

GERIATRICS

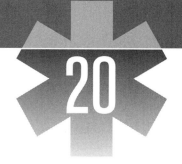

20

1. The fact that by the year 2030, 25% of Americans will be over the age of 65 and represent more than 70% of EMS transports is referred to as:
   a. the "Aging of America"
   b. the "Graying of America"
   c. the "Gray Panthers"
   d. the "Old American"

2. Which of the following is not an important patho-physiological consequence of aging that affects the need for EMS care by the elderly?
   a. The elderly have more falls as a result of less mobility.
   b. Poor eyesight results in lowered perception and accident avoidance.
   c. The elderly have fixed incomes that limit their use of EMS.
   d. Pain perception is decreased with aging and is associated with higher injury rates.

3. Common physiological changes seen in the elderly include all of the following *EXCEPT*:
   a. decreased reaction time
   b. increased prevalence of cataracts
   c. decreased hearing acuity
   d. less fluent and understandable speech patterns

4. One of the greatest fears that must be recognized by the EMT while assessing the elderly patient is:
   a. fear of disfigurement
   b. fear of pain
   c. fear of financial impact
   d. fear of losing autonomy

5. While assessing your elderly patient you get the impression that he does not understand what you are saying. Which of the following should you do to improve communication with him?
   a. Locate hearing aids, eyeglasses, and dentures if needed.
   b. Speak at eye level so that the patient can see you.
   c. Speak slowly, distinctly, and respectfully.
   d. All of the above are correct.

6. Which of the following is not an appropriate and professional manner in which to address an elderly patient?
   a. "sweetheart"
   b. "sir"
   c. "Mr."
   d. "yes ma'am."

7. The single most important aspect of assessing the elderly is:
   a. being patient
   b. obtaining a complete list of their medications
   c. keeping the patient dressed
   d. keeping the patient warm

8. While assessing your 85-year-old patient, you notice that she appears quite thin and frail. Important questions to ask would include:
   a. "How much weight have you lost this year?"
   b. "Doesn't your family take good care of you?"
   c. "Are you receiving 'meals on wheels,' and if so, are you eating?"
   d. "Why don't you live in a nursing home where the food is good?"

9. All of the following COMMONLY affect the manner in which an elderly patient presents with a complaint *EXCEPT:*
   a. presence of intoxication
   b. minimization or denial of symptoms by elderly patients
   c. presence of more than one disease
   d. presence of polypharmacy

10. Which portion of the physical exam of the elderly patient is the most difficult to perform accurately?
    a. blood pressure monitoring
    b. lung auscultation
    c. mental status exam
    d. abdominal exam

11. Kyphosis, minimal body fat over bony areas, and arthritis are all common findings in the elderly, which should prompt you to do which of the following during transport?
    a. ensure adequate padding and protection between the patient and the cot or backboard
    b. keep the patient covered with additional blankets to protect against hypothermia
    c. ensure that the patient is restrained in the correct anatomical position to promote circulation
    d. never physically restrain an elderly patient to a backboard

12. The condition that represents the leading cause of death in the elderly is:
    a. coronary artery disease
    b. cerebrovascular disease
    c. pneumonia
    d. trauma

13. The elderly are predisposed to pneumonia for all of the following reasons *EXCEPT:*
    a. decreased immune response to infection
    b. increased incidence of smoking
    c. reduced pulmonary function
    d. increased exposure to pathogens

14. The signs and symptoms of pneumonia in the elderly patient are usually identical to that of the younger patient.
    a. true
    b. false

15. During your physical assessment of the geriatric patient suspected of having pneumonia, the most sensitive indicator may be the presence of:
    a. tachypnea
    b. fever
    c. rhonchi
    d. hypoxia

16. While assessing a 72-year-old man with shortness of breath and a history of COPD, the most important feature of his medical history is:
    a. history of prior hospitalizations
    b. recent use of antibiotics
    c. prior need for intubation
    d. history of recurrent pneumonia

17. Viruses are the most common cause of upper respiratory illness and are just as common in the elderly as in the younger patient. Therefore the elderly patient with a cough and fever is more likely to have a viral infection.
    a. true
    b. false

18. Which of the following is the most common symptom of acute myocardial infarction in the elderly patient?
    a. fatigue
    b. chest pain
    c. neck pain
    d. arm pain

19. Which of the following is a normal change to the aging cardiovascular system?
    a. decreased peripheral resistance due to atherosclerosis
    b. increased blood flow to all organs
    c. widened pulse pressure
    d. increased incidence of postural hypotension

20. Because "silent" myocardial infarctions are more common in the older patient, the most common physical finding is:
    a. diaphoresis
    b. hypotension
    c. dyspnea
    d. bradycardia

21. After deciding to administer lidocaine to an 80-year-old man suffering a heart attack and exhibiting multifocal PVCs, you must take into consideration all of the following *EXCEPT:*
    a. interaction with other medications he is taking
    b. slower metabolism in the elderly
    c. less lean body mass
    d. the presence of a living will

22. Heart failure in the elderly is almost always due to a heart attack.
    a. true
    b. false

23. The most common dysrhythmia in the elderly is:
    a. atrial flutter
    b. atrial fibrillation
    c. first-degree AV block
    d. bigeminal PVCs

24. Your elderly patient has no complaints of chest pain. Her vital signs are normal, and her oxygen sats are 92%. The monitor shows a sinus rhythm with unifocal PVCs alternating between every sixth and eighth beat. These types of PVCs should:
    a. be expected
    b. always be treated
    c. usually be treated
    d. never be treated

25. Electrolyte abnormalities in the elderly can lead to dysrhythmias from which of the following causes?
    a. diuretic use
    b. potassium supplement use
    c. impaired renal function
    d. all of the above

26. An 82-year-old man with a history of hypertension complained of sudden onset of severe back pain before passing out. Which of the following physical findings would you look for?
    a. pulsatile abdominal mass
    b. unexplained hypotension
    c. diminished distal pulses
    d. all of the above

27. The management of the suspected aortic dissection would include all of the following *EXCEPT:*
    a. gentle handling of the patient
    b. calming of the patient
    c. large-bore IV administration and fluid boluses to establish normotension
    d. administration of morphine

28. Hypertension in the elderly is associated with the same causes and risk factors as in the younger patient.
    a. true
    b. false

29. The most common presenting symptom of chronic hypertension in the elderly is:
    a. anxiety
    b. chest pain
    c. altered mental status
    d. headache

30. Your 72-year-old patient has broken her hip. Her blood pressure is 210/110. What is the most appropriate treatment for her hypertension?
    a. administration of morphine for pain
    b. administration of nitroglycerin
    c. administration of labetalol
    d. no treatment is necessary

31. Which of the following is true regarding the mental status exam in the elderly?
    a. It is normal and appropriate to expect cognitive deterioration with aging.
    b. Impairments in hearing or sight can affect cognitive ability.
    c. Cognitive function relates to ability to hear and see accurately.
    d. Fatigue and changes in sleep pattern usually do not affect the mental status exam in the elderly.

32. Your 69-year-old female patient presents with sudden onset of left facial drooping, slurred speech, and left hemiparesis. Each of the following is true regarding cerebral vascular disease in the elderly *EXCEPT:*
    a. stroke is the third leading cause of death in the elderly
    b. transient ischemic attacks are more common than strokes
    c. minimizing time in the field is critical to outcome
    d. all stroke patients should be given high-flow oxygen

33. Which of the following is the most accurate description of the difference between dementia and delirium in the elderly?
    a. Dementia results in disorientation to time and place, whereas delirium results in the inability to remember past events.
    b. It is usually easy to differentiate the two in the prehospital setting.
    c. Delirium is acute in onset, whereas dementia is slow and progressive.
    d. Delirium is rarely caused by organic brain dysfunction from tumors, metabolic disorders, fever, or drug reactions.

34. A 78-year-old man complains of chest pain. When asked how long he has had it he says, "I don't know." He continues to give the same answer to all questions. Which of the following is the *MOST CORRECT* statement regarding his dementia?
   a. He probably has atherosclerosis, which has reduced cerebral blood flow and resulted in dementia.
   b. Alzheimer's dementia occurs much earlier than this, and therefore an organic process must be excluded.
   c. Chronic infections, toxic metal poisoning, and reduction in certain brain chemicals are the known causes of Alzheimer's dementia.
   d. Alzheimer's dementia is irreversible.

35. Patients with dementia are likely to act in which of the following manners?
   a. They will confabulate, or make up, stories to fill in the gaps from their memory loss.
   b. They will tend to be paranoid because they believe that others know things they do not.
   c. They rarely become agitated or violent.
   d. All of the above are characteristic of a person with dementia.

36. An 89-year-old woman complains of abdominal pain, constipation, and nausea. Which of the following should be considered possible causes?
   a. gastrointestinal hemorrhage
   b. bowel obstruction
   c. aortic aneurysm
   d. all of the above

37. Gastrointestinal bleeding in the elderly is usually a benign symptom of diverticulosis and rarely results in death.
   a. true
   b. false

38. All of the following are causes of bowel incontinence in the elderly *EXCEPT:*
   a. fecal impaction
   b. normal and expected changes with aging
   c. dementia
   d. spinal cord injury from spinal stenosis

39. You are transporting a 76-year-old man with pneumonia from the nursing home and notice pressure ulcers on his back, buttocks, and the heels of both feet. Which of the following is true?
   a. This is a clear sign of neglect and should be reported.
   b. Pressure ulcers result from occlusion of major blood vessels to the area.
   c. Once the skin breaks down the potential for infection is high.
   d. Nutrition plays little role in the etiology.

40. Which of the following statements about common eye problems in the elderly is correct?
   a. Cataracts result in clouding of the cornea to the point of total blindness.
   b. Glaucoma leads to blindness.
   c. Cataracts are treated with surgical replacement of the lens.
   d. Glaucoma results from destruction of the retina as a result of increased intraocular pressure.

41. Geriatric patients are at increased risk for adverse drug reactions because of changes in the body's ability to metabolize and distribute the drug in the body. All of the following drugs commonly cause toxicity in the geriatric patient *EXCEPT:*
   a. antidysrhythmics such as lidocaine and digitalis
   b. antibiotics such as penicillin and tetracycline
   c. antidepressants and psychotropics
   d. antihypertensives and diuretics

42. The same amount of alcohol is required for clinical intoxication to occur in both the elderly and younger patient because of its rapid absorption kinetics.
   a. true
   b. false

43. Which of the following is true regarding hypothermia and the elderly?
   a. Hypothermia is more likely due to environmental conditions than to hyperthermia.
   b. Medications are more likely to cause hypothermia than hyperthermia.
   c. The potential for hypothermia is greater because of the physical characteristics of the older adult.
   d. Medical causes of hypothermia are rare.

44. Which of the following statements is true regarding trauma in the elderly?
    a. Trauma is the fifth leading cause of death for persons over the age of 65.
    b. In persons over the age of 80, falls account for 50% of injury-related deaths.
    c. The risk of fatality from multiple trauma is three times greater at age 70 than at age 20.
    d. All of the above are correct.

45. Because of stiffening of the cranial attachments and intolerance to space-occupying lesions, the elderly patient is more likely to present with early signs of increased intracranial pressure from head trauma.
    a. true
    b. false

46. A 79-year-old man is involved in a head-on collision in which he is not restrained. He complains of pain in his neck, chest, and back. You find no apparent injuries on exam, and his vital signs are normal. The most appropriate treatment would consist of oxygen, IVs, and rapid transport because:
    a. the elderly will often not tell you if they are injured
    b. the elderly usually have normal vital signs until they deteriorate
    c. the mechanism of injury must be considered over physical findings
    d. increased elasticity and cardiovascular reserve increase the potential for life-threatening thoracic injuries

Questions 47 through 49 refer to the following scenario:

An 89-year-old woman falls down while leaving church. She complains of left hip pain and is unable to walk. She has a history of COPD and HTN.

47. Each of the following is true regarding trauma in the elderly *EXCEPT*:
    a. falls are often the result of some underlying medical condition
    b. morbidity and mortality from trauma are higher because of the increased incidence of operative and postoperative complications
    c. abdominal injuries may be less apparent, requiring a high degree of suspicion
    d. elderly patients with hip fractures typically do well after surgery and rehabilitation.

48. As it relates to her vital signs and need for IV administration, which of the following is most correct?
    a. Elderly patients are more likely to be tachycardic from pain and anxiety.
    b. Rapid IV fluid administration is rarely harmful if the patient is hypotensive.
    c. Cardiac ischemia can result as both the cause of the fall and the result of the fall.
    d. All of the above are correct.

49. Her COPD history is likely to play a role in her treatment for all of the following reasons *EXCEPT*:
    a. COPD results in decreased vital capacity and chest wall compliance
    b. high-flow oxygen usually used in multiple trauma is not indicated
    c. stress may exacerbate her COPD
    d. airway management may be more difficult because of dentures

50. You respond to the home of an elderly woman who lives with her children and are met by a young woman who tells you her grandmother is unconscious in the bedroom. You find her lying in her bed covered in feces, her skin covered in sores, and responsive to verbal stimuli only. The granddaughter tells you her parents left for the weekend and placed food at the side of the bedridden woman's bed. Which of the following are true?
    a. Treatment should consist of IV fluid for hydration, cardiac monitoring, and blood glucose analysis.
    b. You are legally mandated to report what appears to be elder abuse.
    c. Elder abuse is classified as physical, psychological, or financial.
    d. All of the above are true.

ANSWERS TO CHAPTER 20: GERIATRICS

1. b. The "Graying of America" highlights the importance of expanded education, training, and understanding of the special needs of the geriatric patient.

2. c. Although it is true that the elderly tend to live on fixed incomes, this is a social issue and not a result of the physical changes of aging. Each of the other listed changes is related to increased EMS needs of the elderly.

3. a. Reaction time increases with age and contributes to elderly persons' inability to avoid accidents. Cataracts, a condition that clouds the cornea, results in decreased visual acuity leading to falls. Decreased hearing acuity impairs their ability to communicate, as do changes in their speech patterns, which accompany aging.

4. d. Elderly patients fear that their illness or injury will result in no longer being able to care for themselves independently. Although all fears must be addressed, it is vital that the EMT recognize the role of the patient's autonomy. This can done by allowing the patient the greatest latitude in how your treatment is rendered and by respecting their ability to make choices.

5. d. Because of the deficits in vision, hearing, and speech, each of the listed actions will improve communication with the elderly. Speaking at eye level and maintaining eye contact are key to successful communications with the elderly. Additionally, turning on lights will assist the visually impaired patient.

6. a. Although it is easy for us to identify the elderly patient with one of our family members, it is disrespectful to address him or her using terms of endearment unless given permission to do so.

7. a. From the manner in which the history is taken to the performance of the physical exam and transport, patience is the key to successful interaction with the elderly.

8. c. The social and living conditions of your patient should be assessed so that this information can be passed along to the medical staff because it may affect the ability of the patient to return home independently. This information should be obtained in a respectful manner.

9. a. The elderly often have several diseases, which can confuse the issue of which one is chronic and which one acute. Denial plays a major factor and must be addressed. Although alcoholism is on the rise in the elderly, it is less common than the other listed causes. Polypharmacy results in drug-drug interactions, which influence how the patient's disease process will manifest itself.

10. c. In performing the mental status exam on the elderly patient you may be required to enlist the help of family, friends, and caregivers to obtain an accurate determination not only of the patient's mental status but also of any acute change from the norm.

11. a. Kyphosis, or curvature of the spine, along with the other listed conditions will require you to provide additional padding for the patient to fill the voids created by their posture. Attempting to place the elderly patient in what is considered the "correct" position will inflict pain and may worsen the underlying condition. Additional blankets should be used according to the patient's level of comfort.

12. c. Pneumonia is the most common cause of death in the elderly. It usually occurs as a complication of various conditions including underlying lung disease, cerebrovascular accidents, and trauma.

13. b. Decreased ability to fight infection, age-related reduction in pulmonary functions such as the ability to cough, and increased exposure to the bacteria that cause pneumonia, while living in the institutional setting, all contribute to an increased incidence of pneumonia in the elderly.

14. b. Because the elderly frequently do not develop significant fever, have the ability to cough forcibly, or mount a typical immune response to pneumonia, they rarely present with the classic signs and symptoms associated with the younger patient.

15. a. Elderly patients with pneumonia may not be able to cough or take a deep breath, which may preclude you from hearing rhonchi. They may have underlying COPD or other causes of hypoxia, which are not specific to pneumonia. The presence of tachycardia and tachypnea may be the only signs and symptoms of pneumonia. However, tachycardia may be blunted by the presence of beta-blocker medications. Fever is often absent in the elderly patient.

16. **c.** The prior need for intubation is one of the most sensitive indicators to the potential seriousness of the patient's condition. Recent use of steroid therapy increases the potential need for more aggressive intervention.

17. **b.** With age, the incidence of viral infection declines and the bacterial infection increases. This is a result of immunity from long-term exposure to viral infections, which rarely cause debilitating infection.

18. **a.** Pain is an uncommon complaint in geriatric heart attack victims. They usually complain of shortness of breath, fatigue, and other vague symptoms. This occurs as a result of changes in the nervous system combined with the prevalence of the "silent" MI, which then presents with decompensation.

19. **d.** As the cardiovascular system ages, the slow but steady buildup of atherosclerosis causes the vessels to become rigid, resulting in increased resistance and decreased blood flow, which is evidenced by the narrowing of the pulse pressure. Increased vagal tone results in the inability of the heart rate to increase with position changes, resulting in postural hypotension.

20. **c.** Following an unrecognized heart attack the heart decompensates and congestive heart failure develops resulting in dyspnea, rales, and tachycardia.

21. **d.** Any drug administration to the older patient must take the following into consideration to reduce the potential for negative side effects. Reduced lean body mass, slower metabolism, impaired renal and hepatic function, and the possibility of drug interactions must be considered. Whether she has a living will or even a DNR order should not affect your decision to treat significant PVCs as long as the treatment does not violate her requests.

22. **b.** As the heart ages it becomes increasingly prone to cardiomyopathies, which result in cardiomegaly. Congestive heart failure eventually develops without the involvement of myocardial infarction.

23. **b.** Atrial fibrillation is the most common dysrhythmia in the elderly. It results from impairment in the conduction pathways in the atria, which often become enlarged with age.

24. **a.** PVCs in an elderly patient are usually due to hypertensive heart disease. They only should be treated once the underlying precipitator such as hypoxia, pain, or hypoperfusion is dealt with and only then if they are hemodynamically significant.

25. **d.** Dysrhythmias in the elderly can occur from electrolyte disturbances. Hyperkalemia and hypokalemia are the most likely causes.

26. **d.** Abdominal aortic aneurysm rupture is associated with a high mortality rate and should be suspected in all cases of syncope in the elderly. The patient will typically complain of severe nontraumatic back pain and may have one or more of the listed physical findings.

27. **c.** Although the patient with a dissecting aortic aneurysm may be hypotensive, the administration of fluid may worsen the bleeding. Therefore fluid resuscitation should be performed only for severe hypotension with altered mental status. Gentle handling, sedation, and pain medication administration will lessen the likelihood of further dissection.

28. **a.** Atherosclerosis, diabetes, and obesity have the same contributing factors to the development of hypertension in the elderly as they do in the younger patient.

29. **c.** Memory loss and an altered mental status are common presenting symptoms of hypertension in the elderly. Other common symptoms include epistaxis, tremors, and nausea and vomiting. All of these are associated with chronic and often unrecognized hypertension.

30. **a.** Systolic hypertension in the elderly is usually a result of pain and anxiety, and their treatment will be most effective in lowering the blood pressure. The use of nitrates and labetalol would be appropriate in the presence of an acute coronary syndrome.

31. b. Cognition is the ability to reason and understand and requires proper function of both the brain and perception organs. Any impairment in perception such as poor eyesight or hearing can give the incorrect impression that the patient does not understand you. Elderly patients are very susceptible to fatigue, and this should be taken into consideration when assessing their mental status.

32. d. Transient ischemic attacks, or mini strokes, are more common than strokes but herald the potential for a devastating event. With the advent of cerebral thrombolytics, the adage "time is brain" underscores the importance of delivering a patient to an appropriate facility within 3 to 6 hours for definitive care. Studies show that unless the patient is hypoxic, no supplemental oxygen is needed, and in fact, high-flow oxygen may worsen the ischemia around the stroke.

33. c. The primary difference between delirium and dementia is in speed of onset. Both can impair orientation, but dementia tends to be more dramatic with illusions and hallucinations. In the absence of good historians it is very difficult to tell the difference between the two. Delirium is often caused by an organic process that can be life threatening.

34. d. Alzheimer's disease is a condition in which the nerve cells of the cerebral cortex die and the brain shrinks. It is irreversible. It is not related to atherosclerosis, and its cause is unknown, although many theories exist.

35. a. The patient with dementia recognizes that he should know the answer to your questions and will attempt to "cover up" the memory loss with stories. He may often regress to a childlike state requiring total care for feeding, toileting, and physical activities. As the disease progresses he may become agitated and violent as abstract thinking becomes impaired, interfering with work and social interactions.

36. d. Abdominal pain is a serious complaint in the elderly, and the potential for life-threatening conditions such as those listed should always be considered.

37. b. GI bleeding most often affects patients between the age of 60 and 90 and has a mortality rate of 10%. It has a higher risk because the elderly are less able to compensate for the blood loss, less likely to feel the symptoms, and more likely to take aspirin, which causes ulcers.

38. b. Bowel incontinence is abnormal at any age and should not be relegated to the expected physical findings in the elderly.

39. c. Pressure ulcers generally occur over the bony prominences of the back and buttocks due to decreased fat in the skin. They become easily infected because of poor circulation and immune response and are caused by local ischemia to the tissues and are worsened with poor nutrition, with constant exposure to irritants such as urine, and in conditions of poor sensation such as stroke and diabetes.

40. b. Almost everyone over the age of 65 has some degree of cataract, which is clouding of the lens and rarely results in total blindness. It is corrected by surgery. Glaucoma, which results in increased intraocular pressure, damages the optic nerve resulting in blindness and is easily prevented with proper screening exams and medical therapy.

41. b. Antibiotics are not known to have age-related incidence of adverse reactions. Intolerance to cardiac and psychiatric medications results in more toxicity in the elderly.

42. b. Because of impaired liver function, lower amounts of alcohol result in intoxication in the elderly, who also have less tolerance to its effects.

43. c. Hypothermia is more common than hyperthermia because of the physical characteristics of the geriatric patient, such as less body water to store heat and poor compensatory mechanisms. Medication reactions, particularly antidysrhythmics, beta blockers, and cyclic antidepressants will cause hyperthermia rather than hypothermia. Many medical conditions can result in hypothermia and should be considered.

44. d. All of the list statements are true. This underscores the importance of understanding the need for aggressive management of the elderly trauma patient.

45. b. Because of cerebral atrophy, there is the potential for more damage to bridging veins stretched by the movement of the brain. However, the extra space within the cranial vault often allows a geriatric patient to develop significant extradural hemorrhage before symptoms are manifested.

46. c. Because of poor cardiovascular reserve and increased stiffness of the thorax, the potential for life-threatening injuries is much higher. Unless there is some underlying dementia the patient will be just as truthful as the next patient. However, when the mechanism of injury is present the paramedic must give it greater consideration than for the younger patient.

47. d. Falls should be suspected to indicate an underlying medical condition until proven otherwise. Syncope, altered mental status, and hypotension are just some examples. Because of poor lung compliance and cardiovascular reserve, the elderly patient does not tolerate surgery well, and poor immune response increases postoperative complication rates. Hip fractures have a high morbidity rate in that often the geriatric patient is unable to return to full and independent activity.

48. c. Cardiac ischemia with dysrhythmia and syncope must be considered in the differential for the cause of the fall and may also be caused by the stress of the injury. Because of poor cardiovascular reserve, rapid fluid administration, even if hypotensive, can result in congestive heart failure. Beta-blocker use and decreased responsiveness to hypovolemia may blunt the tachycardic response and if present indicate the potential for severe hypovolemia.

49. b. Because of the possibility of impairing the hypoxic drive, the application of high-flow oxygen to the elderly trauma patient with COPD should be performed with judicious administration guided by pulse oximetry and exam. However, this should not preclude the use of oxygen because hypoxia in multiple trauma increases mortality significantly. COPD results in decreased lung compliance and vital capacity, which impairs respiration and ventilation. Although it is true that dentures make airway management more difficult, they are not a result of COPD.

50. d. Elder abuse is a growing problem in the United States, affecting more than 1 million adults yearly. Warning signs of abuse or neglect include an upset or agitated state, dehydration, malnutrition, and unsafe and unsanitary living conditions.

SPECIAL CHALLENGES AND HOME HEALTH CARE PATIENTS

21

1. You are dispatched to an MVC where a vehicle has been rear-ended at high speed. The driver of the struck vehicle is your patient. As you make contact with the patient, your partner enters the back seat and takes manual c-spine stabilization. You start to talk with the patient who is alert and has no signs of head trauma when she pulls away from you. You tell her to calm down and follow your instructions but she continues to struggle. Your patient may be:
   a. suffering an unrecognized head injury
   b. intoxicated
   c. unable to understand your actions because she is deaf
   d. all of the above

2. Your 75-year-old patient complains of difficulty hearing, which came on suddenly after he began taking a new medication. Some medications can cause hearing loss. This form of hearing impairment would be described as:
   a. conductive deafness
   b. Meniere's disease
   c. sensorineural deafness
   d. natural degeneration

3. En route to a call for chest pain, your dispatcher notifies you that your patient lives alone and is hearing impaired. The patient contacted the 911 center by means of a special telephone that receives typed messages. You arrive and find a 55-year-old male who is pale, is diaphoretic, and is clutching his chest. While you are assessing the patient, you find it difficult to communicate your intentions for caring for his problem. He is becoming more anxious. Your actions should include which of the following?
   a. Just load and go to the hospital with this patient; he is having a heart attack and needs immediate interventions.
   b. Have your partner retrieve the patient's hearing aid and in the meantime communicate with him in writing.
   c. Speak very loudly to the patient and exaggerate your words so that he can read your lips.
   d. All of the above are correct.

4. Your patient is a 36-year-old female who slipped on some water in the kitchen and twisted her ankle. Your assessment of the patient's history reveals that she is blind as a result of a previous head injury. She lives alone and is aided by a guide dog to perform her daily activities. She has a possible fracture/dislocation of the ankle, and the patient needs to be transported to the hospital for further care. Which of the following is the most appropriate action in dealing with the patient's guide dog?
   a. Leave the dog plenty of water and food because this injury may require a lengthy visit in the emergency department.
   b. Tell the patient that she should have family bring the dog upon her discharge.
   c. Have the dog accompany the patient to the hospital.
   d. Family pets are not your concern; you have the patient's needs to care for.

5. Patients who stutter are referred to as having which of the following?
   a. fluency disorder
   b. delayed development
   c. articulation disorder
   d. voice production disorder

6. Your patient is a 60-year-old female found on the floor. Your general impression is that she is awake, alert, in no obvious distress, and has an estimated weight of over 375 pounds. She apologizes for calling you and states that her knees gave out when she was walking up the back stairs from outside. She states she pulled herself this far to reach the phone to call for help. Her husband is disabled and cannot help lift her. She denies injury but states she needs assistance to get up. Which of the following is the most appropriate plan of care for this patient?
   a. Do your best to assist the patient to a chair or a standing position and have a release for nontransport signed.
   b. Perform an assessment of the patient before moving her even though she denies injury.
   c. Inform her of recent advances in weight loss.
   d. The patient chose to eat and gain weight to this amount, and it is not your responsibility to get her up because you may hurt yourself while trying.

7. Dispatch advises that you are to respond to a 7-year-old male patient having seizures. When you arrive you find the patient postical sitting in a wheelchair. You note he is in a brace with a halo traction device. His mother advises the child is recovering from an MVC in which he sustained head and spinal injuries. The patient has been home for 1 week and was doing well until this seizure. Your primary concern at this time is:
   a. ensuring that the halo device and brace stay in position
   b. arranging some kind of padding for the posterior pins in the occipital area
   c. airway management even though you know there is a spinal injury
   d. getting the patient out of the chair and onto the cot to treat him with medications

8. Patients that fall under the category of "mentally ill" include all of the following *EXCEPT:*
   a. schizophrenia
   b. manic-depressive disorder
   c. Down syndrome
   d. obsessive-compulsive behavior

Questions 9 through 12 refer to the following scenario:

Robert is a 42-year-old mentally handicapped man who also suffers from manic-depressive disorder. He works full-time at a fast-food restaurant. Robert has not gone to work for several days because he just didn't feel well. The employer, who knows Robert personally, calls you because he is concerned about him. On arrival at Robert's residence, you find the door unlocked. Robert calls from a back room and tells you to come in. You find the house in disarray and Robert in bed under a heavy quilt. Robert tells you that he has felt nervous for the past few days, which made him feel tired, and he didn't feel like getting out of bed. He says he has a "fluttery" sensation in his chest. His skin is pale and moist, but he says he is "OK."

9. Which of the following statements regarding the patient's history is false?
   a. Noncompliance with prescribed medications may be the cause.
   b. Robert should be asked about the use of alcohol or other drugs.
   c. Questions regarding the use of herbal products such as St. John's wort should be asked.
   d. It is not important to ask Robert about his mental illness.

10. Based on Robert's history of mental illness, complaints of fatigue and nervousness are common to his disorder, and it is safe to assume that this is just a somatization process.
   a. true
   b. false

11. You ask Robert about his medical history, and he tells you that he has no pertinent medical history and sees his psychiatrist only to have his mental condition evaluated and medications prescribed. He has not felt the need to seek medical attention for any problems. Which of the following would be the most helpful in determining if Robert is at risk for medical problems?
   a. asking, "Do you have any family history of high blood pressure or heart disease?"
   b. asking, "What were you doing when the chest fluttering and nervousness began?"
   c. telling Robert, "You need to get up and go to work," and then seeing if he is able to get up and move around
   d. assessing vital signs, obtaining a thorough history, and performing a comprehensive physical exam

12. If Robert would suddenly become aggressive and combative, yelling for you to get out, what is the single most important step for the rescuers to take?
   a. Use medical restraint devices to control his movement.
   b. Determine whether the scene is safe and immediately exit the residence if it's not.
   c. Administer 1 mg Ativan IM to sedate Robert.
   d. Just leave; Robert didn't call you and doesn't want your help.

13. Which of the following debilitating diseases is autoimmune in nature?
   a. multiple sclerosis
   b. cystic fibrosis
   c. cerebral palsy
   d. muscular dystrophy

14. Poliomyelitis is an infectious disease caused by a virus that is spread through direct and indirect contact with infected feces and by airborne transmission. Since the vaccines (Salk and Sabin) were made available in the 1950s, this disease is no longer a concern for EMS providers.
   a. true
   b. false

15. Your ambulance is dispatched to a residence where a 45-year-old male is having chest pain. He says his wife called, but he doesn't want an ambulance. He states he can't afford an ambulance and can't miss work. He asks you to leave. You see that his color is poor, his breathing is labored, and he is clutching his chest. His wife is crying, asking him to go with you. Your best action would be to:
   a. tell his wife that because the patient won't give you permission to treat, there is nothing you can do. Advise dispatch that the patient was a refusal.
   b. call law enforcement to have the patient put in protective custody so that you can treat and transport him
   c. advise him of the need for early intervention, call Medical Control, and have the patient talk with the physician
   d. while the patient's wife drives him to the hospital, follow them in the ambulance in case something happens

Questions 16 through 20 refer to the following scenario:

You're called to the home of a child with cerebral palsy. He is ventilator dependent, and the home health aid tells you his tracheostomy tube has malfunctioned. He appears to be in respiratory distress with audible stridor.

16. The initial management would be to:
   a. remove the tracheostomy tube
   b. ventilate him with a bag-valve-mask
   c. assess the tracheostomy tube for obstruction
   d. none of the above

17. On examination the tube appears to be dislodged from the stoma. It is appropriate to make an attempt at pushing it back in.
   a. true
   b. false

18. What would be the appropriate treatment if the tracheostomy tube was lost and could not be found?
   a. rush the patient to the hospital for an X-ray to see where it is lodged in his lung
   b. insert an appropriately sized ET tube into the tracheostomy
   c. perform rapid sequence intubation
   d. place the patient on a nonrebreather mask

19. Once the airway has been secured what is the next step?
   a. transport to the hospital
   b. contact the parents to consent for treatment
   c. perform a thorough history and physical exam
   d. contact medical control for further orders

20. After contacting the parents you learn that the child has a Do Not Resuscitate order. You have violated that order with your actions.
   a. true
   b. false

Questions 21 through 25 refer to the following scenario:

A 46-year-old man with metastatic lung cancer has become unresponsive at home. His wife and family are gathered around the bed. He is cyanotic and appears to be in pain, and there is vomit in his mouth.

21. An appropriate question would be:
   a. "Does the patient have a Living Will or Do Not Resuscitate order?"
   b. "What would you like us to do?"
   c. "Why did you call an ambulance?"
   d. "Don't you have hospice care?"

22. The family states he is a No Code, but they want you to help him. Appropriate interventions COULD include all of the following *EXCEPT:*
   a. suction the airway
   b. position him for comfort
   c. perform endotracheal intubation
   d. administer morphine for pain

23. After the airway has been cleared and morphine has been administered, he is breathing easier. The next steps in treatment include all of the following *EXCEPT:*
   a. have the family sign the treat and release form
   b. perform a thorough history and physical examination
   c. consult the family as to their desire for transport
   d. assist them in contacting their physician or hospice nurse

24. After administering 2 mg of morphine to the patient his respirations drop to four per minute. You should immediately:
   a. administer naloxone to reverse respiratory suppression
   b. ask the family what they want you to do
   c. intubate him because it is your fault he quit breathing
   d. contact medical control for orders

25. You learn that the patient does not have hospice care and that the family is totally unprepared for his death. Despite his DNR status it would be appropriate to transport him to the hospital.
   a. true
   b. false

Questions 26 through 28 refer to the following scenario:

You are called to the home of a Cambodian family who has a 4-year-old child with a fever. On exam he is resting comfortably and is in no distress. While listening to his lung sounds you notice a pattern of red welts on either side of the spine from the upper to lower back in a symmetrical pattern.

26. You should consider the possibility of abuse and notify law enforcement.
   a. true
   b. false

27. No one in the family speaks English. Therefore:
   a. you cannot obtain consent to treat the child
   b. you must wait until an interpreter arrives before treating the child
   c. you should assume implied consent since they called 911
   d. none of the above

28. When interviewing the family you notice that the women do not talk and the men will not look you in the eyes. You should suspect they are lying.
   a. true
   b. false

29. Patients requiring long-term home care can develop emergent needs. Which of the following leads the list of causes for 911 assistance?
   a. plugged gastric feeding tube
   b. malfunctioning Foley catheter
   c. inability to administer medication through a vascular access device
   d. respiratory distress

30. It is not uncommon to have home care patients connected to a ventilator. Ventilators are of three basic types. Which is not one of them?
   a. timed-cycle
   b. volume
   c. positive pressure
   d. negative pressure

31. The volume ventilator is triggered to deliver a given volume of air. It will stop delivery when:
   a. the machine is disconnected from the patient
   b. the respiratory rate increases
   c. extreme airway pressures are reached
   d. none of the above

32. The pressure ventilator is triggered to deliver a set tidal volume:
   a. when the preset time interval occurs
   b. when the machine senses the negative pressure of inspiratory effort
   c. immediately after expiration has occurred
   d. all of the above

33. Regardless of the type of ventilator used, the machine will turn itself off if the flow of oxygen is interrupted.
   a. true
   b. false

34. You are called to the home of a ventilator-dependent patient. His wife states that she dropped a book on the front panel of the machine and some of the knobs were turned, and now the alarms are going off. While contacting medical control for orders, what would be the appropriate initial ventilator settings for a man weighing 70 kg?
a. FiO_2 of 0.4
b. tidal volume of 700 cc
c. rate of 24 breaths per minute
d. 15 cm of PEEP

35. While assessing the patient connected to a ventilator, the high pressure alarm goes off. All of the following could cause this *EXCEPT*:
a. secretions in the ET tube
b. patient anxiety
c. leak in the ET tube cuff
d. coughing by the patient

36. An indwelling vascular access device (VAD) may be used to provide long-term vascular access for which of the following reasons?
a. dialysis
b. fluid and nutritional administration
c. chemotherapy and antibiotic administration
d. all of the above

37. Vascular access devices always enter the central venous system of the vena cava.
a. true
b. false

38. The most common complication of the VAD is:
a. infection
b. occlusion
c. embolus
d. infiltration

39. Because the VAD is prone to infection it should never be used to administer prehospital medication.
a. true
b. false

40. There are several types and brands of central venous catheters. The primary difference between a peripherally inserted central catheter (PICC) line and others such as a Hickman, Groshong, or Mediport is:
a. the PICC line is shorter than the others
b. the PICC line enters directly into the central venous system
c. the PICC line enters the peripheral vein and extends into the central venous system
d. there is no difference

41. While administering medication through a VAD, you meet resistance. You should suspect what condition and perform what action?
a. air embolus and position the patient in the left lateral decubitus position with the head down
b. occlusion by a thrombus and attempt to gently aspirate the clot with a 10-cc syringe
c. occlusion of the catheter from a kink and push harder on the syringe
d. none of the above

Questions 42 through 45 refer to the following scenario:

You are called to the home of 36-year-old paraplegic man complaining of abdominal pain. He is bedridden, and on exam you find his lower abdomen to be distended. He states he usually performs self-catheterization three times a day but has run out of supplies.

42. You should suspect what condition?
a. drug-seeking behavior because the paraplegic cannot sense abdominal pain
b. acute urinary retention
c. urinary tract infection
d. bowel obstruction

43. The most common serious complication of chronic indwelling urinary catheters is:
a. obstruction
b. accidental removal
c. infection
d. rupture of the catheter balloon

44. Medical control has ordered you to insert a Foley catheter. After passing the catheter 6 inches into the penis, there is no urine return and you begin to inflate the balloon with saline. While doing so you meet resistance. You should:
a. push harder because the first few cc of water require greater pressure to start the inflation
b. stop and pull the catheter back 1 or 2 inches and try again
c. deflate the balloon and advance the catheter a few more inches, watching for urine return
d. consult medical control immediately

45. While inserting the catheter gross blood enters the drainage tube. This may indicate which of the following?
a. placement of the catheter into a false urethral passage
b. the patient has hemorrhagic cystitis
c. the patient is on anticoagulants
d. all of the above

46. You are called to examine a patient complaining of abdominal pain. He has a history of bladder cancer, and on exam you find a plastic pouch connected to an ostomy in the right lower quadrant draining clear yellow fluid. This is characteristic of what condition?
a. ileostomy from an opening in small intestines
b. urostomy, which is an artificial bladder created with a section of small intestines
c. colostomy from an opening in the large intestines
d. bowel obstruction

47. The administration of nutrition and fluid may require the use of a feeding tube. What is the most common serious complication of these devices?
a. occlusion with material
b. perforation of the gastric wall
c. infection at the entrance site
d. aspiration of gastric contents

Questions 48 through 50 refer to the following scenario:

An 87-year-old woman complains of abdominal pain and vomiting. On exam you find her experiencing waves of colicky pain and actively vomiting. She has a colostomy bag, which she says has been empty for 2 days.

48. All of the following are likely causes for her condition *EXCEPT:*
a. bowel obstruction
b. fecal impaction
c. gastroenteritis
d. stenosis of the ostomy

49. Appropriate treatment for her would consist of:
a. IV access and fluid resuscitation
b. administration of an antiemetic such as Tigan
c. administration of an opiate analgesic
d. all of the above

50. It is never acceptable to insert a nasogastric tube into an awake patient.
a. true
b. false

ANSWERS TO CHAPTER 21: SPECIAL CHALLENGES AND HOME HEALTH CARE PATIENTS

1. **d.** Many conditions could explain her behavior. However, always consider the possibility that your patient may be hearing impaired and unable to understand why someone is holding her head. It is important to make eye contact with patients to gain consent and a level of communication to properly assess injuries or illnesses.

2. **c.** In sensorineural deafness, sounds that reach the inner ear fail to be transmitted to the brain because of damage to the structures in the ear or to the acoustic nerve, which connects the inner ear to the brain. It is often incurable. Conductive deafness refers to faulty transportation of sound from the outer to the inner ear. It can result from infection or even an accumulation of earwax. Meniere's disease is a form of sensorineural deafness that affects the inner ear with nerve deafness, vertigo, or tinnitus. Natural degeneration of the cochlea can occur with age and develops slowly.

3. **b.** It is important to communicate with your patient. He may be in critical condition and needs to understand this. By relieving his anxiety, you may lessen his chest pain. If he has a hearing device available, get it and have him use it, even if it takes a minute. By communicating in writing you can be sure that you understand the signs and symptoms the patient is experiencing. Performing a load and go would only increase his anxiety and does not allow you to obtain consent for treatment. Eighty percent of hearing loss is related to the loss of high-pitched sounds. Raising your voice or shouting brings your voice to a higher pitch making it more difficult to understand.

4. **c.** A guide dog is the patient's visual aid. The dog is used for more than just ambulatory needs. Patients who are unimpaired and live alone may have concerns for their family pets. Therefore it is important when possible to attempt to make arrangements for the care of those pets.

5. **a.** Fluency disorders are not well understood. They are marked by repetitions of single sounds or whole words, and by the blocking of speech. Articulation disorder is an inability to produce speech sounds due to damage to nerve pathways passing from the brain to the muscles of the larynx, mouth, or lips. Voice production disorders are characterized by hoarseness, harshness, inappropriate pitch, and abnormal nasal resonance. They often result from disorders of the vocal cords. Some can be caused by hormonal or psychiatric disturbances or hearing loss.

6. **b.** Obese patients often have an extensive medical history. It is associated with an increased risk for hypertension, stroke, heart disease, diabetes, and some cancers. Osteoarthritis also is aggravated by increased body weight. Because of these concerns it is important to reassure the patient that you are there to help her, treat her professionally, and perform an appropriate assessment using appropriate equipment. The potential for injury or underlying medical causes for the fall is great. Caloric intake that exceeds calories burned is only one cause of obesity. Do not assume that the patient's weight problem is totally an eating disorder. It may be caused by low basal metabolic rate or by genetic predisposition for obesity.

7. **c.** Accommodations may have to be made for medical devices such as halo traction devices. Whether a patient is a paraplegic or quadriplegic, in a wheelchair, or at home connected to a ventilator, basic principles of care still apply. Airway management with spinal precautions still take priority.

8. **c.** Down syndrome is a form of developmental disability. A person who is developmentally disabled has impaired or insufficient development of the brain. Mental illness refers to any form of psychiatric disorder. Two broad categories of mental illness are psychosis and neurosis.

9. **d.** When dealing with the mentally ill a complete history including their mental illness should be explored regardless of the nature of their complaint. The use of over-the-counter herbal preparations is common among the mentally ill and can be a sign of manic behavior.

10. **b.** Manic-depressive disorder, also known as *bipolar disorder*, is marked by periods of mania and depression. Although it is not uncommon for patients to sleep for long periods of time during depression, a thorough search for a medical cause should be undertaken.

11. d. All patients with chest discomfort should be evaluated for heart problems. A focused patient assessment needs to be completed to rule out any possibility of cardiac origin.

12. b. Once Robert becomes combative, the scene is unsafe. Law enforcement should be contacted to witness any behavior that appears to be dangerous to Robert or others. Neither medical nor chemical restraints are appropriate at this point, and both violate his civil rights. Leaving the residence without any follow-up could be a negligent action. Robert may be experiencing a life-threatening medical problem. Contacting law enforcement will provide witness that Robert was able to make a reasonable decision to refuse care.

13. a. Multiple sclerosis is a progressive and incurable autoimmune disease of the CNS, whereby scattered patches of myelin in the brain and spinal cord are destroyed. Cystic fibrosis is an inherited metabolic disease of the lungs and digestive system that manifests in childhood. Cerebral palsy is a general term for nonprogressive disorders of movement and posture. The disease results from damage to the fetal brain during later months of pregnancy, during birth, during the newborn period, or in early childhood. Muscular dystrophy is an inherited muscle disorder that results in a slow but progressive degeneration of muscle fibers.

14. b. While the incidence of polio has declined since the 1950s, the disease may affect those not immunized, such as foreigners and indigent children.

15. c. Patients with life-threatening medical conditions may be in denial of the severity of the situation. Financial challenges of medical care without insurance and the possibility of loss of income can affect the reasoning behind refusing care. Often the patient will listen to the physician on the phone, and this action is in the rescuer's best interest in the event something untoward would occur after the ambulance leaves. Leaving the scene without receiving informed consent from the patient is not professional and can be negligent. The patient has the right to refuse care, and law enforcement will just increase the patient's anxiety. Allowing the family to transport a critical patient in a personal vehicle risks not only the family but also the lives of others in the event of an accident.

16. c. The most common cause of tracheostomy malfunctions are related to mucous plugging of the tube. This can be alleviated by using a small suction catheter to remove the material. Sometimes it is helpful to instill some saline into the tube to loosen the plug before suctioning.

17. a. True. The length of the tracheostomy's existence will determine the likelihood of easily replacing the tube. Long-standing tracheostomies have a well-healed opening, and the tube can usually be easily reinserted.

18. b. The reason the patient has a tracheostomy is because of his inability to ventilate sufficiently without mechanical support. Often these patients will have difficulty controlling their secretions leading to aspiration. An appropriately sized endotracheal tube can be inserted 2 to 3 cm, the balloon inflated, and the extra length cut off. An X-ray is not needed because tracheostomy tubes are larger than the bronchi and it probably fell out on the floor.

19. c. After correcting the obvious life threat, you must complete the history and physical exam to ensure that no injury has occurred and that no other potentially serious conditions exist. Depending on the situation, the patient may or may not require transport to the hospital once the guardians have been contacted. On-line medical control should be consulted regarding disposition if there is any question.

20. b. False. Do Not Resuscitate orders pertain to actions to be taken in the event that breathing stops or the heart ceases to function. Procedures to maintain an airway are not heroic and do not constitute a violation of such an order.

21. a. Families of terminally ill patients often panic when death is near and regardless of their support structure or preparation may be unfamiliar with the process. Your questions should be directed toward the most appropriate care for the patient and not judgmental in any way.

22. c. Do Not Resuscitate does not mean do not care. Basic airway maintenance consists of opening the airway and providing supplemental oxygen and does not violate the DNR order. Comfort measures include appropriate positioning and analgesic administration.

23. a. The decision to leave such a patient at home should only occur once a thorough history and physical has been performed to rule out the potential for acute deterioration. Despite his DNR status the family may wish for him to be transported. Consultation with their personal physician or hospice nurse can facilitate this decision.

24. d. It is highly unlikely that such a small dose of morphine would result in respiratory arrest. The administration of naloxone may precipitate acute withdrawal because he is probably taking opiate analgesics. Intubation would not be indicated. Medical control should be contacted for advice.

25. a. True. Families of the terminally ill require significant counseling and support. Unless this has been prearranged it is best handled in the hospital. Medical control should be notified prior to arrival to coordinate the necessary staff.

26. b. False. These marks are consistent with the ritual called *coining*, where a hot coin is rubbed vigorously across the skin in the hopes of releasing the bad omens causing the illness. This represents an accepted cultural diversity. However, if any question remains, it is appropriate to bring it to the attention of medical control.

27. c. Implied consent pertains to this case because 911 was called by someone who had a reasonable belief that an emergency existed. This may have been from a family member elsewhere. When dealing with children in particular, it is prudent to err on the side of treatment.

28. b. Cultural mannerisms must be taken into consideration when dealing with both the family and the patient. Many Asian cultures will regard you as their elder regardless of age, and looking down is a sign of respect. Though the families tend to be maternal in nature, it is common for the man of the house to do the talking with strangers. Seemingly benign actions such as patting the head of the patient may be viewed as a sign of disrespect.

29. d. Despite the reason for long-term home care, respiratory distress leads the reasons for summoning emergency assistance. This distress may be related to either an acute or a chronic condition, and the rescuer must be prepared for both. The other listed causes must also be prepared for when dealing with the chronically ill patient.

30. a. Ventilators are of three types though only two are routinely encountered. They are volume, positive pressure, and negative pressure. Negative pressure ventilators are rarely used but may be seen in the care of the polio patient.

31. c. The volume ventilator cycles once the preset tidal volume is delivered. It will not sense that it has become disconnected from the patient. Despite this, extremely high-peak pressures will set off alarms and stop the flow of air.

32. b. The pressure ventilator is triggered by the negative pressure of inspiration. It will have preset tidal volume but will stop inspiration if a preset pressure is reached. The period of inspiration and expiration are usually timed in a 1:3 ratio.

33. b. False. Ventilators are run on air with oxygen bled into the mixture to deliver a specific concentration. The flow of oxygen does not power the machine itself.

34. b. The usual initial ventilator settings are FiO_2 of 100%, which can be lowered later once pulse oximetry has been obtained. Tidal volume is 10 to 15 cc/kg. Respiratory rate should be set at 10 to 15 breaths/minute with an inspiratory flow of 40 to 60 L/sec. The inspiratory pressure to trigger delivery should be set at 12 cm H_2O. PEEP should not be used unless ordered by medical control. Often, the proper settings will be listed somewhere on the machine as recorded by the home health nurse or respiratory therapist.

35. c. The most common cause of a high pressure alarm is obstruction of the tubing from secretions, mucous plugging, water, or a kink. If patients are anxious or coughing they will "buck" the ventilator and not allow it to deliver the inspiration. Calming and clearing of mucus will alleviate this. Cuff leaks, disconnections from the patient, or dislodgment of the tracheostomy will result in low pressure alarms.

36. d. Various medical conditions such as diabetes, gastrointestinal resection, cancer, and chronic infection may require long-term vascular access. The VAD allows continuous access to the blood stream without the inconvenience of repeated venipuncture.

37. b. The renal dialysis shunt is completely located in the peripheral venous system and connects the venous system to the arterial system.

38. a. Infection of the VAD site is the most common complication and usually results in its removal. Occlusion occurs from clotting of blood in the catheter or precipitation of the medications being administered through it. Emboli may break off from a thrombus or the catheter tip may shear away and travel to the heart. Infiltration occurs when fluid leaks around the puncture site of the vein into the surrounding tissue.

39. b. False. Often the reason a patient has a VAD is because of poor peripheral vein access. If aseptic technique is used the VAD can be used to administer prehospital therapy. However, if a suitable peripheral IV can be established, that is preferred.

40. c. The PICC line is usually inserted into a peripheral arm vein and threaded up and into the superior vena cava. The other listed devices are inserted directly into the central venous system at the subclavian vein. This is important in that more fluid is required to flush the PICC line than the other devices.

41. b. Occlusion of the catheter by thrombus is met with resistance when attempting to use the VAD. Attempting to dislodge the clot with irrigation could result in an embolus. If gentle aspiration does not relieve the obstruction the patient may require the administration of thrombolytics to dissolve the clot.

42. b. Acute urinary retention may occur from many causes, but in the long-term home care patient it is usually due to some neuromuscular disorder or cancer. The pain from bladder distension is carried via the autonomic nervous system, which is usually functional in the paraplegic.

43. c. Urinary tract infections, which may lead to urosepsis, represent the most serious complication of chronic indwelling urinary catheters and is usually the result of improper handling during insertion and cleaning.

44. c. Lack of urine in the drainage tube indicates that the bladder has not been entered. Significant resistance to inflation of the balloon further indicates that the tip of the catheter is not properly positioned. Either advance the catheter or remove it and try again.

45. d. Any bleeding as a result of urinary catheter passage is cause for concern and should receive prompt transportation to the hospital for evaluation.

46. b. As a result of bladder cancer the patient has had his bladder removed. The ureters are connected to a small segment of ileum removed from the small intestines and connected to the surface by an opening in the abdominal wall. The fluid is urine colored but may have some mucus from intestinal secretions.

47. d. Aspiration of gastric contents can result from improper positioning, overfilling of the stomach, and bowel obstruction. It can result in respiratory distress and pneumonia. Occlusion is the most common reason for their replacement but is not serious. Gastric perforation and infection are uncommon.

48. c. Previous abdominal surgery predisposes this patient to bowel obstruction from adhesions. Fecal impaction can occur from constipation and inadequate water intake. Stenosis of the ostomy could occlude the opening. Gastroenteritis would produce significant discharge from the ostomy.

49. d. The patient will require IV access because she is unable to tolerate fluid orally. An antiemetic such as Tigan, Compazine, or Zofran would be indicated. The myth that the administration of opiate analgesics to patients with abdominal pain has been refuted with excellent research that indicates that the surgical abdominal examination is actually enhanced by reduction in the patient's pain and anxiety with narcotic administration.

50. b. False. If properly trained the insertion of a nasogastric tube can relieve the pain and suffering associated with gastric distension and will reduce the likelihood of vomiting and aspiration during transport.

Miscellaneous and Special Operations

22

Legal Aspects

1. A contractual or legal obligation that may exist that requires EMS personnel to provide emergency medical care is the:
   a. Good Samaritan act
   b. medico-ethical act
   c. statute to act
   d. duty to act

2. Deviating from the accepted standard of care that a reasonable, prudent EMS provider would render is:
   a. abandonment
   b. breach of contract
   c. negligence
   d. breach of duty

3. Assistance may be rendered to an unconscious patient or to an ill child whose parents or guardians cannot be reached under the principle of:
   a. actual consent
   b. informed consent
   c. implied consent
   d. minor's consent

4. Terminating care of a patient without ensuring continuation of care at the same level or higher, or without the patient's consent to stop rendering care is:
   a. breach of contract
   b. assault and battery
   c. breach of consent
   d. abandonment

5. The four elements necessary to prove negligence are:
   a. duty to act, breach of duty, damage, and proximate cause
   b. actual consent, breach of duty, damage, and breach of confidentiality
   c. duty to act, breach of contract, injury, and abandonment
   d. lack of informed consent, duty to act, breach of contract, and damage

6. An EMS report or record:
   a. should be thorough and accurate
   b. cannot be changed after the patient is transferred to the hospital
   c. is of little value if an EMS provider is sued
   d. cannot be used in court

7. Guidelines for EMS providers that are established by local and state laws or protocols, professional organizations or societies, and acceptable case law precedents make up the:
   a. patient's bill of rights
   b. standard of care
   c. local tort laws
   d. civil EMS code

8. Generally, if there are no written Do Not Resuscitate (DNR) orders present, you should:
   a. attempt to contact the family doctor before starting CPR
   b. begin resuscitation efforts
   c. consult law enforcement officers on the legality of starting CPR
   d. accept the family's word that DNR orders exist

9. To refuse medical care, the patient must:
   a. refuse any and all care the EMS personnel may provide
   b. be 15 years of age or older
   c. not have received any medical care prior to the point of refusing
   d. be mentally competent

10. EMS personnel may be required to report a suspected situation involving:
    a. child abuse
    b. commission of a crime
    c. abuse of the elderly
    d. all of the above

Ambulance Operations

11. The recommended number of feet an ambulance should be parked from wreckage is:
    a. 50
    b. 100
    c. 150
    d. 200

12. Generally, ambulances should be escorted by police or other emergency vehicles:
    a. only if the crew is unfamiliar with the location of the patient or receiving facility
    b. whenever possible
    c. whenever responding to a potentially violent situation
    d. only when a operator with minimal experience is driving

13. A helicopter landing zone should ideally:
    a. be a maximum of 90 feet by 90 feet square
    b. be in a fenced area to keep onlookers away
    c. be at least 100 feet by 100 feet square
    d. have no more than a 15-degree slope

14. A medical helicopter should initially be approached:
    a. from the rear
    b. immediately after it lands
    c. from the front
    d. in a standing position

15. The "2-second rule" refers to:
    a. the amount of time the ambulance should remain stopped at a traffic light before proceeding
    b. the length of time a driver should look in the sideview mirror
    c. the maximum amount of time it should take the driver to make a driving decision
    d. the safe distance that should be maintained between the ambulance and a vehicle it is following

16. Before crossing an intersection, the emergency vehicle driver should:
    a. look to the left, then to the right, and then again to the left
    b. turn off the siren and listen for other emergency vehicles
    c. look to the right, and then the left
    d. turn on the vehicle's 4-way flashers

Multiple Casualty Situations

17. The five major components of FEMA's Incident Command System (ICS) organization are:
    a. command, finance, logistics, operations, planning (C-FLOP)
    b. fire, rescue, EMS, police, HazMat (FREPH)
    c. medical, triage, treatment, transportation, staging (M-TTT-S)
    d. safety, liaison, information, command, staging (SLICS)

18. A unified command structure would be useful at all of the following types of incidents *EXCEPT*:
    a. an incident that affects more than one jurisdiction
    b. an incident involving multiple agencies within a jurisdiction
    c. an incident involving a structure fire that requires multiple engine and ladder companies to control
    d. an incident that has an impact on multiple geographical and functional agencies

19. The three Command Staff positions in the Incident Command System are:
    a. Triage Unit Leader, Treatment Unit Leader, and Transportation Unit Leader
    b. Fire Officer, EMS Officer, and Law Enforcement Officer
    c. Branch Director, Group Supervisor, and Unit Leader
    d. Safety Officer, Information Officer, and Liaison Officer

20. The responsibility of the first arriving EMS unit at a mass casualty incident is to:
    a. immediately transport the most critical patients to the nearest hospital
    b. assume command, assess the situation, and not perform any patient care
    c. start extricating patients
    d. start caring for the most critically injured victims

21. A yellow triage tag signifies:
    a. a second-priority patient
    b. a patient who has minor injuries
    c. an obviously dead patient
    d. a lowest-priority patient

22. The position of triage officer should be assigned to:
    a. the highest ranking EMS officer
    b. the EMS provider with the most seniority
    c. the most qualified EMS provider
    d. a nurse, if available

23. A green triage tag signifies a patient:
    a. with moderate-priority injuries
    b. with low-priority injuries
    c. who is suffering psychological problems because of the incident
    d. who is ready to be transported

24. Match the following sectors/groups/units with their primary responsibilities: extrication, transportation, treatment, triage, staging, supply.

    _____ sorts patients based on medical priority

    _____ obtains and distributes resources such as medical equipment and personnel

    _____ ascertains capabilities of receiving hospitals and coordinates loading of ambulances

    _____ rescues patients who are trapped at the scene

    _____ organizes incoming ambulances and coordinates the movement of ambulances to the loading zone

    _____ coordinates medical care for injured patients after they have been sorted and moved

25. Using the following descriptions to prioritize patients at a mass casualty scene, categorize them as first, second, third, or fourth. (NOTE: If you normally use the color system, mark the patients as red, yellow, green, or black.)

    _____ severe head injury, no pulse or breathing

    _____ severe burns

    _____ multiple bone or joint injuries

    _____ minor soft tissue injuries

    _____ unconscious, unknown cause

    _____ back injury without spinal damage

    _____ a severe medical problem

    _____ shock

    _____ extremity fracture accompanied by minimal pain

    _____ multiple traumatic injuries accompanied by full cardiac arrest

    _____ burns without airway problems

    _____ active labor with a breach presentation

26. A red triage tag signifies a patient who is:
    a. bleeding
    b. a delayed transport patient
    c. burned
    d. a highest-priority patient

27. Your unit is dispatched to a shooting in a school. While responding, you are advised that there are multiple persons injured. You are also advised to use caution because the perpetrator has not yet been apprehended and a serious fire is burning in one of the classrooms. You would likely expect this incident to be managed using:
    a. strategic command
    b. unified command
    c. roving command
    d. single command

28. When using the START triage system, the three primary parameters that are assessed are:
    a. airway, breathing, and circulation (ABC)
    b. appearance, respiration, mentation (ARM)
    c. pulse, perfusion, performance (PPP)
    d. respiration, perfusion, mentation (RPM)

29. The difference between primary and secondary triage is:
a. primary triage uses paper tags to indicate a patient's condition, but secondary triage uses color-coded tape or ribbon
b. primary triage is performed at the incident site to rapidly categorize patients condition for treatment, and secondary triage is performed in the treatment area
c. primary triage categorizes patients based on their airway-breathing-circulation status, whereas secondary triage is based on pulse rate, blood pressure, and respiratory rate
d. primary triage is performed at the incident site to rapidly categorize patient's condition for treatment, and secondary triage is performed in the treatment area

Hazardous Materials

30. The primary responsibility of EMS responders at an incident involving hazardous materials is:
a. identifying the hazardous material
b. controlling any spills or leaks
c. the safety of self, the public, and any patients
d. removing patients in the immediate vicinity of the hazardous material

31. Hazardous material transported by motor vehicles may be identified by:
a. calling CHEMTREC
b. obtaining a sample and sending it to a laboratory
c. referencing the ID number on the placard
d. contacting the local poison control center

32. Information about a hazardous material used at an industrial or commercial site is best obtained:
a. from the NFPA 704 symbol on the building
b. from a Material Safety Data Sheet (MSDS)
c. by interviewing plant employees
d. by reading the label on the container from which the substance came

33. Generally, EMS personnel should enter an area where hazardous materials are found:
a. any time a patient's life is in danger
b. if the EMS provider has completed a hazmat "Awareness" course
c. whenever firefighting turnout gear is available
d. only if the EMS provider has proper training in wearing hazmat equipment and SCBA

34. EMS vehicles and personnel at a scene involving hazardous materials should be positioned:
a. upwind from the incident and at a safe distance
b. downwind from the incident
c. close enough to quickly reach anyone who is sick or injured as a result of the incident
d. downhill from the incident

35. Match the following placard or label colors to the corresponding type of hazardous material: blue, green, black/white, orange, red, red/white, white, yellow.
_____ flammable/combustible (liquid or gas)
_____ flammable solid
_____ water reactive
_____ poison (solid, liquid, or gas)
_____ oxygen/oxidizer
_____ explosive
_____ nonflammable gas
_____ corrosive

36. The blue triangular area containing a "W" with a line through it, situated in the upper corner of the placard in Figure 22-1, means:
a. the material is not a waste product
b. wearing protective suits is not necessary
c. the material is not affected by weather conditions
d. water should not be placed on the material

Figure 22-1

37. The small number "2" at the bottom of the placard in Figure 22-2 indicates the material is a:
a. gas
b. liquid
c. solid
d. high explosive

Figure 22-2

38. When the NFPA 704 system is used, the blue diamond within the placard relates to the material's:
a. flammability hazard
b. reactivity hazard
c. health hazard
d. special hazard

39. The decontamination corridor is found within the:
a. cold zone
b. warm zone
c. hot zone
d. red zone

40. Hazardous materials that damage the liver are classified as:
a. cardiotoxins
b. hemotoxins
c. hepatotoxins
d. nephrotoxins

41. The two primary goals of rapid decontamination are to:
a. remove the patient from danger and then provide gross decontamination
b. perform gross decontamination followed by administration of specific antidotes
c. isolate the hazardous environment and perform a rapid patient assessment
d. wash the patient with a neutralizing agent and then provide a thorough rinse with clean water

ANSWERS TO CHAPTER 22: MISCELLANEOUS AND SPECIAL OPERATIONS

Legal Aspects

1. d. Duty to act refers to the responsibility of an EMS provider, either by statute or function, to provide patient care when the opportunity presents itself.

2. c. A deviation from the accepted standard of care that a reasonable, prudent EMS provider would render is considered negligence.

3. c. Implied consent allows medical care providers to assist an unconscious patient or a minor child if a true emergency situation exists. The basis of implied consent is that a rational and reasonable person who is similarly ill or injured but able to communicate would want medical care.

4. d. Abandonment is inappropriate termination of care or turning care over to personnel who do not have training and expertise appropriate for the medical needs of the patient. An example would be a paramedic passing the care of a patient needing advanced life support care to an EMT-Basic.

5. a. In most states, four elements must be proved for negligence to exist: (1) there was a duty to act; (2) there was a breach of duty (i.e., actions were performed at a level below the standard of care); (3) there was damage to the patient or other individual; and (4) the breach of duty was the proximate cause of the damage.

6. a. Because they are important safeguards, EMS reports and records must be thorough and accurate. No one has a memory good enough to remember everything about a call, and lawsuits may occur years later. The EMS report is a legal document that is admissible in court. The document, if sloppy and incomplete, can be detrimental because it implies that the EMS provider's abilities are also sloppy and incomplete. Testimony from memory may not be enough; the court will generally view a procedure or action not documented as not having been performed.

7. b. The standard of care is established by local and state laws or protocols, professional organizations and societies, and acceptable case law precedents.

8. b. Although EMS providers should honor written DNR orders, it is generally recommended that resuscitation efforts be started if the DNR orders are not physically present. In many areas, if DNR orders are produced while resuscitation efforts are being performed, the efforts may be ceased.

9. d. To refuse medical care, the patient must be mentally competent. A patient is allowed to refuse a particular form of therapy or one aspect of care. The patient can refuse further care even after treatment procedures have been started. Although there are some exceptions, patients generally must be at least 18 years of age to refuse treatment.

10. d. In most areas, EMS personnel are required to report a situation that they suspect involves abuse of a child or the elderly, or the commission of a crime. Check your local protocols and laws for reporting guidelines and procedures.

Ambulance Operations

11. b. It is generally recommended that an ambulance be parked at least 100 feet from wreckage.

12. a. If the crew is unfamiliar with how to get to the location of the patient or how to get to the receiving facility, it is generally acceptable for the police or other emergency vehicles to escort an ambulance. Even in these cases, however, escorts should be avoided if possible because of the dangers involved in escort situations. In these cases, it is best if an experienced driver is operating the ambulance.

13. c. Ideally, a helicopter landing zone should be at least 100 feet by 100 feet. For larger helicopters, 125 feet by 125 feet is desirable (consult local air medical services for recommended size). The ground should have no more than a 10-degree slope and should be clear of wires, fences, or other obstructions.

14. c. Most medical helicopters should initially be approached only from the front and approached only after being directed to do so by the pilot or flight crew. Stay low when approaching the helicopter because rotor blades can dip low to the ground and cause injury.

15. d. The "2-second rule" refers to the distance that should be maintained between an emergency vehicle and the vehicle in front of it. Using a fixed object as a reference point, it should take the emergency vehicle at least 2 seconds to reach the object after the vehicle ahead has passed the object. This following distance should be increased if driving conditions are hazardous or if the emergency vehicle is a large fire or rescue truck.

16. a. Before crossing an intersection, the emergency vehicle driver should look to the left, then the right, and then again to the left.

Multiple Casualty Situations

17. a. The five major components of FEMA's Incident Command System (ICS) organization are command, finance, logistics, operations, planning. The acronym C-FLOP can be used to remember the components.

18. c. A unified command structure would most likely be used at incidents that affect more than one jurisdiction, that involve multiple agencies within a jurisdiction, or that have an impact on multiple geographic and functional agencies. An incident such as one involving a structure fire that requires multiple engine and ladder companies to control is more likely to be managed with a singular command structure with a fire officer assuming the position of Incident Commander.

19. d. The three Command Staff positions are the Safety Officer, Information Officer, and Liaison Officer.

20. b. The first EMS unit to arrive at a multiple casualty incident should assume medical command, assess the situation, start calling for additional aid, and direct incoming units. Patient care should not be started by this unit. Clear command must be established early if the incident is to be managed in an orderly fashion. If enough EMS personnel are present, triage may also be started.

21. a. A yellow triage tag signifies a second-priority or moderately injured patient.

22. c. The most qualified and competent EMS provider should assume the role of triage officer. Rank and seniority are unimportant at the scene of a multiple casualty incident. Nurses, unless specially trained, lack the experience and expertise necessary to properly triage patients in the field.

23. b. A green triage tag signifies a patient with minor injuries. These are delayed-priority patients. Patients with green tags are sometimes referred to as the "walking wounded." This is not an accurate term because some walking patients may have severe injuries, and some patients with minor injuries may not be able to walk.

24. Match the following sectors/groups/units with their primary responsibilities: extrication, transportation, treatment, triage, staging, supply.

triage sorts patients based on medical priority

supply obtains and distributes resources such as medical equipment and personnel

transportation ascertains capabilities of receiving hospitals and coordinates loading of ambulances

extrication rescues patients who are trapped at the scene

staging organizes incoming ambulances and coordinates the movement of ambulances to the loading zone

treatment coordinates medical care for injured patients after they have been sorted and moved

25. Using the following descriptions to prioritize patients at a mass casualty scene, categorize them as first, second, third, or fourth. (NOTE: If you normally use the color system, mark the patients as red, yellow, green, or black.)

fourth (black) severe head injury, no pulse or breathing

first (red) severe burns

second (yellow) multiple bone or joint injuries

third (green) minor soft tissue injuries

first (red) unconscious, unknown cause

second (yellow) back injury without spinal damage

first (red) a severe medical problem

first (red) shock

third (green) extremity fracture accompanied by minimal pain

fourth (black) multiple traumatic injuries accompanied by full cardiac arrest

second (yellow) burns without airway problems

first (red) active labor with a breach presentation

26. d. A red triage tag signifies a critical, first-priority patient.

27. b. Because this type of an incident involves operations of multiple agencies (EMS, law enforcement, and fire), it would best be managed with a unified command structure.

28. d. The three primary parameters that are assessed when using the START triage system are respiration, perfusion, and mentation. These parameters can be remembered with the acronym RPM. The parameters are a respiratory rate of 30, whether capillary refill is under or over 2 seconds or whether a radial pulse is present, and whether the patient can follow basic commands (mentation).

29. b. Primary triage is performed at the incident site to rapidly categorize patients' condition for treatment. Triage tags, labels, or tape/ribbon may be used and the focus is to sort patients quickly. Secondary triage is performed in the treatment area. The goal is to retriage patients to assign priorities of care and transport.

Hazardous Materials

30. c. The primary responsibility of EMS responders at a hazardous materials incident is their own safety and the safety of the public and any patients. Access to patients should be accomplished only after personnel are properly protected with appropriate gear and breathing apparatus. Although early identification of the substance is important, it does not take priority over safety considerations. Identification is usually the responsibility of the fire department or hazardous materials team. Controlling the actual incident is not usually the job of EMS personnel.

31. c. Identification of hazardous materials transported by motor vehicles is best made by referencing the four-digit guide number found on placards and shipping information. Keep in mind, however, that the ID number on the placard may not provide exact identification because the number may be used to identify more than one chemical in a closely related group. The vehicle operator may not know what is being carried, and laboratory testing is a time-consuming process. Never smell or touch a potentially hazardous material. Identification should always be made while the EMS personnel remain at a safe distance from the incident.

32. b. Information about a hazardous material used at an industrial or commercial site is best obtained by referencing a Material Safety Data Sheet (MSDS). Plant employees may not be familiar with the material or may provide inaccurate information, and the container may be misleading.

33. d. Generally, only EMS personnel with proper training in wearing hazmat equipment and SCBA should enter an area where hazardous materials are found.

34. a. EMS vehicles and personnel at a scene involving hazardous material should be positioned upwind and uphill from the incident at a safe distance. Shouting distance is normally much too close because fumes may quickly reach EMS personnel. In most instances, patients should be brought to EMS personnel, unless the EMS provider is properly trained and protected to enter the scene.

35. Match the following placard or label colors to the corresponding type of hazardous material: blue, green, black/white, orange, red, red/white, white, yellow.

red flammable/combustible (liquid or gas)

red/white flammable solid

blue water reactive

white poison (solid, liquid or gas)

yellow oxygen/oxidizer

orange explosive

green nonflammable gas

black/white corrosive

36. d. A blue triangular area containing a "W" with a line through it, situated in the upper corner of a placard, signifies that the material is reactive to water and water should not be placed on it.

37. a. A small number "2" at the bottom of a placard indicates that the material is a gas. This number is known as the class or division number. The numbering system is as follows: 1: explosive, 2: gas, 3: flammable liquid, 4: flammable solid, 5: oxidizer, 6: poisons, 7: radioactive materials, 8: corrosives, 9: miscellaneous.

38. c. When the NFPA 704 system is used, the blue diamond within the placard relates to the material's health hazard. The red diamond relates to the material's flammability hazard, the yellow diamond to the reactivity hazard, and the white diamond shows any special hazards. The numbers 0 through 4 appear within the blue, red, and yellow diamonds and relate to the degree of hazard.

39. b. The decontamination corridor is located within the warm or yellow zone. This is the buffer zone between the hot or red zone where contamination is present and the cold or green zone, which is safe.

40. c. Hepatotoxins are substances that damage the liver. Cardiotoxins are hazardous materials that may induce myocardial ischemia and cardiac rhythm disturbances. Hemotoxins are hazardous substances that may cause the destruction of red blood cells resulting in hemolytic anemia, and nephrotoxins are especially destructive to the kidneys.

41. a. Rapid decontamination is a two-step process that consists of removing the patient from danger and then providing gross decontamination.

CASE PRESENTATIONS

23

1. Your unit responds to assess a 58-year-old female patient with a history of diabetes. She states she just doesn't feel right and is having nonspecific pain in her upper back under her left shoulder blade. She denies having sustained any recent injuries. Vital signs are pulse 88 and regular, blood pressure 146/82, respirations 16, and oxygen saturation of 97% on room air. Appropriate management would include:
   a. backboard, cervical collar, and morphine
   b. 12-lead ECG, oxygen, and IV
   c. albuterol, Lasix, and high-flow oxygen
   d. diazepam, D_{50}, and cervical immobilization device

2. It is an icy winter morning, and a compact car has been struck by a van. The 23-year-old driver of the car, who was unrestrained, has been thrown into the passenger seat by the force of the collision. There is minor entrapment, but the door is quickly forced. The patient, who already has a cervical collar on, is carefully but rapidly removed to a backboard and to the warm ambulance. The patient's primary complaint is some dyspnea accompanied by some belly pain. The patient has a pulse of 132, blood pressure of 114/72, respiratory rate of 24, and oxygen saturation of 92%. You expose his chest and listen to breath sounds. The left side is clear. When listening to the right side, you clearly hear breath sounds on the upper right, but can hear no breath sounds below the nipple line. You suspect this patient has a:
   a. herniated diaphragm
   b. tension pneumothorax
   c. hemothorax
   d. pulmonary contusion

3. A 54-year-old male has substernal chest pain radiating to his left arm, has dyspnea, and is pale and diaphoretic He has a history of heart problems and has already taken a nitroglycerin tablet with no relief. Your pharmacological management is most likely to include:
   a. aspirin and morphine only because the patient has already taken his nitroglycerin and received no relief
   b. oxygen, Lasix, and nitroglycerin
   c. morphine, diazepam, and adenosine
   d. additional nitroglycerin, aspirin, and morphine

4. Your patient is a 28-year-old female in her eighth month of pregnancy. Her family called because she had been complaining of a severe, persistent headache and was vomiting. As you begin your evaluation, you notice that her face and hands appear swollen. She is somewhat confused and disoriented, and vital signs reveal a blood pressure of 162/100. Further questioning of the family reveals the patient experienced sudden weight gain prior to the onset of the other complaints. While caring for this patient, be alert for:
   a. a sudden drop in blood pressure
   b. sudden respiratory arrest
   c. seizures
   d. uncontrolled vaginal bleeding

5. A medication that may be needed while managing this patient is:
   a. proparacaine
   b. oxytocin
   c. dopamine
   d. magnesium sulfate

6. After arriving home from work, a man finds his wife unconscious in bed. Your patient is a 28-year-old woman. She is responsive only to painful stimuli. Her pulse is 128, and she is pale and sweating. The husband tells you she is an insulin-dependent diabetic. Management of this patient would likely include starting an IV and administering:
   a. adenosine
   b. D$_{50}$
   c. naloxone
   d. diphenhydramine

7. If you were unable to start an IV, an option would be to:
   a. administer glucagon IM
   b. administer naloxone through an ET tube
   c. administer epinephrine subcutaneously
   d. administer nebulized albuterol

8. You have been summoned to the local shopping mall to examine a pregnant female experiencing an "unknown problem." She is pale, her pulse is rapid and weak, and she is complaining of severe, localized abdominal pain. She is in her eighth month of pregnancy. Physical examination reveals some bleeding from the vagina. The patient denies any previous episodes of bleeding. This presentation most likely indicates:
   a. ectopic pregnancy
   b. spontaneous abortion
   c. postpartum hemorrhage
   d. abruptio placentae

9. Management of this patient would include:
   a. administering oxytocin
   b. rapid transport to the closest hospital
   c. starting two IVs using large-bore needles
   d. monitoring for seizure activity and administering magnesium sulfate

10. You are dispatched to a "sick person" at a local restaurant. Upon arrival, you find a female patient reclining in a booth. Friends say she was talking but suddenly became unresponsive. She is breathing and responds somewhat to verbal stimuli but can only utter sounds. Upon examination you notice that she is unable to move her extremities on the left side, and her mouth tends to droop on the left side. Her vital signs are within normal range. Based on the clinical presentation, you likely the suspect the patient is experiencing:
    a. a myocardial infarction
    b. an allergic reaction to food
    c. a stroke
    d. seizure activity

11. This patient is best transported:
    a. in a supine position with the head elevated 15 degrees
    b. in a prone position
    c. on her right side with her feet elevated
    d. sitting upright

12. The patient is a full-term pregnant female in labor. When you examine the vaginal area, you notice a section of the cord protruding from the vaginal opening. As part of your management, you may need to:
    a. tell the patient to push as hard as possible to assist with delivery
    b. use two gloved fingers to push the presenting part of the fetus away from the cord
    c. attempt to reposition the cord
    d. tell the patient to cross her legs and not to push

13. The patient should be transported:
    a. on her knees with her buttocks up in the air and her chest lower than her pelvis
    b. on her back with her head and shoulders slightly elevated
    c. on her left side with her head slightly elevated
    d. sitting upright with her knees flexed and a pillow underneath the knees to provide support

14. Proper care of the exposed umbilical cord includes:
    a. attempting to push the cord back into the birth canal
    b. wrapping the cord in a dry trauma dressing
    c. covering it with a moist, sterile dressing
    d. placing cord clamps on the exposed section

15. For the second time in the day, you are dispatched to the same local retirement home. Your patient is an active and independent 72-year-old woman. She is not pleased that her neighbors summoned you, but she is obviously having a lot of difficulty breathing. She states she has been short of breath for about the past 4 hours, but did not want to bother anyone. She has no chest pain. Her pulse is 96 and irregular, her blood pressure is 144/82, her breathing rate is 26 and labored, and her oxygen saturation is 89% on room air. When you listen to her chest, you note wheezing on both inspiration and expiration. Questioning about medical history reveals she has a history of emphysema. The medication of choice for this patient is:
    a. furosemide IV
    b. nebulized albuterol
    c. epinephrine SQ
    d. nitroglycerin sublingually

16. Your unit is called to a feed store for a person injured in the storeroom. Your patient is a 15-year-old teenager who was moving inventory when a shelf containing unmarked bags of dry powder fell over. Many of the bags have burst, and your patient is covered with the unknown powder. He is complaining of nausea, abdominal cramps, and moderate difficulty breathing. While performing your examination, you notice that he is sweating and salivating profusely and his eyes are watery. There is some uncontrolled muscle twitching present. The patient's symptoms are most likely related to:
    a. a possible intracranial bleed
    b. partial seizures
    c. organophosphate poisoning
    d. hypoxia caused by inhaling a powder

17. Early management of the patient would include:
    a. placing the patient in shock position and conserving body heat
    b. wiping off the powder with a damp rag
    c. wrapping the patient in a plastic sheet
    d. brushing off as much powder as possible and washing off the rest

18. A medication that would likely be administered to this patient is:
    a. naloxone
    b. dopamine
    c. D$_{50}$
    d. atropine

19. It is a typical Friday night at the local knife and gun club, better known as "The East End Bar and Grill." Your patient was on the losing end of a disagreement and received multiple stab wounds to the chest. The knife is still in place. The patient is conscious and complaining of dyspnea. His pulse is rapid and weak. A Level I trauma center is about 8 minutes away. Management of this patient will likely include:
    a. removing the knife because it may interfere with breathing
    b. starting two large-bore IVs and running them wide open until reaching the hospital
    c. leaving the knife in place and stabilizing it with a bulky dressing
    d. calling for a helicopter to provide air evacuation

20. The other chest wounds should be:
    a. covered only if bleeding is severe
    b. covered with a loose, bulky dressing
    c. left uncovered to allow rapid evaluation by hospital personnel
    d. covered with an occlusive dressing

21. On the way to the hospital your patient develops severe respiratory difficulty. You listen to breath sounds and note that they are severely diminished on the right side. Your next action would be to:
    a. insert a large gauge needle in the second intercostal space, midaxillary line, going over the top of the rib
    b. insert a large gauge needle in the fifth intercostal space, midclavicular line, going under the bottom of the rib
    c. insert a large gauge needle in the second intercostal space, midclavicular line, going over the top of the rib
    d. insert a large gauge needle in the fifth intercostal space, midaxillary line, going under the bottom of the rib

22. It is a sunny fall day. The patient is a 9-year-old girl who was outside playing in the leaves at a friend's house when she began having difficulty breathing. Her friend's parents tell you that she has a history of asthma, but this attack seems much worse than others. When assessing the patient you note that she is restless and very anxious and that auscultation of breath sounds reveals pronounced wheezing, primarily on expiration. Attempts to contact the parents have been unsuccessful. Ideally, part of the management of this patient would include administering:
    a. 0.05 to 0.15 mg/kg albuterol via nebulizer
    b. 1 mg epinephrine 1:10,000 IV
    c. 5 mg diazepam IM
    d. 20 mg Lasix IV

23. This incident was likely precipitated by:
    a. an emotional stress
    b. an infection
    c. an allergic reaction
    d. a drop in the patient's blood sugar level

24. If this patient's parents were not available to give permission to treat and transport the patient, EMS personnel:
    a. can transport, but only if a police officer places the child in protective custody
    b. can treat and transport under the principle of implied consent
    c. have to wait to transport until another close relative could be contacted
    d. can transport but are not legally permitted to treat the patient without parental consent

25. Your patient is a 39-year-old male who has been experiencing persistent abdominal pain for the last 12 hours with no relief. He has a history of alcoholism but takes no medications. He states he has been vomiting and that it "looks funny." You notice the vomitus in a trash can, and it resembles coffee grounds. His abdomen is generally tender. Vital signs reveal a slightly rapid pulse and breathing, but blood pressure is normal. You suspect this patient has:
   a. alcohol poisoning
   b. appendicitis
   c. gastrointestinal bleeding
   d. cardiac compromise

26. The patient states that he is extremely thirsty. You should:
   a. start a large-bore IV to provide the patient some fluid
   b. give the patient water to drink, but less than one cup
   c. encourage the patient to drink as much as possible to replenish lost fluids
   d. start two large-bore IVs and run them both wide open

27. A patient is in active labor. Upon your arrival, you follow all the local protocols for handling imminent delivery. Everything seems to be going routinely, but immediately after moving your patient to your cot, her bag of waters breaks. You notice that the fluid is thick and resembles pea soup. You become concerned because you are now dealing with:
   a. abruptio placentae
   b. a meconium emergency
   c. preeclampsia
   d. toxemia of pregnancy

28. If the baby is delivered before reaching the hospital and is depressed (e.g., poor respiratory effort, decreased muscle tone, or heart rate less than 100 beats per minute), your primary action should be to:
   a. immediately cut the cord
   b. immediately get an APGAR score
   c. warm, dry, and stimulate the infant
   d. aggressively suction the baby's airway

29. You are dispatched to the city park for a person with difficulty breathing. Upon arriving, you encounter a distraught 19-year-old girl who has been stung by a bee. She is complaining of diffuse itching and a tightness in her throat and chest. Physical exam reveals a generalized rash accompanied by hives and a weak, rapid pulse. Wheezing is noted when you listen to the chest. This patient is experiencing:
   a. status asthmaticus
   b. mild allergic reaction
   c. an anaphylactic reaction
   d. status epilepticus

30. You note that the stinger is still imbedded in your patient's arm. You should:
   a. remove the stinger with a pair of tweezers
   b. leave the stinger in place
   c. cover the stinger with a cold pack
   d. scrape the stinger out using the edge of a card

31. Medications that may be used in the management of this patient include:
   a. albuterol, atropine, and adenosine
   b. atropine, epinephrine, and lidocaine
   c. albuterol, epinephrine, and diphenhydramine
   d. D_{50}, diphenhydramine, and naloxone

32. Your unit is sent to the scene of a person who has fallen down a flight of steps at a college dormitory. The patient is a 20-year-old male who fell approximately three fourths of the way down a long flight of steps. The patient is unconscious and lying on his back at the bottom landing. Assessment of the patient reveals he has a blood pressure of 76/40 and a weak, regular pulse with a rate of 64. His skin is dry and flushed. You suspect he is suffering from:
   a. psychogenic shock
   b. neurogenic shock
   c. anaphylactic shock
   d. septic shock

33. Your patient is an 82-year-old woman with severe difficulty breathing. As you enter the house, you hear gurgling breathing from the back bedroom. She is sitting upright in bed and coughing up frothy sputum. When you listen to her breath sounds, you hear rales and rhonchi bilaterally. She has difficulty speaking, but denies any pain. You notice her neck veins are distended, and examination of her ankles and feet reveal marked swelling. This patient's primary problem is most likely related to:
    a. chronic obstructive pulmonary disease (COPD)
    b. an acute asthma attack
    c. an acute myocardial infarction
    d. congestive heart failure (CHF)

34. Pharmacological interventions for this patient would include:
    a. albuterol, atropine, and furosemide
    b. nitroglycerin, furosemide, and morphine
    c. dopamine, adenosine, and nitroglycerin
    d. diphenhydramine, lidocaine, and morphine

35. Your patient was recently released from the hospital after undergoing abdominal surgery. The patient had a coughing spell, which caused his stitches to rupture. Upon your arrival you find part of the man's intestines protruding through the open incision. Management would include:
    a. replacing the organs in the abdominal cavity
    b. covering the organs with a moist, sterile dressing
    c. applying direct pressure on the organs to prevent internal bleeding
    d. covering the organs with a dry, sterile dressing

36. The patient should be transported:
    a. on his left side with his knees and hips flexed
    b. sitting up with his knees straight
    c. on his back with his knees and hips flexed
    d. on his right side with his knees and hips straight

37. It's another Friday night at the local high school football game. As usual, your team is losing. You and your partner are standing by at the game trying to make the best of the last 10 minutes before returning to the station when spectators nearby start yelling that someone has "passed out." It takes you only about a minute to reach a 58-year-old man who is in cardiac arrest. Your first action is to:
    a. begin two-rescuer CPR
    b. intubate the patient
    c. attach the patient to an ECG monitor/defibrillator
    d. establish IV access

38. When analyzing the patient's ECG, you see the rhythm shown in Figure 23-1. Your partner confirms that pulses are absent. At this point, your next action is to immediately:
    a. try to identify a correctable cause of the rhythm
    b. defibrillate the patient
    c. intubate the patient
    d. initiate transcutaneous pacing

39. After inserting an endotracheal tube in the patient and verifying placement, an IV is initiated. Medications that may be included in protocols to manage this patient include:
    a. vasopressin, epinephrine, and amiodarone
    b. epinephrine, atropine, and lidocaine
    c. adenosine, amiodarone, and atropine
    d. nitroglycerin, morphine, and procainamide

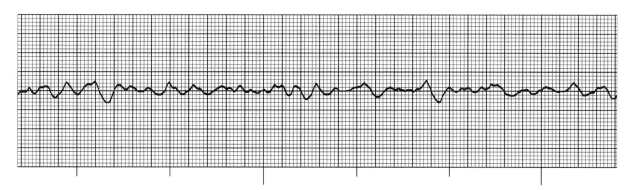

Figure 23-1

40. You are dispatched to a possible behavioral emergency. When you enter the house, police are already on the scene arguing with a 43-year-old male. You notice the inside of the house has been demolished prior to your arrival. The patient tells you that foreign agents are trying to kill him by letting tarantulas loose in his house. From time to time the patient claims to see one going under a piece of overturned furniture. He also tells you that he is convinced that the agents operate out of the local hospital and that he is not going to be taken alive. Discussion with the patient's family reveals that he has a long history of behavioral problems and he has not been taking his prescribed medication. He also has a history of violence. You should:
    a. offer to help the patient kill all the tarantulas if he goes with you to the hospital
    b. tell him you are just taking him to see his family doctor
    c. join the police in arguing with him about going to the hospital
    d. consider restraining the patient

41. While returning from the hospital, you and your partner notice a crowd gathered on a downtown street corner. A man is lying on the ground actively seizing. Bystanders say he was jogging down the street when he suddenly fell to the sidewalk and started to jerk violently. You notice blood coming from the vicinity of the left side of his head. Your first action in assisting the patient is to:
    a. protect him from further injury
    b. intubate the patient to protect the lungs from aspirate
    c. control the bleeding from his scalp
    d. establish an IV

42. While managing the patient, you note that the seizure activity is continuing without any intervening periods of consciousness. The most appropriate first-line drug of choice for this patient is:
    a. D_{50}
    b. diazepam
    c. magnesium sulfate
    d. lidocaine

43. The dose indicated for this patient is:
    a. 1 mg/kg IV
    b. 1 to 4.0 mg IM
    c. 5 to 10 mg IV
    d. 2 g IM

44. A 62-year-old male has gone into cardiac arrest while at work in a fabricating plant. He is currently one level above the main floor lying on a metal grate deck. Co-workers are doing CPR. The first priority in this situation is to:
    a. defibrillate the patient
    b. move the patient off of the metal decking
    c. intubate the patient
    d. administer epinephrine

45. When analyzing the patient's ECG, you see the rhythm shown in Figure 23-2. Your partner confirms that pulses are absent. A critical component of managing this patient includes:
    a. trying to identify a correctable cause of the rhythm
    b. administering 0.5 mg of epinephrine every 3 to 5 minutes for the duration of the arrest
    c. alternating doses of epinephrine and atropine
    d. early initiation of transcutaneous pacing

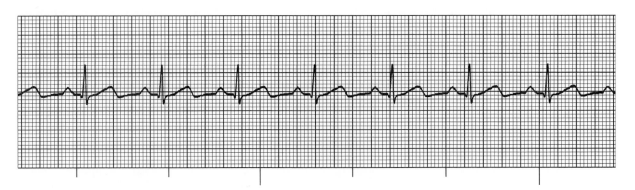

Figure 23-2

46. After inserting an endotracheal tube in the patient and checking for breath sounds, you note that breath sounds are only heard on the right side. Your next action would be to:
   a. deflate the cuff, pull the tube out, and reattempt intubation
   b. deflate the cuff and pull the tube back slightly
   c. deflate the cuff and insert the tube slightly further into the lungs
   d. leave the tube in place and ventilate at a faster rate

47. IV access is difficult. While continuing to try to gain IV access, your crew can:
   a. administer 1 mg of atropine down the ET tube
   b. administer 2 mg of epinephrine down the ET tube
   c. administer 40 units of vasopressin down the ET tube
   d. administer 300 mg of amiodarone down the ET tube

48. A 26-year-old woman went into active labor at home. Just prior to your arrival, police advise you the infant has been born. When you reach the scene, you find a newborn who is limp and has a heart rate of 88. Your first action is to:
   a. begin ventilating the infant with 100% oxygen
   b. begin chest compressions
   c. intubate the newborn
   d. administer oxygen by nonrebreather mask

49. When you reassess the newborn, you find the infant's heart rate has now dropped to 56. At this point, you should:
   a. ventilate the infant but not perform chest compressions
   b. attempt to stimulate the baby by flicking the soles of its feet
   c. begin chest compressions
   d. suction the infant

50. There has been a serious motor vehicle crash on the expressway. You and your partner have just removed an injured patient who is 7 months pregnant. Your assessment reveals that she has a pulse rate of 132 and a blood pressure of 82/58. During transport, it is best to position your patient:
   a. on her right side with her head slightly elevated
   b. flat on her back
   c. in a position of comfort
   d. on her left side

51. A man has been injured in a boiler explosion at a local factory. He has partial-thickness burns over 50% of his body. Your exam reveals that he has a pulse of 116 and a blood pressure of 90/68. The likely reason for this patient's rapid pulse and low blood pressure is:
   a. the patient has a spinal injury with accompanying neurogenic shock
   b. the patient has another serious injury causing blood loss
   c. a large volume of fluid has been lost through seepage from the burns
   d. hypothermia has developed because of heat loss through the area of the burn

52. It is mid-December. You and your partner respond to a report of an unconscious man in the park. You find a male who appears to be in his mid-40s lying on a park bench partly covered with newspapers. An almost empty alcohol bottle is next to the bench. The patient responds only to painful stimuli, he has a slow breathing rate, and his extremities look cyanotic. The most likely serious condition responsible for this situation is that he is:
   a. postictal following a seizure
   b. suffering from a stroke
   c. hypothermic
   d. intoxicated

53. Treatment of the patient on the park bench would include:
   a. gently handling the patient when moving him to the ambulance
   b. trying to get the patient to drink warm fluids
   c. gently massaging the patient's arms and legs
   d. applying heat packs to the arms and legs

54. While moving the patient into the ambulance, he suddenly goes into cardiac arrest. A quick look at the ECG reveals ventricular fibrillation. Initial management of this patient would be to:
   a. start CPR but do no ALS procedures until the patient can be rewarmed
   b. immediately start CPR and initiate overdrive pacing with a transcutaneous pacemaker
   c. defibrillate at 200 J, 300 J, 360 J; intubate; and consult medical control for further instructions
   d. defibrillate at 200 J, 300 J, 360 J; start core rewarming procedures; and follow standard guidelines for managing ventricular fibrillation

55. It's 3:00 A.M., and a local resident awoke when she heard the sound of metal hitting a solid object. A car has struck a large tree head on, and now you and your crew must take care of the severely injured 23-year-old driver. He is unresponsive and was obviously unrestrained. The steering wheel of the car is severely bent. Your patient is having obvious trouble breathing, and his breathing is shallow and slow. He is also cyanotic. Your partner listens to breath sounds and advises you that they are present on the left side but absent on the right. However, neck veins are not distended. The patient's vital signs are pulse 134, blood pressure 74/56, respirations 32 and labored, and oxygen saturation of 88% on room air. Based on your observations, your major concern is that this patient may have:
a. a pelvic fracture
b. a tension pneumothorax
c. a closed-head injury
d. cardiac tamponade

56. The reason for the absence of distended neck veins is most likely that
a. mediastinal shift has obstructed the great vessels in the chest
b. blood is pooling in the pulmonary capillary beds
c. the patient is experiencing widespread vasodilation
d. the patient is hypovolemic

57. Treatment of this patient would likely include:
a. performing a needle decompression of the chest
b. performing a needle cricothyroidotomy
c. starting an IV with an 18-gauge catheter and running it TKO
d. inserting a nasopharyngeal airway

58. There has been an explosion at a local industry with reports of a man burned. On arrival, you find a 31-year-old male patient with burns on the front of his body that are red and blistered. He is complaining of severe pain and respiratory difficulty. You notice that blisters and reddening are also present on his face and his hands. Referring to Figure 23-3, you calculate the approximate percentage of burned area to be:
a. 9% to 13%
b. 16% to 18%
c. 22% to 24%
d. 30% to 32%

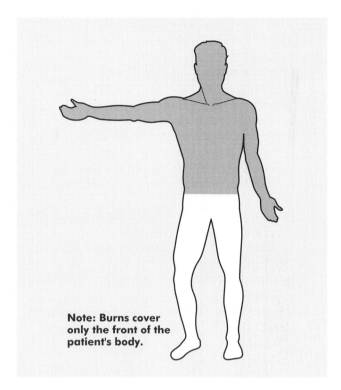

Note: Burns cover only the front of the patient's body.

Figure 23-3

59. Considering the description of the burns, you would classify them as:
a. superficial
b. partial thickness
c. medium thickness
d. full thickness

60. Based on the type, percentage, and location of the burns, this patient is considered to have a:
a. minor burn
b. superficial burn
c. moderate burn
d. critical burn

61. Your patient was stranded on a rural road when her car broke down in a freezing rainstorm. Although she is wearing a winter coat, the shoes she had on were a pair of open-toed high heels. The patient had to walk to a distant farmhouse to find help. On examination, you note her feet are cold to the touch and her toes appear white and waxy. She is also complaining of excruciating pain. You are mainly dealing with:
a. a late or deep local cold injury
b. a superficial local cold injury
c. an early local cold injury
d. a generalized cold injury

62. The local hospital is only about 9 minutes away. While en route to the hospital:
   a. apply heat to the injured areas of her feet and toes and administer diphenhydramine to decrease itching and redness
   b. break any blisters that may have formed and administer lidocaine for pain control
   c. rub or massage the affected toes and administer nitroglycerin to promote vasodilation, which will enhance circulation in the extremities
   d. cover the affected areas with dry dressings and administer morphine for pain control

63. You are caring for an unconscious patient with an obvious head injury due to trauma. The patient's medical history is unknown. During your assessment, you note the patient has a blood pressure of 76/48 and pulse rate of 130. You should:
   a. start an IV and administer D_{50} in case the patient is hypoglycemic
   b. suspect other injuries or bleeds and start two large-bore IVs
   c. intubate the patient and hyperventilate at a rate of 30 breaths per minute
   d. start a dopamine drip and titrate to desired blood pressure

64. During your examination of a 4-year-old child experiencing breathing difficulty, you note wheezing on expiration. The wheezing is most likely caused by:
   a. throat inflammation
   b. upper airway obstruction
   c. constriction of the lower airways
   d. dilated bronchioles

65. Your patient is semiconscious and having difficulty maintaining an airway but still has a gag reflex. The airway you would consider using is the:
   a. oropharyngeal airway
   b. nasopharyngeal airway
   c. dual lumen airway
   d. endotracheal tube

66. Following delivery of a healthy infant, you prepare to cut the umbilical cord. The first clamp should be placed about:
   a. 4 inches from the mother
   b. 4 inches from the baby
   c. 10 inches from the mother
   d. 10 inches from the baby

67. Your patient has a history of violent behavioral problems and is extremely agitated. Your best course of management is to:
   a. approach the patient alone to gain his confidence
   b. surprise the patient and overpower him
   c. leave the patient for the police to deal with
   d. approach the patient only with backup assistance

68. You and your partner are dispatched to a middle-class residential neighborhood for a male patient with abdominal pain. The patient is reluctant to discuss his problem, but when you question him about his recent medical history, he finally informs you that he has been vomiting what looks like coffee grounds. This patient should be suspected of having:
   a. appendicitis
   b. gastrointestinal bleeding
   c. diverticulitis
   d. gall bladder problems

69. A 38-year-old man got lost while out hunting. Upon examination, you find he has pale, cold, dry skin, and is shivering. He is alert and responding appropriately. Care for the patient would include:
   a. rewarming him by applying heat packs to the groin, armpits, and neck areas
   b. having him walk vigorously
   c. massaging his arms and legs to stimulate circulation
   d. giving him hot coffee or alcohol to drink

70. Your patient is a 16-year-old female who experienced a seizure while in bed. She is still unresponsive. Because your assessment reveals no reasons to suspect spinal injury, the position of choice when transporting this patient is:
   a. prone
   b. supine
   c. the recovery position
   d. the shock position

71. A young male patient is found in an alley. He is unresponsive, and his respirations are slow and shallow. Pulses are slow and weak. When assessing the patient, you note bruising around his eyes and behind his ears in the mastoid region. You suspect the patient has a:
   a. narcotics overdose
   b. history of diabetes
   c. basilar skull fracture
   d. seizure disorder

72. While transporting this patient, care providers should be particularly alert for the development of:
    a. hypoglycemia
    b. a myocardial infarction
    c. difficulty breathing
    d. seizures

73. A high school student was accidentally hit in the head with a baseball bat during a practice game. He is bleeding from an area of what you suspect to be an open or depressed skull injury. The bleeding is best controlled by:
    a. applying firm pressure to the wound
    b. applying digital pressure to both carotid arteries
    c. packing the wound with gauze
    d. using a loose, bulky dressing

74. A 56-year-old male patient with a history of heart problems is complaining of chest pain that is similar to what he has previously experienced with his angina. He does not have his nitroglycerin with him, and your protocols allow you to administer nitroglycerin in these cases without consulting medical direction. Prior to administering the nitroglycerin you should:
    a. verify the patient's blood pressure is above 120 systolic
    b. question the patient regarding what medications he takes
    c. check the patient's ECG and preferably obtain a 12-lead ECG
    d. start an IV

75. Your patient has fallen from a roof. He has open fractures to both legs and an angulated fracture of the right forearm. His pulse is 132 and his blood pressure is 76/58. He also complains of dyspnea. Initial management would be to:
    a. splint all injuries prior to moving the patient to prevent further blood loss
    b. perform full body immobilization with a backboard and immediately transport
    c. splint only open musculoskeletal injuries prior to moving the patient
    d. quickly move the patient to the ambulance cot in whatever way necessary and rapidly transport

76. Along with the administration of oxygen, management on the way to the hospital is likely to include:
    a. placing the patient in the PASG and inflating all three compartments
    b. starting one large-bore IV and running it wide open
    c. placing the patient in the PASG and inflating only the legs
    d. starting two large-bore IVs and contacting medical control

77. Your patient has a history of bronchitis and is complaining of shortness of breath and a productive cough, which brings up thick, greenish mucus. While being transported, this patient should generally be placed:
    a. flat on his back
    b. on his left side
    c. in a position of comfort
    d. in Trendelenburg position

78. A 32-year-old female is found unconscious in a garage with a car still running. After ensuring personal safety, donning appropriate personal protective equipment, and reaching the patient, the first step in caring for her is to:
    a. apply a cervical collar and remove her on a backboard
    b. remove her from the hazardous environment
    c. determine the type of toxic gas involved
    d. open her airway and assess breathing

79. You suspect this patient's primary problem is that she:
    a. is suffering from carbon monoxide poisoning
    b. is experiencing a hypoglycemic episode
    c. is postictal following a seizure
    d. has a possible head injury from a fall in the garage

80. Management of this patient would include all of the following *EXCEPT*:
    a. placing the patient on a cardiac monitor
    b. initiating an IV at a TKO rate
    c. attaching the patient to a pulse oximeter to ascertain oxygen saturation
    d. administering high-flow oxygen by nonrebreather mask

81. A 22-year-old male has suffered a severe laceration to the forearm as a result of an industrial accident. Direct pressure is not adequately controlling the bleeding. The pressure point of choice for controlling this patient's bleeding is over the:
a. temporal artery
b. popliteal artery
c. brachial artery
d. tibial artery

82. You encounter a 42-year-old male patient who is complaining of minor respiratory distress, a tight feeling in the throat, and itching. Your exam reveals some wheezing in the lungs and hives all over the patient's arms. The patient has a pulse rate of 98 and a blood pressure of 126/72. You suspect this patient is experiencing:
a. cardiac problems
b. a drug overdose
c. an allergic reaction
d. a diabetic emergency

83. Pharmacological intervention will most likely include administration of:
a. albuterol and diphenhydramine
b. epinephrine 1:10,000 SQ and albuterol
c. diazepam and lidocaine
d. diphenhydramine and furosemide

84. Your patient was working on his car when the battery blew up in his face. He has obvious chemical burns to his face and is complaining of burning in his eyes. The patient's eyes should be irrigated:
a. with a neutralizing solution
b. for not more than 15 minutes
c. until the patient reaches the hospital
d. only while on the scene of the incident

85. A 34-year-old male has had a finger amputated in an industrial accident. The proper way to package the finger for transportation to the hospital is to:
a. pack it in ice
b. wrap it in a sterile dressing and keep it cool
c. immerse it in sterile water
d. wrap it in a wet, sterile dressing and keep it warm

86. You are preparing to transport a child with a gastrostomy tube. The two positions in which the patient may be transported are:
a. lying on the back or lying on the left side with the head lower than the trunk
b. in a position of comfort or prone with the head lower than the trunk
c. sitting or lying on the right side with the head elevated
d. supine or prone with the head elevated

87. You and your partner are sent to evaluate a female patient experiencing a behavioral emergency. A sign that she may potentially become violent would be if she is:
a. sitting on the edge of a seat
b. lying on a bed or couch
c. using monotone speech
d. exhibiting open hands

88. While assessing a 65-year-old man who is complaining of shortness of breath, you hear wheezes. The patient is a smoker and has a history of chronic obstructive pulmonary disease. He is visiting relatives and forgot to bring all his medication with him. He tells you he normally has a "puffer" with him that he "sucks on when it is hard to breathe." Your pharmacological interventions for this patient are likely to include:
a. Proventil 0.4 mg/kg IM
b. albuterol 2.5 mg via nebulizer
c. Ventolin 5.0 mg via metered dose inhaler
d. epinephrine 0.3 mL 1:1,000 SQ

89. Three 11-year-old boys were playing with a pile of tree limbs and brush, gasoline, and matches. The combination did not go together well. One boy's t-shirt caught fire and burned completely off him before neighbors could come to his assistance and put the fire out. Referring to Figure 23-4, you calculate his percentage of burns to be:
a. 14% to 16%
b. 18% to 20%
c. 24% to 26%
d. 30% to 36%

90. When examining the burns, you notice that there are some areas of burn that appear dry, white, and leathery. Based on the description of the burns, you would classify them as:
a. superficial
b. partial thickness
c. moderate thickness
d. full thickness

91. Based on the type, percentage and location of the burns, this patient is considered to have a:
a. minor burn
b. superficial burn
c. moderate burn
d. critical burn

92. Treatment of these burns would include:
a. covering the patient with clean, dry burn sheets
b. wrapping the patient in moistened sterile bandages
c. wrapping the patient with a nonporous dressing
d. starting two large-bore IVs of normal saline and running them wide open

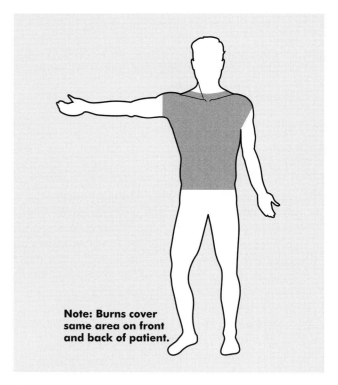

Note: Burns cover same area on front and back of patient.

Figure 23-4

93. A 74-year-old male is found in cardiac arrest in his room on the third floor of an apartment building. Upon reaching the patient, your first action is to:
a. start CPR
b. attempt to start an IV
c. check his ECG rhythm
d. intubate him

94. When analyzing the patient's ECG, you see the rhythm shown in Figure 23-5. Your partner confirms that pulses are absent. This patient is in:
a. asystole
b. electromechanical dissociation
c. pulseless electrical activity
d. ventricular fibrillation

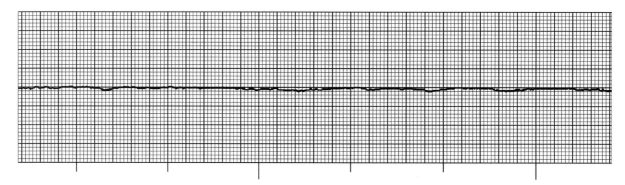

Figure 23-5

95. The next step in managing this patient is:
 a. trying to identify a correctable cause of the rhythm
 b. administering 0.5 mg of epinephrine every 3 to 5 minutes for the duration of the arrest
 c. checking the rhythm in multiple leads
 d. early initiation of transcutaneous pacing

96. Medications that are indicated for the management of this cardiac arrest include:
 a. a single dose of 40 units of vasopressin initially and 10 minutes later 1.0 to 1.5 mg of epinephrine, which is then repeated every 3 to 5 minutes
 b. 1.0 mg of epinephrine every 3 to 5 minutes and 1.0 mg of atropine every 3 to 5 minutes up to 0.04 mg/kg
 c. a single dose of 40 units of vasopressin and a single dose of 300 mg of amiodarone
 d. a single dose of 300 mg of amiodarone and 0.5 mg of atropine every 3 to 5 minutes up to 3.0 mg

97. A procedure that may be indicated in managing this patient is:
 a. synchronized cardioversion
 b. early initiation of transcutaneous pacing
 c. pleural decompression in case a tension pneumothorax is the underlying cause of the arrest
 d. initiation of a second, large-bore IV line run wide open

98. You are dispatched for a sick child with a high fever. Upon arrival, you find a 5-year-old female sitting on the edge of her bed. She is leaning slightly forward and drooling because she says it "hurts too much to swallow." Her mother tells you she started complaining of a sore throat just a short time earlier in the day and that she now has a 103°F fever. You are concerned because you suspect the child may have:
 a. bronchiolitis
 b. status asthmaticus
 c. epiglottitis
 d. meningitis

99. An important part of your management of this patient would be to:
 a. lay her flat on her back during transport
 b. have appropriate-sized emergency airway equipment selected and immediately available
 c. initiate an IV line
 d. examine her throat for signs of redness and swelling

100. An unusual incident has taken place at a local shopping mall. A number of patrons have become ill and have excess salivation, tearing, and gastrointestinal discomfort, and some are vomiting. A few patients are unresponsive and seizing. You never thought you would see it happen in your area, but you realize these people are victims of a terrorist attack. You suspect this incident involves a:
 a. biological warfare agent
 b. mustard agent
 c. blister agent
 d. nerve agent

101. Medications used to treat these patients include:
 a. albuterol, diphenhydramine, and epinephrine SQ
 b. atropine, diazepam, and pralidoxime chloride (2-PAM chloride)
 c. furosemide, albuterol, and dopamine
 d. lidocaine, phenergan, and naloxone

102. It's Saturday night and you respond to a call for an unresponsive patient at a local pool hall. Upon your arrival, you are guided to a men's restroom, where you find an unresponsive male who appears to be in his mid twenties. He does not respond even to deep painful stimuli, and his respirations are extremely slow and shallow. Pulse rate is about 70, and his oxygen saturation is 84%. Pupils are equal and constricted. There is no sign of trauma to the head. At this point you suspect this patient:
 a. is hypoglycemic
 b. has taken too many tricyclic antidepressants
 c. has overdosed on narcotics
 d. is postictal following a seizure

103. The most appropriate initial management of this patient would be to:
   a. insert an endotracheal tube to protect the airway
   b. start an IV with a crystalloid solution at a TKO rate
   c. place the patient on a cardiac monitor and look for the presence of dysrhythmias
   d. start ventilating with a bag-valve-mask

104. The pharmacological intervention most likely to make a difference for this patient is:
   a. naloxone
   b. sodium bicarbonate
   c. diphenhydramine
   d. D_{50}

105. An acceptable IV dose of this medication would be:
   a. 1.0 to 1.5 mEq/kg
   b. 0.4 to 2.0 mg
   c. 12.5 to 25 mg
   d. 25 to 50 g

ANSWERS TO CHAPTER 23: CASE PRESENTATIONS

1. **b.** Diabetic patients, especially females, may have an atypical presentation when suffering a myocardial infarction. These are often referred to as "silent" MIs. Obtaining a 12-lead ECG is critical in such cases. There is no reason to suspect neck and back injury, so a cervical collar and backboard are not warranted. Checking a blood glucose level is also indicated.

2. **a.** Although rare, blunt force trauma may result in a herniated diaphragm and shifting of abdominal contents into the thoracic cavity. Breath sounds are critical to recognizing this. If the patient had a pneumothorax or hemothorax, breath sounds may be diminished on one side, but this would be a diffuse finding. The clear breath sounds in the upper part of one side of the chest, coupled with a total absence of breath sounds below a certain point, indicates something in the chest cavity is interfering with lung function. In some cases, if part of the GI tract has migrated into the thoracic cavity, bowel sounds may be heard when auscultating the chest.

3. **d.** This patient has classic signs of acute coronary syndrome. Aspirin, morphine, and additional nitroglycerin are indicated in the management of this patient. In cases where a patient has already taken his own nitroglycerin, additional doses are indicated since nitroglycerin acts as an antiischemic. Also, EMS personnel cannot guarantee the age or efficacy of the patient's personal prescription.

4. **c.** This patient is showing signs and symptoms of preeclampsia. EMS personnel should be alert for the sudden occurrence of seizures.

5. **d.** Magnesium sulfate may be used in the management of seizures associated with eclampsia.

6. **b.** From the history and physical presentation, personnel should suspect a hypoglycemic emergency. Although a blood glucose check is warranted, this should be obvious to EMS personnel even before the check. Early administration of D_{50} is warranted.

7. **a.** If an IV cannot be established on a patient experiencing serious hypoglycemia, glucagon can be administered IM. Glucagon stimulates the liver to break down glycogen so that glucose is released into the blood. The normal adult dose is 0.5 to 1.0 mg IM and the dose may be repeated in 7 to 10 minutes if needed. Always follow local protocols.

8. **d.** Vaginal bleeding that occurs during the third trimester of pregnancy is usually associated with a problem with the placenta, such as abruptio placentae or placenta previa. In this case, the single attack of bleeding coupled with the presence of pain indicates abruptio placentae. Vaginal bleeding may be minimal and often is out of proportion to the degree of shock displayed by the patient because much of the bleeding may be concealed.

9. **c.** Because serious signs of shock are already present, initiation of two IVs with large-bore needles is indicated. This should be done while en route to the hospital. Fluid administration should be guided by medical command or local protocols. The patient should be transported to a hospital capable of dealing with serious obstetrical emergencies. This may not be the closest hospital.

10. **c.** This patient appears to be experiencing a stroke.

11. **a.** If the patient's condition permits, she should be kept supine with her head elevated 15 degrees to facilitate venous drainage.

12. **b.** Management of a prolapsed cord may include inserting two gloved fingers into the vagina to push the presenting part of the fetus away from the cord, thereby taking pressure off the cord. When pressure is taken off the cord, it may spontaneously retract. However, EMS personnel should not attempt to reposition the cord.

13. a. The patient should be transported in the knee-chest position. To accomplish this, the patient positions herself on her elbows and knees with her buttocks facing up in the air and her chest lower than her pelvis. This position allows gravity to assist in taking some pressure off the cord. The patient may also be transported on her back with her buttocks elevated. Because this is a true emergency situation, transport should be done using lights and sirens unless contraindicated by local protocols.

14. c. Proper care of the exposed umbilical cord includes covering it with a moist, sterile dressing. This can minimize temperature changes that may cause umbilical artery spasm.

15. b. The management plan for this patient should include the early administration of albuterol. Albuterol is useful in treating wheezing because it relaxes smooth muscles of the bronchial tree by stimulating adrenergic receptors of the sympathetic nervous system. Because there are no signs of pulmonary edema, neither nitroglycerin nor furosemide is indicated. Although epinephrine also acts as a bronchodilator, its administration is contraindicated as it can cause serious cardiac complications.

16. c. This patient is displaying the classic signs and symptoms of organophosphate poisoning. Organophosphates are used in many pesticides and organophosphate poisoning causes increased sympathetic tone. The signs and symptoms can be remembered with the acronym SLUDGE: Salivation, Lacrimation, Urination, Defecation, GI cramping, and Emesis.

17. d. Because the poison is entering the skin through absorption, it must be removed. Brush off as much of the chemical as possible, then wash off any remaining chemical with copious amounts of water. The patient's clothing should be removed. Wrapping the patient in a plastic sheet would keep the poison near the patient and allow continued absorption. Personnel treating the patient should also be careful not to become contaminated.

18. d. Administration of atropine is indicated for organophosphate poisoning. However, the dose needed to counteract the effects of the organophosphate is much higher than the typical dose used to treat cardiac emergencies. Doses of 2 to 5 mg IV may be given every 5 to 15 minutes as required.

19. c. Management of this patient would include leaving the knife in place and stabilizing it with a bulky dressing. Removing it could cause further hemorrhage and complications. Although IVs may be initiated, because EMS personnel cannot control the hemorrhaging within the chest cavity, running them wide open may be contraindicated as it can make the bleeding worse. With a trauma center being so close, time should not be wasted waiting for a helicopter to arrive.

20. d. The other chest wounds should be covered with occlusive dressings to prevent air from entering the thoracic cavity.

21. c. The patient has developed a tension pneumothorax. Pressure must be relieved or the patient will die. Your course of action is to perform pleural decompression. This can be accomplished by inserting a large-gauge needle in the second intercostal space, midclavicular line. The needle should be inserted over the top of the rib. Some areas may allow the fifth or sixth intercostal space, midaxillary line to be used as an alternate site. Consult local protocols.

22. a. Pharmacological intervention for this patient would include the administration of 0.05 to 0.15 mg/kg albuterol via nebulizer.

23. c. This incident was likely precipitated by an allergic reaction. Emotional stress and an infection can also precipitate an asthma attack.

24. b. Even if the parents are not present, care and transport can proceed under the principle of implied consent. A police officer need not be present.

25. c. This patient likely has a gastrointestinal bleed. The fact that the vomitus looks like coffee grounds indicates that the bleed is in the stomach because the coffee groundlike material is partially digested blood.

26. a. Although it is appropriate to start an IV on this patient, large amounts of fluid are likely not needed in the prehospital setting. It may be best to consult with medical direction regarding the amount of fluid administration, which will help replenish lost fluid while not overloading the patient.

27. b. Discharge of amniotic fluid that resembles thick, green pea soup indicates a meconium emergency and potential fetal distress.

28. d. If the baby is delivered before reaching the hospital and is distressed (e.g., poor respiratory effort, decreased muscle tone, or heart rate less than 100 beats per minute), aggressive suctioning is a must. Pay particularly close attention to the baby's airway to keep the meconium from entering the lungs.

29. c. Signs and symptoms indicate your patient is experiencing an anaphylactic reaction. This is a severe allergic reaction, not a mild one.

30. d. Scrape the stinger out using something like the edge of a card or something similar. Using tweezers may force more poison into the wound. Do not leave the stinger in place because muscles around the poison sac may continue to constrict, thereby forcing more poison into the patient.

31. c. Albuterol, epinephrine, and diphenhydramine may all be useful in the management of this patient.

32. b. Neurogenic shock is associated with spinal injuries. Damage to the spinal cord produces loss of sympathetic tone to the vessels, which results in dilation of the blood vessels. This causes the "container" to be too large for the normal amount of blood in the system. The patient will present with low blood pressure, but the pulse rate remains normal and the typical signs of cool, clammy skin are not present because catecholamines are not released.

33. d. Your patient's difficulties are related to congestive heart failure (CHF). Acute pulmonary edema, dyspnea, jugular vein distention, and peripheral edema are prime clues that CHF is the problem.

34. b. This patient will probably benefit from administration of nitroglycerin, furosemide, and morphine. All have a vasodilatory effect that reduces cardiac preload thereby helping to reduce pulmonary congestion. In addition, furosemide is a potent diuretic and therefore facilitates elimination of excess fluid from the body.

35. b. Eviscerations should be covered with moist, sterile dressings that are then covered with an occlusive dressing. The organs should not be replaced, and direct pressure should not be applied to the area.

36. c. If there is no accompanying spinal or leg injuries, transport an evisceration patient on his or her back with the hips and knees flexed to decrease abdominal pressure.

37. c. Early defibrillation is the key in managing this patient. Defibrillation takes priority over airway and CPR. It is therefore critical that the patient's ECG rhythm be ascertained early in the incident. This may be done using through-the-paddle monitoring or by attaching electrodes to the patient. In many cases, the patient can be attached directly to the monitor just as quickly as using through-the-paddle monitoring. The advantage to this is that the ECG tracing will be much clearer in many cases. If two EMS personnel are present, one can start one-rescuer CPR while the other analyzes the ECG.

38. b. This patient is in ventricular fibrillation (VF). EMS personnel should immediately defibrillate the patient.

39. a. Vasopressin, epinephrine, and amiodarone are all medications that may be used to manage ventricular fibrillation.

40. d. Because of the violent nature of this patient's behavior, restraints will probably be needed to protect him and the rescuers. In most cases, police assistance should be available prior to applying restraints. Do not argue with or lie to the patient, and do not go along with his hallucinations.

41. **a.** Your first action in assisting the patient is to protect him from injury. The violent uncontrolled jerking associated with seizures can cause the patient to harm himself. It may be necessary to place padding between the patient and any hard objects while the seizure runs its course. It will be impossible to obtain an accurate blood pressure while the patient is seizing. Also, do not attempt to place anything in the patient's mouth while seizures are still actively occurring.

42. **b.** Diazepam raises the seizure threshold in the motor cortex and is therefore indicated to control grand mal seizure activity.

43. **c.** The adult dose of diazepam is 5 to 10 mg given slow IV push.

44. **b.** Although early defibrillation is critical, in this case it cannot be accomplished while the patient is still on the metal decking because this may cause injury to the rest of the rescuers. Therefore the first priority in this case is to quickly remove the patient from the metal decking.

45. **a.** This patient is in Pulseless Electrical Activity (PEA). This is a serious situation with a high mortality rate. EMS personnel should attempt to identify a correctable cause of the rhythm as early as possible in the arrest management, and then take steps to correct the cause.

46. **b.** If breath sounds are only heard on the right side, this is likely a right main-stem intubation. Deflate the cuff and pull the tube back slightly until lung sounds are heard on both sides.

47. **b.** When administering medications down the ET tube, 2 to 2½ times the IV dose should be given. Therefore 2 mg of epinephrine should be administered down an ET tube. Vasopressin and amiodarone should not be given via the endotracheal route.

48. **a.** A heart rate of less than 100 in a newborn is not adequate. Because slow heart rates are often associated with hypoxia, the baby should be ventilated with 100% oxygen. This will often help to improve the heart rate.

49. **c.** Any time a newborn infant's heart rate is below 60 beats per minute despite effective positive-pressure ventilation with 100% oxygen for approximately 30 seconds, chest compressions should be started.

50. **d.** This patient should be transported on her left side to relieve pressure on the vena cava and abdominal organs. The patient should still be secured on a backboard, but the board and patient can be tilted as a unit so as not to compromise spinal immobilization.

51. **b.** The most likely cause of shock in this patient is hypovolemia due to other injuries. Burns, even those that cover a rather large area of the body, do not cause a rapid development of hypovolemia and shock. Because burns look serious, they can often lead caregivers to overlook other less obvious but more severe injuries. A thorough patient exam and assessment will minimize the possibility of missing other injuries.

52. **c.** This patient is most likely hypothermic. Alcohol ingestion can especially predispose a patient to hypothermia, as can the use of drugs and various medical conditions.

53. **a.** Severely hypothermic patients should be handled gently. Rough handling can send cold, acidotic blood, which has pooled in the extremities to the patient's core and cause ventricular fibrillation. Massaging the arms and legs or applying heat packs or hot water bottles to the extremities can do the same. Patients who are not responsive should not be given anything to drink.

54. **c.** A hypothermic heart usually does not respond well to ALS procedures, especially medications. Some medications may even produce the opposite effect than that expected or desired. Generally, if a hypothermia patient goes into ventricular fibrillation, three defibrillations should be administered and an airway secured. Further attempts at ALS procedures are best guided by medical control. Field rewarming of hypothermia patients is generally not indicated. Always follow local protocols and guidelines.

55. **b.** Your major concern is that the patient may have a tension pneumothorax. Based on mechanism of injury, the patient may also have a closed injury or a pelvic fracture, but these injuries, while life-threatening, will not cause death as quickly as the tension pneumothorax and cannot be adequately managed in the field by EMS personnel.

56. **d.** Although distended neck veins may be a sign of tension pneumothorax, there must be sufficient blood volume in the system to allow the distention to occur. If the patient is hypovolemic, distended neck veins will not be present.

57. **a.** Because this patient appears to have a tension pneumothorax, a needle decompression is indicated. Because he is unresponsive, endotracheal intubation is also indicated. Two large-bore IV lines should be initiated and medical control should be contacted for direction regarding fluid administration.

58. **c.** With the use of the rule of nines for adults, the percentage of burns for this patient is approximately 22% to 24%, as shown in Figure 23-3. The fronts of the arms are approximately 4.5% each, the front of the chest is approximately 9%, and the front of the face is 4.5%.

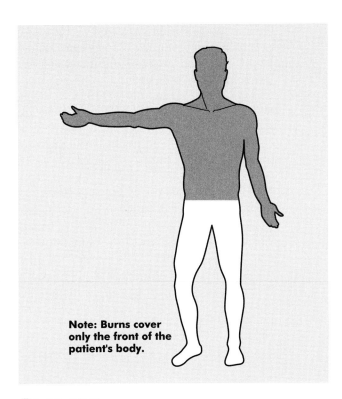

Note: Burns cover only the front of the patient's body.

Figure 23-3

59. **b.** A burn characterized by reddened skin, blister formation, and intense pain is classified as a partial thickness burn.

60. **d.** Based on the percentage of burns and the fact that the patient's face and hands are involved, these burns would be considered critical.

61. **a.** This patient has a late or deep local cold injury.

62. **d.** The patient's injured areas should be protected by covering them with dry dressings. When dressing the patient's toes, make sure they are separated. Do not massage the areas and do not break any blisters that may have formed. In most cases, the injured parts should not be rewarmed. Morphine is also indicated for pain management. Always follow local protocols regarding management of late or deep local cold injuries, including frostbite.

63. **b.** Isolated head injuries normally do not cause hypotension and other signs of shock. In this case, other injuries that would lead to significant blood loss should be suspected. Two large-bore IVs are indicated. However, caution must be exercised when administering fluid. Enough fluid should be given so that cerebral perfusion can be maintained; however, too much fluid may exacerbate cerebral edema. Medical control may provide valuable guidance in such situations. D_{50} administration should be guided by blood glucose readings because increasing blood glucose levels can cause increased cerebral swelling. Intubation may be indicated, but arbitrary hyperventilation in the absence of clear signs of brain swelling is contraindicated. Dopamine should not be used to raise the blood pressure of a hypovolemic patient.

64. **c.** Wheezing is a result of constriction of the lower airways. In children it is often associated with asthma or bronchiolitis.

65. **b.** Patients in need of an airway but who still have a gag reflex present are best managed with a nasopharyngeal airway.

66. **b.** The first clamp should be placed approximately four (4) inches or four (4) fingers width from the infant. The second clamp is placed approximately two (2) inches away from the first clamp toward the mother.

67. **d.** When a violent patient is encountered, the best course is to approach the patient only with backup assistance, preferably from police. Because the patient may also be in need of medical care, EMS personnel should not just leave the patient for police to deal with. This may be considered abandonment.

68. **b.** Partially digested blood has a coffee-ground appearance. Therefore a patient vomiting coffee-ground emesis should be suspected of having gastrointestinal bleeding.

69. **a.** Because the patient is alert and responding appropriately, active rewarming may be accomplished with warm blankets and/or with the application of heat packs to the groin, armpits, and neck areas. Always follow local protocols concerning the management of generalized cold exposure patients. The patient should not be given caffeine-containing beverages because these cause vasoconstriction and diuresis. Alcoholic beverages should not be given because alcohol produces peripheral vasodilation and increases heat loss from the skin.

70. **c.** In the absence of spinal injuries, seizure patients may be transported in the recovery position, lying on the left side.

71. **c.** Bruising around the eyes (raccoon's sign) or over the mastoid process (Battle's sign) is indicative of a basilar skull fracture.

72. **d.** When transporting a patient with a severe head injury, always be prepared to manage seizures should they develop. Related to this is the need to maintain and guard the patient's airway. If paramedics are trained to perform rapid sequence intubation, this patient may benefit from the procedure if he appears to have difficulty maintaining his airway.

73. **d.** Bleeding from an open or depressed skull injury is best controlled with a loose, bulky dressing. Caution should be exercised because applying direct pressure may force bone fragments into brain tissues.

74. **b.** Prior to administering nitroglycerin, it is important to ask the patient what medications he or she is taking. If a patient is taking a medication such as Viagra, nitroglycerin administration can produce severe and even fatal hypotension. Female patients as well as male patients should be asked about this, and it is best to ask specifically about Viagra use because some patients may be reluctant to mention it when simply asked about their medications. Generally, a patient's blood pressure should be greater than 100 mm Hg systolic before giving nitroglycerin. It is not necessary to start an IV or check the patient's ECG prior to nitroglycerin administration, but obtaining a 12-lead ECG as soon as possible is desirable.

75. **b.** Although this patient needs to get to a trauma center as quickly as possible, spinal immobilization still needs to be performed. Your best course of action is to perform full body immobilization with a backboard and then rapidly transport to the closest appropriate facility.

76. **d.** Trauma care is challenging. Much must be considered before fluid resuscitation is initiated. Although two large-bore IVs are indicated, fluid administration should be guided by medical control. It is best to avoid using PASG because the dyspnea may be the result of a hemothorax, which may be exacerbated by raising blood pressure and increasing the intraabdominal pressure.

77. **c.** Patients experiencing breathing difficulty are generally best transported in a position of comfort. This will normally be in a sitting position.

78. **b.** Although assessing the airway and breathing are important, the patient should be removed from the hazardous environment and placed in a safe area prior to starting an assessment.

79. **a.** This patient most likely has carbon monoxide poisoning.

80. **c.** Pulse oximeter units cannot differentiate whether hemoglobin is saturated with oxygen or with carbon monoxide. Therefore

readings from a pulse oximeter will be useless because they will not truly indicate the patient's status.

81. **c.** Pressure should be applied to the brachial artery, which supplies blood to the arm.

82. **c.** Based on the patient's signs and symptoms, he is most likely experiencing an allergic reaction.

83. **a.** Pharmacological intervention will most likely include administration of albuterol to relieve respiratory difficulty and diphenhydramine to control the itching and hives. If epinephrine is administered subcutaneously, a 1:1000 concentration is used.

84. **c.** The patient's eyes should be irrigated until the patient reaches the hospital.

85. **b.** Generally, the proper way to package an amputated finger for transportation to the hospital is to wrap the finger in a sterile dressing and keep it cool. Do not immerse it in water, moisten it, or pack it in ice because this can cause tissue damage. Always follow local protocols regarding packaging of amputated body parts.

86. **c.** Children with gastrostomy tubes should normally be transported either sitting or lying on the right side with the head elevated. This reduces the risk of aspiration.

87. **a.** Sitting on the edge of her seat may be a signal that the patient is posturing herself for action that may become potentially violent. Potentially violent patients may also appear agitated, pace, or be unable to sit still, speak in loud, fast speech, and clench their fists. Obtaining a thorough history may also reveal that the patient has displayed violent behavior in the past.

88. **b.** Pharmacological intervention for this patient will likely include administering 2.5 mg of albuterol via nebulizer.

89. **d.** With the use of the rule of nines for children, the front and back of the torso are 18% each, as shown in Figure 23-4. Considering the boy's t-shirt covered most of his torso, you calculate the patient's percentage of burns to be 30% to 36%.

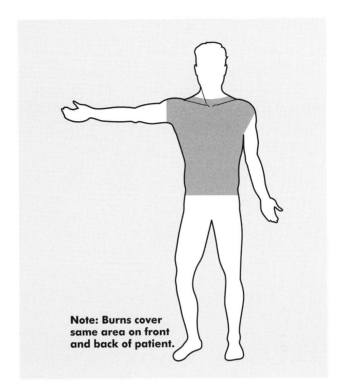

Note: Burns cover same area on front and back of patient.

Figure 23-4

90. **d.** Burns that are dry, white, and leathery skin or that are charred black or brown are classified as a full-thickness burns.

91. **d.** Based on the percentage of burns and the fact that the burns are circumferential, that is, they encircle the torso, these burns would be considered critical.

92. **a.** The burns should be covered with a clean, dry burn sheet. Wet dressings should be avoided because the percentage of burn area is so large that covering them with wet dressings can cause hypothermia. Leaving the burn exposed to the air will increase the pain and chances for infection.

93. **c.** The first action of the arriving EMS crew should be to check the patient's ECG rhythm to ascertain whether he is in a rhythm that should be defibrillated.

94. **a.** The patient is in asystole because there are no complexes indicating any electrical activity.

95. **c.** Asystole should be confirmed in multiple ECG leads to rule out fine ventricular fibrillation.

96. b. Epinephrine and atropine are the two primary medications used to manage asystole. One milligram of epinephrine is administered every 3 to 5 minutes for the duration of the code, and 1.0 mg of atropine is given every 3 to 5 minutes up to a maximum dose of 0.04 mg/kg.

97. b. Transcutaneous pacing may be indicated in the management of asystole. However, for best results it must be initiated early in the arrest.

98. c. This child probably has epiglottitis. With epiglottitis the child's epiglottis swells and can totally obstruct the airway. Clues include a relatively rapid onset of a high fever, sore throat with reluctance to swallow, and a forward-sitting position and drooling.

99. b. Epiglottitis patients are in danger of quickly developing total airway occlusion. Appropriate-sized emergency airway equipment should be selected and immediately available to manage the patient if this occurs. Make no attempt to visualize the airway if the child is still ventilating adequately because placing anything in the child's mouth or throat, such as a tongue depressor to examine the throat, may precipitate complete obstruction. Also, make no attempt to lay the child down. The child should be transported in a position of comfort. Do not attempt to start an IV because this can agitate the child and precipitate airway obstruction.

100. d. Signs and symptoms of a nerve agent exposure are similar to those of an organophosphate poisoning. The mnemonic SLUDGE can be used to remember signs and symptoms. SLUDGE stands for Salivation, Lacrimation (tearing), Urination, Defecation, Gastrointestinal cramping, and Emesis.

101. b. Pharmacological intervention for nerve agent exposure primarily involves administration of atropine and pralidoxime chloride (2-PAM chloride). Dose is usually related to degree of symptoms and the doses of atropine are much higher than that used for cardiac events. Diazepam is indicated for the management of seizures that may occur as a result of nerve agent exposure.

102. c. This patient most likely has overdosed on narcotics. The pinpoint pupils and severe respiratory depression should alert the EMS providers to this possibility.

103. d. Because the patient has slow, shallow respirations and a low oxygen saturation, the patient must be ventilated. However, because you suspect a narcotics overdose and narcotics overdoses can be reversed, it may be best to manage the airway with a bag-valve-mask and then rapidly try to establish IV access to allow administration of medications. If an endotracheal tube is inserted and then the patient regains consciousness following medication administration, EMS providers must try to control a conscious patient with an ET tube in place. For airway control a nasopharyngeal airway may be used.

104. a. Naloxone is a narcotic antagonist and would be indicated as the first medication to administer to this patient.

105. b. The adult IV dose for naloxone is usually 0.4 to 2.0 mg. Naloxone administration may be titrated to keep the patient responsive and free from respiratory depression but somewhat docile during transport.

SAMPLE FINAL EXAM

24

This chapter contains a 150-question sample test with a mix of knowledge-based and scenario-based questions. Should the user wish to only review scenario-based questions, he or she should go to Chapter 23.

1. Several things can lead to accumulation of fluid in the interstitial space. During an immune response the primary mechanism is:
   a. increased capillary hydrostatic pressure
   b. decreased oncotic pressure
   c. increased capillary permeability
   d. lymphatic vessel obstruction

2. Information contained in the Patient Care Report is:
   a. not discoverable
   b. confidential
   c. judgmental
   d. not considered part of the patient medical record

3. The most important factor to determine when evaluating patients with serious musculoskeletal trauma is:
   a. whether there is vascular compromise in the injured extremity
   b. whether they have any life-threatening conditions
   c. whether there is a fracture or merely a simple sprain
   d. whether they can bear weight on the injured extremity

4. Your patient is a 76-year-old female who is in a nursing home. Upon your arrival, you notice she is semiconscious. Her pulse is 120, her respirations are rapid, and her blood pressure is 88/60. She is slightly warm to the touch. There are no signs of internal bleeding. According to the staff, her only history is that of a recent urinary tract infection. You suspect her low blood pressure to be related to:
   a. hypovolemic shock
   b. septic shock
   c. cardiogenic shock
   d. neurogenic shock

5. To package an amputated part for transportation to the hospital, the EMS provider should:
   a. pack it in ice
   b. immerse the part in sterile water
   c. wrap it in a sterile dressing and keep it cool
   d. wrap it in a wet, sterile dressing and keep it warm

6. A man reports a sudden pain in his right calf after going up for a rebound while playing basketball. He complains of pain with weight bearing, and on examination you feel a depression at the back of his ankle distal to the calf muscle. You suspect what condition?
   a. ankle fracture
   b. deep venous thrombosis
   c. rupture of the Achilles tendon
   d. fracture of the talus of the foot

7. Prevention of high-altitude illness includes all of the following *EXCEPT*:
   a. eating a high-protein diet
   b. taking steroids
   c. using a gradual ascent (days)
   d. sleeping at lower altitudes each night

8. Acute pulmonary edema occurs when:
   a. the right ventricle cannot pump enough blood into the lungs
   b. the alveolar capillary beds become blocked
   c. the left ventricle fails to function effectively as a pump and blood backs up into the pulmonary circulation
   d. the right atrium is unable to adequately manage the blood it is receiving from the vena cava

9. In compensated shock, the body:
   a. reduces venous capacitance in response to blood loss
   b. is hemodynamically unstable and shows pronounced symptoms of shock
   c. can no longer maintain preload
   d. is incapable of meeting its metabolic needs

10. A pelvic fracture results in severe bleeding from disruption of:
    a. the periosteum, which is rich in blood vessels
    b. the symphysis pubis, causing a rupture of the urethra
    c. the sacroiliac joint, causing rupture of the iliac arteries
    d. the posterior attachment of the aorta, resulting in aortic rupture

11. Pharmacological therapy for all of the obstructive airway diseases is aimed at:
    a. providing positive airway support
    b. increasing oxygenation by decreasing interstitial fluid
    c. reversal of bronchiole spasm and reduction of mucus production
    d. removing the offending agent that precipitated the event

12. When managing a patient with a crush syndrome:
    a. avoid IV fluid administration to prevent development of pulmonary edema
    b. aggressively hydrate the patient to manage hypovolemia and maintain urine output
    c. consider administering furosemide to help maintain urine output
    d. always administer calcium chloride to prevent hyperkalemia

13. A 16-year-old football player is tackled, landing on his shoulder. He is able to move the upper arm freely but complains of pain over the top of the shoulder. On palpation you find tenderness and swelling at the distal end of the clavicle. He most likely has:
    a. an anterior shoulder dislocation
    b. a shoulder separation
    c. a humerus fracture
    d. a posterior shoulder dislocation

14. An acute electrolyte abnormality would most likely be suspected if the ECG shows:
    a. the presence of U waves or peaked T waves
    b. the presence of J waves or ST segment elevation
    c. rounded T waves or a PR interval greater than 0.12 second
    d. ST segment depression or flutter waves

15. Upon examining your patient's ECG, you note wide QRS complexes. The PR interval varies and there is no correlation of P waves to QRS complexes. This best describes a:
    a. first-degree AV block
    b. second-degree AV block Type I (Wenckebach)
    c. second-degree AV block Type II
    d. third-degree AV block

16. If hypoglycemia is suspected in the neonate, appropriate therapy may include administration of:
    a. 2 to 5 mL/kg of dextrose 50% solution given over 10 minutes
    b. 4 to 6 mL/kg of dextrose 5% solution given over 15 minutes
    c. 5 to 10 mL/kg of dextrose 10% solution given over 20 minutes
    d. 10 to 15 mL/kg of dextrose 25% solution given rapid IV push

17. Your COPD patient has quit breathing, and you have intubated the trachea. When you compress the bag, you feel significant resistance and hear wheezes on auscultation. The most effective and immediate treatment would include:
    a. administering IV solumedrol
    b. administering an in-line nebulized albuterol treatment
    c. titrating the oxygen concentration to the patient's pulse oximeter reading
    d. none of the above

18. Kussmaul's respirations are:
    a. an attempt to remove carbon dioxide in response to the metabolic acidosis
    b. an attempt to blow off excess acids secreted into the lung
    c. exemplified by fast and shallow respirations
    d. a response to decreased cerebral glucose metabolism

19. When performing pleural decompression, the proper location for inserting a needle is the:
    a. second or third intercostal space, midclavicular line
    b. second or third intercostal space, midaxillary line
    c. sixth or seventh intercostal space, midclavicular line
    d. ninth or tenth intercostal space, midaxillary line

20. An impaled object may need to be removed if it:
    a. interferes with the airway
    b. is lodged in the ear
    c. is too small to be x-rayed
    d. is lodged in the nose

21. Any expanding lesion within the cranium can result in:
    a. tentorium cerebelli
    b. increased intracranial pressure
    c. decreased intracranial pressure
    d. none of the above

22. After receiving instructions from the on-line medical control:
    a. request confirmation that the orders are actually in your protocol manual
    b. immediately perform them
    c. perform them only if the transmission is recorded
    d. use the "echo" procedure by repeating back what was heard and confirming receipt of the message

23. Each of the following medications acts directly on the bronchiole leading to dilation *EXCEPT*:
    a. atropine
    b. albuterol
    c. metaproterenol
    d. epinephrine

24. Primary differences between adult and pediatric airway anatomy include:
    a. the epiglottis is narrower and longer in children than adults
    b. pediatric patients tend to have larger airways and smaller tongues
    c. the vocal cords of an infant slope from front to back
    d. the cricoid cartilage is the widest part of the airway in the infant and young child and the vocal cords are the narrowest part

25. If a pediatric patient shows signs of significant hypovolemia, appropriate fluid resuscitation should be initiated by administering a:
    a. single fluid bolus of 20 mL/kg of isotonic colloid solution followed by a continuous infusion of crystalloid solution
    b. fluid bolus of 20 mL/kg of isotonic crystalloid solution followed by additional boluses of 20 mL/kg until systemic perfusion improves
    c. rapid 50 mL bolus of colloid solution followed by an IV drip of vasopressor agents to maintain blood pressure
    d. 100 mL bolus of hypertonic crystalloid solution followed by a continuous infusion of crystalloids if signs of shock persist

26. Your patient is a 60-year-old female found on the floor. Your general impression is that she is awake, alert, in no obvious distress, and has an estimated weight of over 375 pounds. She apologizes for calling you, and states that her knees gave out when she was walking up the back stairs from outside. She states she pulled herself this far to reach the phone to call for help. Her husband is disabled and cannot help lift her. She denies injury, but states she needs assistance to get up. Which of the following is the most appropriate plan of care for this patient?
    a. Do your best to assist the patient to a chair or a standing position and have a release for nontransport signed.
    b. Perform an assessment of the patient before moving her even though she denies injury.
    c. Inform her of recent advances in weight loss.
    d. The patient chose to eat and gain weight to this amount, and it is not your responsibility to get her up because you may hurt yourself while trying.

27. Pharmacological treatment and interventions for pulmonary edema consist of diuretics, nitrates, and positive pressure ventilatory support, which result in:
    a. increased oxygen delivery to the lung
    b. decreased blood pressure
    c. increased oxygen to the heart resulting in more efficient contractions
    d. maintenance of alveoli patency and reduction in interstitial fluid

28. When auscultating heart sounds, ensure that the patient is:
    a. in a right lateral recumbent position or lying flat
    b. sitting up and leaning slightly forward or in a left lateral recumbent position
    c. lying flat or sitting up and leaning slightly backward
    d. in Trendelenburg position or a prone position

29. When inserting a needle to decompress the chest, the needle should be inserted:
    a. directly through the rib
    b. below the lower aspect of the rib
    c. above the upper aspect of the rib
    d. either above or below the rib depending on wound location

30. Conscious thought, personality, voluntary motor control, and tactile perception are the function of the:
    a. brain stem
    b. medulla oblongata
    c. cerebellum
    d. cerebral hemispheres

31. The blood supply to the brain is delivered by two carotid arteries and two vertebral arteries. Which of the following is true regarding this blood supply?
    a. The two vertebral arteries supply 80% of the blood flow.
    b. The two vertebral arteries join to form the basilar artery.
    c. The anterior circulation from the carotid arteries is joined to the posterior circulation of the vertebral arteries by the circle of Willis.
    d. There is excellent collateral blood flow between the lobes of the brain and deep in the brain structure.

32. Four medications that may be administered by the endotracheal route include:
    a. atropine, Benadryl, cordarone, dopamine (ABCD)
    b. adenosine, Benadryl, lidocaine, epinephrine (ABLE)
    c. glucagon, adenosine, morphine, epinephrine (GAME)
    d. lidocaine, atropine, naloxone, epinephrine (LANE)

33. You are transporting a patient to a local burn center that is 35 minutes away and are ordered to start an IV while en route to the hospital. An important consideration when starting an IV on a burn patient is:
    a. if a burned area must be used, avoid cleansing the IV site so as not to disturb or remove any tissue
    b. start the IV using a small-bore catheter to minimize additional tissue damage
    c. if an upper extremity is involved, try to find an IV site in the burned area to leave unburned sites for long-term hospital use
    d. use a large-bore catheter

34. Which of the following is the most common symptom of acute myocardial infarction in the elderly patient?
    a. fatigue
    b. chest pain
    c. neck pain
    d. arm pain

35. While assessing a patient with a respiratory complaint you note an alteration in mental status, stridor, diaphoresis, and tachycardia. These are signs of:
    a. cerebral vascular accident
    b. life-threatening respiratory distress
    c. acute myocardial infarction
    d. typical asthma attack

36. A 25-year-old is hit by a train and sustains a C2 fracture/dislocation resulting in quadriplegia. His blood pressure is 60/P with a pulse of 52. Your understanding of neurogenic shock is that it is:
    a. usually temporary and the result of the loss of sympathetic vascular tone
    b. common and should always be suspected in multiple trauma patients
    c. exhibited by pale, clammy skin associated with hypotension and tachycardia
    d. treated differently than hypovolemic shock with the use of vasopressor agents only

37. When properly placed in an endotracheal tube, the tip of the stylet should:
  a. not protrude from the end of the airway
  b. extend no more than ½ inch out the end of the airway
  c. not extend past the middle of the airway
  d. extend approximately 1 inch out the end of the airway

38. Your patient has a history of congestive heart failure and is presenting with severe dyspnea. Jugular vein distention is present and auscultation of breath sounds reveals bilateral crackles and rhonchi. Among the medications you would consider administering are:
  a. albuterol, epinephrine, lidocaine
  b. adenosine, albuterol, atropine
  c. lidocaine, atropine, naloxone
  d. nitroglycerin, furosemide, morphine

39. Wheezes can be described as a:
  a. harsh, raspy sound created by fluid in the lungs
  b. crowing sound heard on inspiration
  c. fine, crackling sound indicating the presence of fluid in the small airways
  d. high-pitched, whistling sound created as air flows through narrowed airways

40. You are ordered to administer 30 mL of an IV drip medication over a period of 20 minutes. Using a microdrip IV administration set, the necessary flow rate would be:
  a. 30 drops per minute
  b. 60 drops per minute
  c. 90 drops per minute
  d. 120 drops per minute

41. A common sign of tracheobronchial disruption is:
  a. elevated blood pressure
  b. bradycardia
  c. Battle's sign
  d. subcutaneous emphysema

42. Hypersensitivity reactions are divided into four distinct types. Which of the following is the most dramatic and may lead to anaphylaxis?
  a. Type I
  b. Type II
  c. Type III
  d. Type IV

43. While examining a patient who twisted her ankle you check for pulses. Which is correct?
  a. The tibialis anterior pulse is behind the lateral malleolus.
  b. The dorsalis pedis is on the dorsum of the foot proximal to the second and third toes.
  c. The tibialis anterior pulse is anterior to the medial malleolus.
  d. None of the above are correct.

44. Heart murmurs normally indicate:
  a. the presence of an aneurysm
  b. a local blood flow obstruction
  c. a narrowing of a coronary artery
  d. the presence of a valvular defect

45. The sympathetic nervous system primarily dominates during:
  a. periods of emotional calm
  b. periods of physical calm
  c. asystole
  d. stressful events

46. After accidentally inhaling an unknown powder, your patient complains of a headache and dizziness. His heart rate is 40, he is drooling and tearing, and he is incontinent of both urine and feces. This is consistent with what toxidrome?
  a. amphetamines
  b. cholinergic
  c. hallucinogens
  d. opiates

47. You respond to a 52-year-old male construction worker who awoke with severe back pain and is unable to get out of bed. He is healthy and complains of "fire" in his back radiating into his left leg, which is worse with coughing and movement. Which of the following is the most correct statement regarding this patient?
  a. Large-bore IVs should be placed as a precaution against a dissecting aortic aneurysm.
  b. Administration of an analgesic such as morphine may be required to facilitate transport to the hospital.
  c. A complete neurological exam is not necessary because he is awake and alert with no history of trauma.
  d. His pain is consistent with renal colic.

48. Signs and symptoms of a tension pneumothorax include:
   a. narrowing pulse pressure, muffled heart sounds, and distended neck veins
   b. dyspnea, bradycardia, and diminished breath sounds on the uninjured side caused by compression
   c. tachycardia, dyspnea, and diminished breath sounds on affected side
   d. decreasing respiratory rate, increasing blood pressure, and bradycardia

49. Of the following, the scenario that would benefit most from transcutaneous cardiac pacing involves a patient in:
   a. PEA with normal-looking QRS complexes and a rate of 68
   b. sinus bradycardia with a rate of 56 and a blood pressure of 112/66
   c. ventricular fibrillation who is unresponsive to defibrillation and medications
   d. third-degree block who is unresponsive to atropine and then becomes hemodynamically unstable

50. The diaphragm is controlled by the _____ nerve.
   a. vagus
   b. cranial
   c. phrenic
   d. intercostal

51. The management of the suspected aortic dissection would include all of the following *EXCEPT*:
   a. gentle handling of the patient
   b. calming of the patient
   c. large-bore IV administration and fluid boluses to establish normotension
   d. administration of morphine

52. Bradycardia and slowing respiratory rate during a respiratory emergency indicate:
   a. resolution of respiratory distress
   b. exhaustion, hypoxia, and imminent cardiac arrest
   c. expected effects of the medication given to treat the attack
   d. the effects of anxiety and stress

53. When administering medications via the endotracheal route, the medication should normally be:
   a. 2 to 2½ times the IV dose
   b. 5 mL or less in volume
   c. half the IV dose
   d. diluted with lactated Ringer's solution

54. The process by which gas exchange occurs between the air-filled alveoli and the pulmonary capillary bed is called:
   a. osmosis
   b. perfusion
   c. diffusion
   d. dispersion

55. Differences in Type 1 and Type 2 diabetes include all of the following *EXCEPT*:
   a. Type 1 requires life-long use of insulin injections
   b. Type 2 is more common in obese, older patients, whereas Type 1 occurs at an early age
   c. Type 2 never requires the use of insulin
   d. Type 2 is usually managed with diet, exercise, and drugs to improve cellular sensitivity to insulin

56. The most important aspect of the assessment of a child is the:
   a. patient's blood pressure
   b. patient's pulse rate
   c. mother's or father's general reactions
   d. rescuer's general impression of the patient

57. A 26-year-old tree service worker has cut his thigh with a chain saw. There is uncontrolled bleeding from the injury despite the application of direct pressure. The pressure point of choice in this situation is the:
   a. posterior tibial artery
   b. popliteal artery
   c. dorsalis pedis artery
   d. femoral artery

58. Most of the damage to tissue from frostbite occurs when:
   a. ice crystals, which are sharp and damage cells, form in the skin
   b. the skin is rewarmed too quickly
   c. water is drawn out of the cells and electrolyte levels become toxic
   d. the frostbitten tissue is submerged in tepid water

59. All of the following are true regarding spinal cord injury (SCI) *EXCEPT*:
   a. SCI caused by prehospital care is the most common cause of lawsuits
   b. it is more common in men than in women
   c. approximately 40% will have permanent disability
   d. approximately 25% of these injuries may be caused by improper prehospital handling

60. When administering fluids to a patient with an uncontrollable hemorrhage and shock, the goal is to:
 a. administer enough fluid to normalize vital signs
 b. withhold fluids totally to avoid potential for pulmonary edema
 c. administer fluids rapidly to achieve a 3:1 replacement ratio of fluid infused to blood lost
 d. titrate fluids until the patient shows signs of clinical improvement

61. When managing a patient with a pulmonary contusion, special care must be taken not to:
 a. lay the patient flat
 b. intubate the patient
 c. administer too much oxygen, which may affect the patient's hypoxic drive
 d. overload the patient with IV fluids

62. Acute respiratory distress syndrome (ARDS) is:
 a. unlikely to result from pneumonia or sepsis
 b. often associated with stridor and signs of airway obstruction
 c. fluid accumulation in the pulmonary interstitial space resulting from increased permeability of the alveoli capillary membranes
 d. the result of repeated asthma attacks leading to scarring of the alveoli walls and the development of blebs

63. Three pharmacological agents commonly used to manage left ventricular failure include:
 a. epinephrine, atropine, and nitroglycerin
 b. nitroglycerin, furosemide, and morphine
 c. vasopressin, epinephrine, and amiodarone
 d. albuterol, furosemide, and diphenhydramine

64. The IV fluid of choice for a burn patient is:
 a. any crystalloid solution
 b. colloid solution
 c. lactated Ringer's solution
 d. plasma

65. Heat from the body is lost to the environment primarily through:
 a. breathing
 b. skin
 c. urination
 d. perspiration

66. The most important factor affecting the specificity of a hormone's action is:
 a. the receptor number and affinity for that hormone on target organs and tissue
 b. the concentration of the hormone in the body
 c. the speed of secretion
 d. the rate of metabolism

67. Appropriate prehospital management of a stroke patient is most likely to consist of all of the following *EXCEPT*:
 a. administering supplemental oxygen if hypoxic
 b. establishing IV access
 c. checking blood glucose level
 d. administering nitroglycerin or labetalol per protocol to treat hypertension

68. A patient who had a recent injury or blow to the left upper quadrant of the abdomen and who is experiencing pain in the left shoulder should be suspected of having a:
 a. retroperitoneal bleed
 b. ruptured appendix
 c. ruptured spleen
 d. pericardial tamponade

69. Management of an evisceration includes:
 a. replacing the organ within the abdomen
 b. applying a moist, sterile dressing to the area and covering it with an occlusive dressing
 c. applying direct pressure to the evisceration to control bleeding
 d. applying the PASG and inflating the legs and abdominal compartment

70. Effective interviewing techniques for patients with behavioral emergencies include all of the following *EXCEPT*:
 a. active listening to concerns or complaints
 b. being supportive and empathetic
 c. invalidating the patient's intense feelings
 d. respecting a patient's personal space

71. Which of the following is most characteristic of ischemic strokes?
 a. They are less common than hemorrhagic strokes.
 b. They develop more suddenly than hemorrhagic strokes.
 c. They are associated with valvular heart disease and atrial fibrillation.
 d. They usually occur with stress or exertion.

72. In cardiogenic shock, the primary cause of decreased cardiac output is:
    a. vasoconstriction
    b. pump failure
    c. fluid loss
    d. rapid heart rate

73. Your 30-year-old patient complains of acute onset of left flank pain that radiates into his groin. He is restless and vomiting. Vital signs are blood pressure 120/70, pulse 120, respiratory rate 16 and afebrile. His presentation is most consistent with:
    a. acute appendicitis
    b. dissecting aortic aneurysm
    c. pyelonephritis
    d. kidney stone

74. Your ambulance is dispatched to a residence where a 45-year-old male is having chest pain. He says his wife called, but he doesn't want an ambulance. He states he can't afford an ambulance and can't miss work. He asks you to leave. You see that his color is poor, his breathing is labored, and he is clutching his chest. His wife is crying, asking him to go with you. Your best action would be to:
    a. tell his wife that because the patient won't give you permission to treat, there is nothing you can do. Advise dispatch that the patient was a refusal.
    b. call law enforcement to have the patient put in protective custody so that you can treat and transport him
    c. advise him of the need for early intervention, call Medical Control, and have the patient talk with the physician
    d. while the patient's wife drives him to the hospital, follow them in the ambulance in case something happens

75. Vagal stimulation results in:
    a. tachyarrhythmias
    b. decreased ventricular ectopy
    c. positive chronotropic effect
    d. a slowing of the heart rate

76. The highest priority when managing a cardiac arrest patient in pulseless electrical activity (PEA) is:
    a. early defibrillation
    b. rapid IV access to allow administration of medications
    c. searching for a correctable cause
    d. early initiation of transcutaneous pacing

77. When initiating medication administration to control seizure activity, which of the following should be considered?
    a. Lorazepam is associated with less respiratory suppression than diazepam.
    b. Respiratory status must be constantly assessed regardless of agent used.
    c. Seizure activity may continue despite the amount of any agent used.
    d. All of the above are correct.

78. When an ECG strip is examined, the QRS complex corresponds to:
    a. atrial depolarization
    b. ventricular depolarization
    c. septal repolarization
    d. ventricular repolarization

79. The goal when administering medications to a patient in congestive heart failure is to:
    a. decrease contractile function of the myocardium
    b. increase blood pressure
    c. decrease venous return to the heart
    d. increase the workload of the heart

80. The last reflex to stimulate respiration occurs:
    a. when the concentration of oxygen in the alveoli decreases to a critical level
    b. when the peripheral chemoreceptors in the aortic arch and carotid artery sense a decrease in the arterial oxygen level
    c. when the pH decreases to a critical level
    d. when the pH increases to a critical level

81. A 79-year-old man is involved in a head-on collision in which he is not restrained. He complains of pain in his neck, chest, and back. You find no apparent injuries on exam, and his vital signs are normal. The most appropriate treatment would consist of oxygen, IVs, and rapid transport because:
    a. the elderly will often not tell you if they are injured
    b. the elderly usually have normal vital signs until they deteriorate
    c. the mechanism of injury must be considered over physical findings
    d. increased elasticity and cardiovascular reserve increase the potential for life-threatening thoracic injuries

82. A 13-year-old male presents with weight loss and fatigue. His mother states that he has been urinating frequently and drinks water constantly. These symptoms are caused by:
    a. elevated glucose levels in the blood, which lead to cerebral impairment and cause this abnormal behavior
    b. loss of glucose in the urine, resulting in an osmotic diuresis and thirst
    c. polydipsia as a reflex to dilute the blood glucose level
    d. not eating properly (fatigue only)

83. An early sign of shock is:
    a. low blood pressure
    b. red, dry skin
    c. rapid heart rate
    d. lethargy

84. The patient you are about to cardiovert suddenly goes limp. You glance over at the cardiac monitor and notice ventricular fibrillation. Your next action is to:
    a. leave the synchronizer on but increase the output to 360
    b. start CPR and attempt to gain IV access if an IV is not already present
    c. turn off the synchronizer and defibrillate at 200
    d. immediately secure the airway, preferably by performing endotracheal intubation

85. The partial seizure differs from the generalized seizure in that:
    a. the partial seizure is always preceded by an aura
    b. the partial seizure never leads to a generalized seizure
    c. the mental status is relatively normal in the partial seizure
    d. the partial seizure last longer than the generalized

86. Of the various types of shock, the one least likely to present with an increased pulse, sweating, and pallor is:
    a. hypovolemic shock
    b. septic shock
    c. cardiogenic shock
    d. neurogenic shock

87. Which of the following statements most accurately describes the difference between ventilation and respiration?
    a. Respiration is the process of breathing, whereas ventilation concerns only the alveoli.
    b. Ventilation is affected by fluid in the interstitial space, whereas respiration is affected by spasm of the bronchioles.
    c. Ventilation and respiration are the same thing.
    d. Ventilation affects removal of carbon dioxide, and respiration concerns the ability to oxygenate the blood.

88. Cerebrospinal fluid is a solution of nutrients and waste products that circulates through and around:
    a. the spinal cord
    b. the cerebral ventricles
    c. the subarachnoid space and dural sinuses
    d. all of the above

89. The initial step in the neurological exam begins with:
    a. ensuring a patent airway
    b. ensuring the patient is breathing
    c. ensuring the patient has a pulse
    d. determining level of consciousness

90. The primary pacemaker of the heart, where electrical impulses originate, is the:
    a. AV node
    b. bundle of His
    c. SA node
    d. Purkinje fiber

91. When an oropharyngeal airway is used to maintain the airway of a pediatric patient:
    a. insert the airway right side up without using the rotating maneuver that would be used for an adult
    b. ascertain what size airway would reach from the corner of the mouth to the earlobe, then insert the next smaller size airway
    c. insert the airway upside down and rotate it once in the proper position
    d. visualize the oropharynx first with a laryngoscope to check for obstructions

92. Which of the following is true regarding hallucinogens?
    a. Mescaline is derived from mushrooms.
    b. Peyote cactus contains the ingredients for LSD.
    c. MDMA or "Ecstasy" has become one of the most popular "designer" drugs.
    d. Prehospital care consists mainly of keeping the patient awake through various means of stimuli.

93. Typical blood loss in an uncomplicated femur fracture is approximately:
    a. less than 500 mL
    b. 500 to 1000 mL
    c. 1000 to 2000 mL
    d. 2000 to 3000 mL

94. A young mother reports that her child has quit breathing. The child is admitted and observed, and no episodes of apnea appear. The child goes home, and the episodes begin again. The child is admitted and observed with a closed-circuit camera. The mother is witnessed smothering the child with a pillow and calling for assistance when she quits breathing. This is an example of a:
    a. conversion disorder
    b. schizophrenia
    c. somatization disorder
    d. factitious disorder

95. A 5-year-old child who has a shunt is complaining of a headache accompanied by nausea. Parents say the child has also been vomiting. You suspect:
    a. a viral illness
    b. an excess of cerebrospinal fluid in the stomach causing nausea
    c. the child has accidentally ingested a poison
    d. increasing intracranial pressure

96. The energy levels generally used to perform initial defibrillation on an adult patient are:
    a. 100, 200, 300 joules for ventricular fibrillation and 200, 300, 360 joules for pulseless ventricular tachycardia
    b. 200, 300, 360 joules for ventricular fibrillation and 100, 200, 300 joules for pulseless ventricular tachycardia
    c. 200, 300, 360 joules for both ventricular fibrillation and pulseless ventricular tachycardia
    d. 260, 300, 360 joules for both ventricular fibrillation and pulseless ventricular tachycardia

97. Significant neurological emergencies may be associated with abnormal posturing of the limbs. Which of the following is true?
    a. Decorticate rigidity is worse than decerebrate rigidity.
    b. Decorticate rigidity involves an abnormal extension of the arms and flexion of the legs.
    c. Decerebrate rigidity involves an abnormal flexion of the arms and flexion of the legs.
    d. None of the above are correct.

98. Which of the following is an appropriate response for the rescuer in the management of paranoid reactions associated with schizophrenia?
    a. speak quietly with family or bystanders so that the patient does not pick up on their concerns
    b. attempt to gain the patient's confidence through kindness and warmth
    c. do not identify yourself as a paramedic because schizophrenic patients do not feel they need medical attention
    d. maintain an attitude that is friendly, yet somewhat distant and neutral

99. The first place to suction the newborn is:
    a. the right nostril
    b. the left nostril
    c. the mouth
    d. both nostrils, then the mouth

100. A 52-year-old male with no history of heart problems presents with crushing substernal chest pain, which is radiating down his left arm, and shortness of breath. He is diaphoretic and, according to his family, appears paler than normal. Treatment of this patient is likely to include:
    a. adenosine, albuterol, atropine (AAA)
    b. adenosine, Benadryl, cordarone (ABC)
    c. lidocaine, atropine, Narcan, epinephrine (LANE)
    d. morphine, oxygen, nitroglycerin, aspirin (MONA)

101. You are transporting a young boy with an allergic reaction. The on-line medical control physician orders you to administer 100 mg of diphenhydramine while your protocols only allow you to administer 25 mg. You should:
    a. repeat back the order to the physician and confirm his order
    b. indicate to the physician that the order is not contained in your protocols and not perform the order
    c. wait until you arrive at the hospital to address the issue with the physician
    d. all of the above

102. Carbon dioxide diffuses from the pulmonary capillaries into the alveoli because:
    a. the hemoglobin in the capillaries has very little oxygen
    b. the hydrostatic pressure is greater in the capillaries
    c. the oxygen concentration is higher in the alveoli
    d. the partial pressure of carbon dioxide is higher in the capillaries

103. A 19-year-old dives head first into 3 feet of water. Initially he is moving all extremities but begins to develop paralysis. The most likely cause is:
a. primary injury from impingement of a bone fragment into the cord
b. secondary injury as a result of swelling and ischemia of the spinal cord
c. spinal cord transsection
d. spinal shock

104. When managing a victim of a blast injury, *avoid*:
a. aggressive positive pressure ventilation
b. starting an IV
c. covering the ear canal
d. removing contaminating material that may be needed as evidence

105. The most common cause of a pulmonary embolus is:
a. a clot breaking off a deep venous thrombosis in the lower extremity
b. the sheared tip of a central venous catheter
c. introduction of air into the vascular tree during diving-related barotraumas
d. foreign material injected by intravenous drug users

106. All of the following statements about suicide are false *EXCEPT*:
a. When a person's depression lifts, the danger of suicide is gone
b. suicidal people are mentally ill
c. most people plan their suicide, then present clues of their intent
d. suicidal tendencies are inherited

107. Crystalloid solutions include:
a. D_5W, normal saline, albumin
b. lactated Ringer's, D_5W, normal saline
c. normal saline, dextran, lactated Ringer's
d. hetastarch, D_5W, lactated Ringer's

108. Enlargement of the interstitial space with fluid or the thickening of the alveoli wall will result in:
a. increased diffusion leading to hypoxia and hypercarbia
b. decreased perfusion leading to hypoxia and hypocarbia
c. increased perfusion leading to hypoxia and hypercarbia
d. decreased diffusion leading to hypoxia and hypercarbia

109. Which of the following are critical factors that can decrease the death and disability from head and neck trauma?
a. rapid transport to the closest appropriate facility
b. early recognition of signs and symptoms of head and neck injury
c. maintaining a clear airway and providing appropriate ventilation
d. all of the above

110. When problems with diffusion cause respiratory emergencies, the treatment initially consists of:
a. improving perfusion by increasing blood pressure
b. provision of high-flow oxygen and measures to remove the fluid in the interstitial space
c. assisting ventilation with a bag-valve-mask
d. intubation

111. A severe heat injury characterized by nausea, headache, irritability and known as heat exhaustion:
a. is another name for heat cramps
b. is difficult to reverse
c. always results in orthostatic pressure changes
d. can progress to heat stroke if left untreated

112. The rescuer may insert his or her fingers into a pregnant patient's vagina:
a. to support the baby's head during delivery
b. only in the case of a breech delivery or prolapsed cord
c. to assist in delivery of the baby's shoulders
d. to check the baby's pulse in the case of a limb presentation

113. When assessing your patient's chest, you note that the chest wall diameter is noticeably increased. You would expect to find this patient has a history of:
a. congestive heart failure
b. previous flail chest
c. chronic obstructive pulmonary disease
d. hypertension

114. The endocrine cells of the pancreas are contained within the islets of Langerhans. Which of the following is true?
a. Insulin is secreted by the delta cells.
b. Beta cells secrete somatostatin.
c. The islets are connected to the pancreatic duct.
d. The alpha cells secrete glucagon.

115. Which of the following criteria will determine whether cervical spine immobilization is indicated?
a. presence of a positive mechanism of injury
b. presence of a negative mechanism of injury
c. presence of an uncertain mechanism of injury with clinical criteria
d. written protocol

116. When an IV is started, if the first puncture attempt is unsuccessful, the second puncture should:
a. be distal to the first
b. use a larger gauge needle
c. always use a smaller needle
d. be proximal to the first

117. A 46-year-old woman presents with agitation, tachycardia, and delirium. On exam you notice that you can see the whites of her eyes completely around her iris and it appears as if her eyeballs are protruding from the sockets. All of the following are true *EXCEPT*:
a. this is consistent with Graves' disease, an autoimmune disorder
b. generalized enlargement of the thyroid gland is called a "gizzard"
c. the condition of protruding eyes is called exophthalmos
d. you would expect to find swelling of her lower neck

118. Emphysema, unlike asthma and chronic bronchitis, is:
a. defined as a productive cough for at least 3 months per year for 2 or more consecutive years
b. exacerbated by extrinsic factors in children and intrinsic factors in adults
c. characterized by accumulation of fluid in the interstitial space
d. almost always associated with cigarette smoking and has irreversible airway obstruction leading to blebs and the need to breathe through pursed lips

119. The types of shock that are associated with systemwide vasodilation are:
a. cardiogenic, anaphylactic, hypovolemic
b. neurogenic, septic, hypovolemic
c. septic, anaphylactic, neurogenic
d. hypovolemic, cardiogenic, neurogenic

120. Your 16-year-old male patient complains of acute onset of severe left scrotal pain after lifting weights in the gym. He is restless, vomiting, and diaphoretic. Which of the following is most correct?
a. This is most likely due to a hernia and may be treated conservatively.
b. This is caused by twisting of a portion of the testicle called the epididymitis.
c. This is most likely testicular torsion, which requires emergency surgery within 4 to 6 hours.
d. This can be treated with manual reduction in the field.

121. The most appropriate treatment of the hyperventilating patient is:
a. have patient breathe into a paper bag
b. assist ventilations with a bag-valve-mask
c. look for any possible cause of respiratory distress and treat appropriately
d. apply a nonrebreather mask but do not attach to oxygen

122. Bradycardia and cardiac arrest in the neonate are usually the result of:
a. metabolic disturbances
b. hypoxia
c. congenital heart defects
d. intracranial hemorrhage

123. Uncuffed endotracheal tubes should generally be used:
a. only for infants below the age of 1
b. for children between the ages of 1 and 10
c. for children over the age of 5
d. for children under the age of 8

124. Diabetes is a systemic disease with many long-term complications. Which of the following best describes some of these complications?
a. Cardiovascular disease and stroke are increased because of repeated injury to small vessels.
b. Wound infections occur because increased blood sugar promotes bacteria growth.
c. Up to 10% of all diabetics develop some form of kidney disease including renal failure.
d. Blindness occurs from increased cataract formation.

125. When performing a needle cricothyrotomy, the needle should be inserted:
a. through the midline of the membrane at a 90-degree angle
b. to the right or left of the midline to allow insertion of two needles and at a 45-degreee angle toward the patient's vocal cords
c. through the midline of the membrane at a 45- to 60-degree angle toward the patient's carina
d. to the right or left of the midline to allow insertion of two needles and at a 30-degree angle toward the patient's carina

126. Management of hypotension resulting from right ventricular failure may include:
a. placing the patient in the Trendelenburg position to improve cerebral blood flow
b. administering a 250-mL IV bolus of normal saline over 5 to 10 minutes
c. limiting IV fluids to reduce the potential for pulmonary edema to develop
d. immediate initiation of an IV drip of dopamine to raise blood pressure

127. Your chronic renal failure patient is complaining of chest pain, and you suspect an acute myocardial infarction. Important issues to consider when treating him include:
a. avoidance of taking blood pressures and starting IVs on the arm with the dialysis shunt
b. avoidance of volume overloading him with IV fluids
c. administration of the usual and customary nitrates and oxygen
d. all of the above

128. Common pulmonary medications include all of the following *EXCEPT:*
a. prednisone
b. propranolol
c. albuterol
d. theophylline

129. To raise the epiglottis out of the way, insert the tip of a curved laryngoscope blade into the:
a. glottic opening
b. vallecula
c. carotid sinus
d. carina

130. When a pregnant patient with a spinal injury is transported on a backboard, the backboard should be:
a. elevated at the head
b. tilted on its right side
c. tilted on its left side
d. completely flat

131. Two illnesses most often characterized by wheezing in children are:
a. epiglottitis and croup
b. pneumonia and asthma
c. bronchiolitis and epiglottitis
d. asthma and bronchiolitis

132. The most important factor that must be considered when treating a victim of a hazardous material is:
a. removing contaminated material from the patient
b. preventing rescuer contamination
c. giving the correct antidote
d. removing the victim from the contaminated area

133. If after inserting an endotracheal tube and listening to lung sounds, sounds are only heard on the right side:
a. deflate the cuff, pull the tube out, and reattempt intubation
b. deflate the cuff and push the tube in slightly
c. leave the tube in place and ventilate at a faster rate
d. deflate the cuff and pull the tube back slightly

134. In a situation involving a prolapsed cord, breech presentation, or limb presentation, the mother may be placed:
a. in a head-down position with her pelvis elevated
b. on her right side with her legs squeezed together
c. in a prone position
d. on her back with her head higher than her feet

135. If pulmonary circulation is inhibited, the blood leaving the lungs will have:
a. a low oxygen content
b. a lower than normal carbon dioxide content
c. an abnormally high oxygen content
d. a higher than normal pH

136. Delivery should be considered imminent when:
a. contractions are less than 2 minutes apart
b. contractions last longer than 20 seconds
c. it is the mother's first pregnancy and contractions are 5 minutes apart
d. the patient is experiencing lower abdominal pain with no back pain

137. When the decision is made to cut the umbilical cord, the first clamp should be placed:
a. about 4 inches away from the baby
b. about 4 inches away from the mother
c. 10 inches from the baby
d. 10 inches from the mother

138. If signs of hypovolemia are present in a neonate, appropriate fluid resuscitation would include:
a. a fluid bolus of 10 mL/kg of isotonic crystalloid solution followed by a second bolus of 10 mL/kg if signs of shock persist
b. a single fluid bolus of 20 mL/kg of isotonic colloid solution followed by a continuous infusion of crystalloid solution
c. a 50-mL bolus of colloid solution followed by an IV drip of vasopressor agents to maintain blood pressure
d. a 100-mL bolus of hypertonic crystalloid solution followed by a continuous infusion of crystalloids if signs of shock persist

139. If an IV or IO route cannot be established in a seizure patient, diazepam may be administered:
a. orally
b. sublingually
c. subcutaneously
d. rectally

140. When taking the vital signs of a pregnant patient in the second trimester of pregnancy, it is normal for the:
a. heart rate to be faster and blood pressure lower
b. heart rate to be slower and blood pressure higher
c. heart rate to be slower and blood pressure lower
d. heart rate to be faster and blood pressure higher

141. A 16-year-old girl is riding the family four-wheeler at night when she runs into the clothesline, which strikes her across the neck knocking her to the ground. On examination she is awake and alert. Her voice is hoarse and she has pain with swallowing. All of the following are true *EXCEPT*:
a. the presence of subcutaneous emphysema indicates tracheal disruption
b. fracture of the trachea can result in airway obstruction requiring surgical intervention
c. cervical spine precautions should be taken
d. emergent intubation should be considered to preclude the possibility of airway obstruction from swelling

142. Which of the following is true regarding nontraumatic back pain?
a. It is an uncommon reason for prehospital transport.
b. Men are twice as likely to be affected as women.
c. The most common cause is idiopathic and difficult to diagnose.
d. Lack of numbness or weakness indicates drug-seeking behavior.

143. The abnormal condition that may occur in the last 3 months of pregnancy that most often is characterized by sudden, severe, low abdominal pain with or without vaginal bleeding is:
a. abruptio placentae
b. uterine inversion
c. placenta previa
d. eclampsia

144. The three primary components of the Pediatric Assessment Triangle are:
a. airway, breathing, mental status
b. respiratory effort, mental status, muscle tone
c. circulation, respiratory rate, skin color
d. appearance, work of breathing, circulation

145. If a pediatric patient needs to be defibrillated, the recommended energy levels are:
a. the first three defibrillations at 2 J/kg, 4 J/kg, 4 J/kg and subsequent defibrillations at 4 J/kg
b. the first three defibrillations at 5 J/kg and subsequent defibrillations at 10 J/kg
c. the first three defibrillations at 20 J and subsequent defibrillations at 40 J
d. the first three defibrillations at 20 J, 40 J, 60 J and subsequent defibrillations at 60 J

146. EMS personnel should be alert for the possibility of seizures when a pregnant patient presents with:
a. swelling of the face, hands, and feet
b. abnormally low blood pressure
c. sudden loss of weight
d. severe lower abdominal pain

147. Pharmacological intervention for a pediatric patient with hemodynamically unstable bradycardia would normally consist of:
a. administering atropine first, followed by epinephrine if no improvement results
b. administering atropine, followed by dopamine if there is no improvement after the second dose
c. administering epinephrine first, followed by atropine if no improvement results
d. administering epinephrine first, followed by pacing if there is no improvement after 10 minutes

148. A child who presents with a high fever, very sore throat, pain when swallowing, and drooling should be suspected of having:
a. croup
b. bronchitis
c. epiglottitis
d. asthma

149. During hypoventilation carbon dioxide levels rise resulting in:
a. metabolic acidosis
b. metabolic alkalosis
c. respiratory acidosis
d. respiratory alkalosis

150. Which of the following is *not* a function of the liver?
a. iron metabolism
b. storage of reserve blood cells
c. detoxification of the plasma
d. production of bile for digestion

ANSWERS TO CHAPTER 24: SAMPLE FINAL EXAM

1. **c.** Chapter 1, Question 56
2. **b.** Chapter 5, Question 10
3. **b.** Chapter 10, Question 20
4. **b.** Chapter 6, Question 50
5. **c.** Chapter 7, Question 22
6. **c.** Chapter 10, Question 30
7. **a.** Chapter 15, Question 57
8. **c.** Chapter 12, Question 61
9. **a.** Chapter 6, Question 39
10. **c.** Chapter 10, Question 27
11. **c.** Chapter 11, Question 44
12. **b.** Chapter 7, Question 39
13. **b.** Chapter 10, Question 6
14. **a.** Chapter 12, Question 23
15. **d.** Chapter 12, Question 32
16. **c.** Chapter 19, Question 12
17. **b.** Chapter 11, Question 66
18. **a.** Chapter 13, Question 25
19. **a.** Chapter 9, Question 24
20. **a.** Chapter 7, Question 21
21. **b.** Chapter 8, Question 14
22. **d.** Chapter 5, Question 32
23. **a.** Chapter 11, Question 45
24. **a.** Chapter 19, Question 35
25. **b.** Chapter 19, Question 73
26. **b.** Chapter 21, Question 6
27. **d.** Chapter 11, Question 50
28. **b.** Chapter 4, Question 73
29. **c.** Chapter 9, Question 25
30. **d.** Chapter 8, Question 19
31. **b.** Chapter 14, Question 9
32. **d.** Chapter 2, Question 12
33. **d.** Chapter 7, Question 72
34. **a.** Chapter 20, Question 18
35. **b.** Chapter 11, Question 25
36. **a.** Chapter 8, Question 38
37. **a.** Chapter 3, Question 62
38. **d.** Chapter 12, Question 110
39. **d.** Chapter 4, Question 65
40. **c.** Chapter 2, Question 56
41. **d.** Chapter 9, Question 34
42. **a.** Chapter 15, Question 63
43. **b.** Chapter 10, Question 12
44. **d.** Chapter 4, Question 75
45. **d.** Chapter 2, Question 25
46. **b.** Chapter 16, Question 5
47. **b.** Chapter 8, Question 52
48. **c.** Chapter 9, Question 13
49. **d.** Chapter 12, Question 40
50. **c.** Chapter 11, Question 19
51. **c.** Chapter 20, Question 27
52. **b.** Chapter 11, Question 30
53. **a.** Chapter 2, Question 51

54. **c.** Chapter 11, Question 8
55. **c.** Chapter 13, Question 15
56. **d.** Chapter 4, Question 25
57. **d.** Chapter 6, Question 10
58. **c.** Chapter 15, Question 36
59. **a.** Chapter 8, Question 25
60. **d.** Chapter 6, Question 32
61. **d.** Chapter 9, Question 21
62. **c.** Chapter 11, Question 36
63. **b.** Chapter 12, Question 65
64. **c.** Chapter 7, Question 65
65. **b.** Chapter 15, Question 15
66. **a.** Chapter 13, Question 2
67. **d.** Chapter 14, Question 14
68. **c.** Chapter 9, Question 37
69. **b.** Chapter 9, Question 47
70. **c.** Chapter 17, Question 5
71. **c.** Chapter 14, Question 10
72. **b.** Chapter 6, Question 29
73. **d.** Chapter 16, Question 43
74. **c.** Chapter 21, Question 15
75. **d.** Chapter 12, Question 12
76. **c.** Chapter 12, Question 99
77. **d.** Chapter 14, Question 32
78. **b.** Chapter 12, Question 18
79. **c.** Chapter 12, Question 66
80. **b.** Chapter 11, Question 23
81. **c.** Chapter 20, Question 46
82. **b.** Chapter 13, Question 19
83. **c.** Chapter 6, Question 23
84. **c.** Chapter 12, Question 105
85. **c.** Chapter 14, Question 21
86. **d.** Chapter 6, Question 24
87. **d.** Chapter 11, Question 24
88. **d.** Chapter 8, Question 16
89. **d.** Chapter 14, Question 1
90. **c.** Chapter 12, Question 29
91. **a.** Chapter 19, Question 36
92. **c.** Chapter 16, Question 39
93. **c.** Chapter 10, Question 17
94. **d.** Chapter 17, Question 18
95. **d.** Chapter 19, Question 86
96. **c.** Chapter 12, Question 78
97. **d.** Chapter 14, Question 5
98. **d.** Chapter 17, Question 9
99. **c.** Chapter 18, Question 22
100. **d.** Chapter 12, Question 111
101. **d.** Chapter 5, Question 45
102. **d.** Chapter 11, Question 16
103. **b.** Chapter 8, Question 36
104. **a.** Chapter 7, Question 27
105. **a.** Chapter 11, Question 52
106. **c.** Chapter 17, Question 15
107. **b.** Chapter 2, Question 59
108. **d.** Chapter 11, Question 10

109. **d.** Chapter 8, Question 6
110. **b.** Chapter 11, Question 11
111. **d.** Chapter 15, Question 21
112. **b.** Chapter 18, Question 18
113. **c.** Chapter 4, Question 63
114. **d.** Chapter 13, Question 9
115. **a.** Chapter 8, Question 32
116. **d.** Chapter 2, Question 60
117. **b.** Chapter 13, Question 47
118. **d.** Chapter 11, Question 41
119. **c.** Chapter 6, Question 25
120. **c.** Chapter 16, Question 60
121. **c.** Chapter 11, Question 63
122. **b.** Chapter 19, Question 15
123. **d.** Chapter 3, Question 66
124. **a.** Chapter 13, Question 29
125. **c.** Chapter 3, Question 76
126. **b.** Chapter 12, Question 67
127. **d.** Chapter 16, Question 58
128. **b.** Chapter 11, Question 28
129. **b.** Chapter 3, Question 53

130. **c.** Chapter 18, Question 47
131. **d.** Chapter 19, Question 42
132. **b.** Chapter 16, Question 8
133. **d.** Chapter 3, Question 64
134. **a.** Chapter 18, Question 44
135. **a.** Chapter 3, Question 8
136. **a.** Chapter 18, Question 15
137. **a.** Chapter 18, Question 27
138. **a.** Chapter 19, Question 11
139. **d.** Chapter 19, Question 56
140. **a.** Chapter 18, Question 8
141. **d.** Chapter 8, Question 61
142. **c.** Chapter 8, Question 50
143. **a.** Chapter 18, Question 51
144. **d.** Chapter 19, Question 19
145. **a.** Chapter 19, Question 61
146. **a.** Chapter 18, Question 54
147. **c.** Chapter 19, Question 60
148. **c.** Chapter 19, Question 51
149. **c.** Chapter 1, Question 70
150. **a.** Chapter 1, Question 50

ILLUSTRATION CREDITS

Figure 1-1 McSwain N, Paturas J: *The basic EMT,* ed 2, St Louis, 2001, Mosby.

Figures 1-2, 1-3, 1-4, 1-5, 1-6, 1-8, 12-1; ECG Strips 1, 3, 5, 6, 7, 9, 10, 11, 12, 13, 14, 15, 16, 17, 18, 19, 20, 21, 22, 23, 24 Sanders MJ: *Mosby's paramedic textbook,* ed 2 revised, St Louis, 2001, Mosby.

Figure 1-7 Thibodeau G, Patton K: *Structure and function of the body,* ed 11, St Louis, 2000, Mosby.

Figure 4-1 Stoy W: *Mosby's EMT-basic textbook,* St Louis, 1996, Mosby.

Figure 4-2 Seidel H: *Mosby's guide to physical examination,* ed 5, St Louis, 2002, Mosby.

Figures 4-3, 7-1, 7-2, 7-3, 12-2, 12-3, 23-1, 23-2, 23-3, 23-4, 23-5 Mack D: *Mosby's EMT-B certification preparation and review,* ed 3, St Louis, 2002, Mosby.

Figure 12-4 Aehlert B: *ACLS quick review study guide,* ed 2, St Louis, 2002, Mosby.

ECG Strips 2, 4, 8 Huszar R: *Basic dysrhythmias,* ed 3, St Louis, 2002, Mosby.